Case Studies in Pharmacy Ethics

Case Studies in Pharmacy Ethics

SECOND EDITION

ROBERT M. VEATCH
Professor of Medical Ethics
The Kennedy Institute
Georgetown University

AMY HADDAD
Professor of Pharmacy Sciences
School of Pharmacy and Health Professions
Center for Health Policy and Ethics
Creighton University

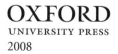

OXFORD
UNIVERSITY PRESS
2008

OXFORD
UNIVERSITY PRESS

Oxford University Press, Inc., publishes works that further
Oxford University's objective of excellence
in research, scholarship, and education.

Oxford   New York
Auckland   Cape Town   Dar es Salaam   Hong Kong   Karachi
Kuala Lumpur   Madrid   Melbourne   Mexico City   Nairobi
New Delhi   Shanghai   Taipei   Toronto

With offices in
Argentina   Austria   Brazil   Chile   Czech Republic   France   Greece
Guatemala   Hungary   Italy   Japan   Poland   Portugal   Singapore
South Korea   Switzerland   Thailand   Turkey   Ukraine   Vietnam

Copyright © 2008 by Oxford University Press, Inc.

Published by Oxford University Press, Inc.
198 Madison Avenue, New York, New York 10016

www.oup.com

Oxford is a registered trademark of Oxford University Press

Library of Congress Cataloging-in-Publication Data
Veatch, Robert M.
Case studies in pharmacy ethics / Robert M. Veatch and Amy M. Haddad. – 2nd ed.
    p. cm.
Rev. ed. of: Case studies in pharmacy ethics / Robert M. Veatch, Amy Haddad. 1999.
Includes bibliographical references and index.
ISBN 978-0-19-530812-9 (pbk.)
1. Pharmaceutical ethics—Case studies. I. Haddad, Amy Marie. II. Veatch, Robert M. Case studies in pharmacy
ethics. III. Title.
[DNLM: 1. Ethics, Pharmacy. QV 21 .V394c 2007]
RS100.5.V43 2008
174.2—dc22   2007014188

9   8   7   6   5   4   3   2   1
Printed in the United States of America
on acid-free paper

Robert Veatch dedicates this book to his father, Cecil R. Veatch, R.Ph., 1905–1978

Amy Haddad dedicates this book to her husband, Steve Martin

Preface

Providing health care increasingly poses ethical choices. Over the past few decades pharmacy has undergone dramatic changes and evolved into a highly patient-oriented profession. The changing role of the pharmacist, development of pharmaceutical care as a practice standard, and complex health and drug distribution systems make it almost impossible to avoid ethical issues. The day is gone (if, indeed, it ever existed) when members of the health care team who are not physicians can consider themselves to be doing their jobs adequately simply by following orders.

In the seven years since the publication of the first edition of *Case Studies in Pharmacy Ethics*, important developments and changes have taken place in the practice of pharmacy. The recent addition of a prescription benefit in Medicare has already led to many changes within the profession. Prescription benefit plans have begun to place limits on the choices of patients and providers. Prescriptions intended to be used by patients to commit suicide have become a legal practice in at least one state. The use of drugs for other morally controversial purposes, including abortion, has forced pharmacists to confront more frequently and more systematically conscientious refusal to dispense. Research medicine also has faced new and complex problems, including the first death of a research subject from an attempt to intentionally manipulate the human genetic code.

Advances in biomedical ethics also have occurred. The National Bioethics Advisory Commission (1996–2001) and, beginning in 2001, the President's Council on Bioethics advanced public discussion of bioethics. New editions of major texts and theories have appeared. New court decisions have reshaped public policy. The teaching of ethics in schools of pharmacy has evolved. For all of these reasons, a new edition is needed.

We have reviewed each case from the first edition, replaced some cases and added others, updated pharmacological, economic, and legal information, and added two new chapters written for this edition. The new Chapter 1 provides our Model for Ethical Problem Solving, a systematic method of dissecting the cases in this volume that will be particularly useful when cases resist less formal analysis. Chapter 13, also entirely new in this edition, acknowledges that the practice of pharmacy is rapidly coming under the influence of formal institutional formularies and drug distribution systems. Hospital and health system formularies are restricting the use of unproven but marginally beneficial and cost-ineffective pharmaceuticals, sometimes forcing pharmacists to cooperate in treatment decisions that are not maximizing the patient's therapeutic interests. Drug distribution systems involve pharmacists in mail-order pharmacies, drug procurement from foreign sources, and Medicare policies. Pharmacists employed in these new and increasingly dominant systems for dispensing as well as pharmacists who are competing with these systems face new and challenging ethical problems, the focus of cases presented in this chapter. While the other chapter titles remain the same, each case in them has been reviewed. New cases replace those that have become dated.

Like all professions, pharmacy imposes ethical standards and obligations on its practitioners. Although pharmacists practice in a variety of settings, such as community pharmacies, hospitals, ambulatory clinics, and home care, there are many problems that all pharmacists share. To begin with, virtually any pharmacist may be asked by a physician, other health care provider, or patient to engage in actions that are not consistent with the pharmacist's conscience. Unless it is supposed that it is best for pharmacists simply to accommodate any and all requests, instances of legitimate moral conflict are bound to occur between the preferences of pharmacists and those of all the other individuals constituting the practice of health care.

Pharmacists may be held accountable for their actions when their professional association has a code, such as the Code of Ethics for Pharmacists of the American Pharmacists Association (APhA). The APhA Code of Ethics calls for certain kinds of conduct. It places the profession (or at least those who are members of the association) on record as viewing the work of its members as people responsible for their actions. The Code of Ethics may conflict, however, with the instruction of the physician, the wishes of the patient, the demands of a third-party payer, or the conscience of an individual caregiver. Codes of various health professions, as we shall see, may actually come into conflict with one another.

Every pharmacist, whether aware of it or not, is constantly making ethical choices. Sometimes these choices are dramatic, life-and-death decisions, but often they are more subtle, less-conspicuous choices that are nonetheless important. One way of seeing the implications of these issues and the moral choices inherent in them is to look at the experiences of one's colleagues, to listen to their stories and the kinds of choices they have had to make in situations like the ones typically faced by pharmacists. This volume is a collection of those situations. It is, we believe, the best way to study the biomedical ethics of the pharmacy profession. Since some teachers of pharmacy ethics may want to use these cases to survey the full range of issues involved in health professional ethics, and given that some courses include practitioners and students from other health professions, we have made an effort to include as many topics in health care as possible, including some that pharmacists face only occasionally (such as genetics and birth technologies), and to include examples of pharmacists interacting with representatives of other health professions.

Pharmacists constitute a significant force in the health care system. Taken together with the many other members of the health care team who daily face difficult moral situations, the instances wherein pharmacists collectively have involvement in the value-based and ethical dimensions of health care are of such magnitude that the exploration of issues contained in this volume is particularly timely.

This collection of cases is based on real situations experienced by practicing pharmacists. Many of the original cases in the first edition were obtained from a national random survey of pharmacists wherein over 400 respondents described ethical problems common to their pharmacy practice.[1] Additional cases were solicited from pharmacy alumni and faculty members as well as clinicians locally and nationally. We have modified details to protect anonymity and to provide clarity in presenting the ethical issues, but in each case some pharmacist has had to face the actual problem presented here. We are grateful to all of the pharmacists who helped us by providing cases.

The writing of this volume has been a truly collaborative effort. Each of the authors has been involved in every case and commentary. In general, Amy Haddad, who is a professor in the Department of Pharmacy Sciences of the School of Pharmacy and Health Professions of Creighton University, drew on her more than 20 years of teaching ethics in the pharmacy program and clinical interactions with pharmacy colleagues as well as the responses of the pharmacists to the above-mentioned survey to prepare first drafts of most of the cases. Robert Veatch, who is a pharmacist and served as a lecturer in pharmacology before pursuing a career in health care ethics, prepared the first draft of much of the introductory material and commentaries, but both participated extensively in all aspects of each chapter and each case.

In addition to the pharmacists who helped by providing case material, we also want to acknowledge the assistance of many others who provided insights about the structure of the book, drug information, research or clinical clarification, including Lee Handke, Pharm.D., Vice President of Pharmacy and Wellness, Blue Cross and Blue Shield of Nebraska; Gary Yee, Pharm.D., University of Nebraska College of Pharmacy; Jennifer Upward, Pharm.D., 2005 graduate, Creighton University School of Pharmacy and Health Professions; Amy Wilson, Pharm.D., and Morgan Sperry, Pharm.D., both faculty members of the School of Pharmacy and Health Professions at Creighton University; and the following Doctor of Pharmacy students from Creighton University: Dua Anderson, Nicole Dunn, Thythu Luu, Katie Normile, Amy Schroeder, Jaclyn Waters, and Erika Zender-Weber. Rebecca Crowell and Justin Herrick of the Center for Health Policy and Ethics at Creighton University also were of particular assistance in the organization of the manuscript.

Robert Veatch also acknowledges the continuing career-long cooperation of the dedicated professional library staff of the National Reference Center for

Bioethics Literature at the Kennedy Institute of Ethics, Georgetown University. Their commitment to careful, systemic mastery of the bioethics literature makes research in the field a joy. He also thanks Moheba Hanif, Sally Schofield, and Linda Powell at the Kennedy Institute of Ethics as well as all the faculty of the Kennedy Institute, many of whom helped provide documentation and clarity for the cases presented here.

In the early stages of this project that resulted in the first edition of this book, Lou Vottero, the former Associate Dean of the Raabe College of Pharmacy at Ohio Northern University, was a full participant. While other responsibilities did not permit him to continue with the writing, we are grateful to him for the role he played in the design of the first edition. While we appreciate the help of all these people, we are, of course, solely responsible for judgments contained in the volume.

In the years since the publication of the first edition, our friend and editor, Jeffrey House, has retired. We are pleased to now be working with Peter Ohlin as editor for this second edition. He has made the transition seamless and resolved many publication problems involved in generating this new edition of the pharmacy case collection as well as developing the companion medical ethics volume.

At the same time that we have prepared this second edition, we have launched preparation of the manuscript of a companion volume, *Case Studies in Medical Ethics*. We have adapted the introductory and theoretical material of this volume for a new collection of cases covering more broadly ethical problems in the various health professions. That volume will provide a much-needed update of the original case study volume in what has now become a series of books presenting cases in the health professions, including nursing, dentistry, and allied health, as well as the more general practice of medicine by physicians and other health professionals. Working with physician and bioethicist Dan English, we expect this companion collection of cases to prove useful for courses in medical ethics that involve students of other health professions in addition to pharmacy as well as undergraduate students of medical ethics.

Note

1. Haddad, A. M. "Ethical Problems in Pharmacy Practice: A Survey of Difficulty and Incidence." *American Journal of Pharmaceutical Education* 55, no. 1 (1991): 1–6.

Contents

Part III   Special Problem Areas

Cases

Case Studies in Pharmacy Ethics

Introduction

Four Questions of Ethics

Biomedical ethics as a field presents a fundamental problem. As a branch of applied ethics, biomedical ethics becomes interesting and relevant only when it abandons the ephemeral realm of theory and abstract speculation and gets down to practical questions raised by real, everyday problems of health and illness. Much of biomedical ethics, especially as practiced within the health professions, is indeed oriented to the practical questions of what should be done in a particular case. Pharmacists, like all health professionals, are, thus, case oriented. Yet if those who must resolve the ever-increasing ethical dilemmas in health care—including not just pharmacists, but patients, physicians, hospital administrators, public policy–makers—treat every case as something entirely novel, they will lose perhaps the best way of reaching a solution, that is, by understanding the general principles of ethics and facing each new situation from a systematic ethical stance.

This is a volume of case studies in pharmacy ethics. It begins by recognizing the fact that one cannot do any ethics, especially health care ethics, in the abstract. It is only in real-life, flesh-and-blood situations that fundamental ethical questions are raised. This volume also acknowledges that a general framework is needed from which to resolve the dilemmas of practicing one's profession. The chapters and the issues discussed within chapters are therefore arranged in order to work systematically through the questions of ethics. Since the main purpose of this book is to provide a collection of case studies from which to build a more comprehensive scheme for health care ethics, the first few pages are addressed to the more theoretical issues. The object is to construct a framework of the basic questions that must be answered in any complete and systematic bioethical system.

We suggest that four fundamental questions must be answered in order for someone to take a complete and systematic ethical position. Each question has several plausible answers that have emerged over 2,000 years of Western thought. For normal, day-to-day decisions made by the pharmacist, it is not necessary to consider each of these questions. In fact, to do so would paralyze the decision-maker. Most decisions are quite ordinary—such as deciding the proper dosing schedule, the most efficacious combination of drugs for a particular disease state, or counseling a patient on drug side effects—and do not always demand full ethical analysis. Other decisions, as in the case of emergency intervention, are not ordinary at all. Still, in both ordinary and emergency situations it is only possible to act without becoming immobilized by ethical or other value because some general rules or guidelines have emerged from previous experience and reflection. If ethical conflict is serious enough, it will be necessary to deal, at least implicitly, with all four of the fundamental questions of ethics.

What Are the Source, Meaning, and Justification of Ethical Claims?

At the most general level, which ethicists call the level of *metaethics,* the first question is: what are the source, meaning, and justification of ethical claims? What is it about a judgment that makes it an ethical judgment?

It may not at first be obvious what counts as an ethical problem for a pharmacist. Pharmacists easily recognize the moral crisis in deciding whether to turn away a patient who cannot afford the prescribed medication, force antipsychotic drugs on an unwilling patient, or dispense the "morning-after pill" for what to the pharmacist seem like trivial reasons or in deciding whether to dispense a lethal medication to help a terminally ill patient in pain end his or her life. These situations clearly involve ethical problems. Yet it is not immediately evident why we call these problems ethical while other choices faced more commonly in the routine practice of pharmacy are not.

To make ethical problems obvious, several steps should be followed:

1. Distinguish Between Evaluative Statements and Statements Presenting Nonevaluative Facts

Ethics involves making evaluations; therefore, it is a normative enterprise. Moving from the judgment that we *can* do something to the one that we *ought to* do something involves incorporating a set of norms—of judgments of value, rights, duties, and responsibilities. Thus, in order to be ethically responsible in pharmacy, it is important to develop the ability to recognize evaluations or value judgments as they are made.

Steps in Identifying Ethical Judgments

1. Distinguish between evaluative statements and statements presenting nonevaluative facts.
2. Distinguish between moral and nonmoral evaluations.
3. Determine who ought to decide.

Pharmacists may believe that normally their professional practice does not involve any evaluations. Value judgments are sometimes hard to recognize, especially when they are not controversial. To develop the ability to identify an evaluation, try the following: Select an experience that at first seems not to involve any particular value judgments such as providing counseling to a patient with a new prescription. Then begin to describe what occurred, keeping watch for evaluative words. Every time a word expressing value is encountered, note it. Among the words to watch out for are such verbs as *want, desire, prefer, should,* or *ought.* These evaluations may also be expressed as nouns, such as *benefit, harm, duty, responsibility, right,* or *obligation,* or in related adjectival forms, such as *good* and *bad, right* and *wrong, responsible, fitting,* and the like.

Terms Signaling Normative Evaluations

Verbs	Nouns	Adjectives
Want	Benefit	Good
Desire	Harm	Bad
Prefer	Duty	Right
Should	Responsibility	Wrong
Feel Obliged	Obligation	Fitting
Ought	Right	Responsible

Sometimes evaluations are made in terms that are not literal, direct expressions of opinion but nonetheless clearly function as value judgments. The Code of Ethics for Pharmacists of the American Pharmacists Association (APhA), for example, states that a pharmacist "respects the autonomy and dignity of each patient."[1] By this statement, the APhA could be describing the way all pharmacists actually behave. Obviously, however, this is not what the statement describes. Rather it is saying that the pharmacist ought to respect the autonomy and dignity of each patient and that the good pharmacist does so.

2. Distinguish Between Moral and Nonmoral Evaluations

This process of distinguishing between moral and nonmoral evaluations can be much harder because often the difference cannot be discerned from the language itself. If one says that the pharmacist did a good job providing information about drug therapy, the statement could express many kinds of evaluations. It could mean the pharmacist did a good job legally, that the pharmacist fulfilled the law. It could also mean the pharmacist did a good job psychologically, that the job was done in a way that produced a good psychological impact on the patient. It could mean the pharmacist did a good job technically, that every relevant piece of information was conveyed accurately. Or it could mean the pharmacist did a good job ethically, that the pharmacist did what was morally required. Conceivably, doing a good job legally or technically could still leave open the question of whether the pharmacist fulfilled every ethical obligation. For example, the pharmacist could fulfill all the laws of the jurisdiction and state all the information in a technically accurate fashion but still fail to convey what the patient needed to know in order to make a substantially autonomous choice about whether to use the medication.

Sometimes value judgments in health care simply express nonmoral evaluations. Saying that the patient ate well does not express a moral evaluation of the way the patient consumed his or her food. Saying that another day of hospitalization will be good for the patient means only that the patient will be helped physically or psychologically, not morally. Even these apparently nonmoral judgments about benefits and harms, however, may quickly lead one into the sphere of ethics. When the patient's judgment of what will be beneficial, for example, differs from the health professional's judgment, ethical dilemmas may emerge. A health professional who is committed morally to doing what will benefit the patient will choose one course while the one who is committed to preserving patient autonomy may reluctantly choose the other.

Ethical or moral evaluations are judgments of what is good or bad, right or wrong, having certain characteristics that separate them from nonmoral evaluations, such as aesthetic judgments, personal preferences, beliefs, or matters of taste. The difference between moral and nonmoral evaluations lies in the grounds on or the reasons for which they are being made.[2]

Moral evaluations possess certain characteristics. They are evaluations of human actions, practices, or character traits rather than of inanimate objects, such as paintings or architectural structures. Not all evaluations of human actions are moral evaluations, however. We may say that a hospital pharmacist is a good administrator or a good clinician without making a moral evaluation. To be considered moral, an evaluation must have additional characteristics. Three characteristics are often mentioned as the distinctive features of moral evaluations. First, the evaluations must be ultimate. They must have a certain preemptive quality, meaning that other values or human ends cannot, as a rule, override them.[3] Second, they must possess universality. Moral evaluations are thought of as reflecting a standpoint that applies to everyone. They are evaluations that everyone in principle ought to be able to make and understand (even if some in fact do not do so).[4] Finally, many add a third, more material, condition: that moral evaluations must treat the good of everyone alike. They must be general in the sense that they avoid giving a special place to one's own welfare. They must have an "other-regarding" focus or, at least, consider one's own welfare no more important than that of another.[5]

Characteristics of Moral Evaluations

1. The evaluations must be ultimate or beyond any further appeal.
2. The evaluations must possess universality. All persons ought to agree (even if they do not).
3. The evaluations must treat the good of everyone alike. One's own welfare should get no special consideration.

Moral judgments possessing these characteristics can sometimes conflict with one another. Conflicts over whether the health care provider ought to care for a patient in the way thought to be most beneficial or most respecting of the patient's autonomy (even though harm may result) can involve conflicts between moral characteristics. Or the caregiver may be faced with the choice between preserving the patient's welfare or that of someone else. He or she may have to choose whether to keep a promise of confidentiality or provide needed assistance for a patient even though a confidence would have to be broken. The caregiver may have to decide whether to protect the interests of colleagues or the institution, whether to serve future patients by striking for better conditions or serve present patients by refusing to strike. These are moral conflicts faced by health care professionals. Chapter 2 presents a series of cases in which both moral and nonmoral evaluations are made in what appear to be quite ordinary health care situations faced by pharmacists. The main task is to discern the value dimensions and to separate them from physiological, psychological, and other facts.

3. Determine Who Ought to Decide

A closely related problem that depends on the question of the source, meaning, and justification of ethical claims is: who ought to decide? This is the focus of Chapter 3. Having learned to recognize the difference between the factual and evaluative dimensions of a case in health care ethics, one will constantly encounter the problem of who ought to decide or where the locus of decision-making ought to rest. The answer will depend, of course, on deciding from where morals come. Chapter 3 presents cases considering a range of sources of moral authority, from professional organizations, health care institutions, patients, families, physicians, and administrators to professional committees and the general public.

   The choice among these decision-makers depends, at least in part, on what it is that ethical terms mean, or more generally, what it is that makes right acts right. Several answers to this question have been offered. One answer recognizes that different societies seem to reach different conclusions about whether a given act is right or wrong. From this perspective, to say that an act is morally right means nothing more than that it is in accord with the values of the group to which the speaker belongs or simply that it is approved by the speaker's group. This position, called social relativism, explains rightness or wrongness on the basis of whether the act fits within the social customs, mores, and folkways of the group. One problem with this view is that it seems to make sense to say that sometimes an act is morally wrong even though it is approved by the speaker's group. That would be impossible if moral judgments were based simply on the values of the speaker's group.

   A second answer to the question of what makes right acts right attempts to correct this problem. According to this position, to say that an act is right means that it is approved by the speaker. This position, called personal relativism, reduces ethical meaning to personal preference. Of course, according to this position, behavior thought to be immoral by some is approved by others. Some say that the reason this can happen is that moral judgments are merely expressions of the speaker's preference.

Such differences in judgment, however, may have another explanation other than that ethical terms refer to the speaker's own preferences. Those disagreeing might simply not be working with the same facts. To claim that two people are in moral disagreement simply because the same act is seen as right by one person or group and wrong by another requires proof that both see the facts in the same way. Differences of circumstances, perspective, or belief about the facts could easily account for many moral differences.

In contrast with social and personal relativism, there is a third group of answers to the question of what makes right acts right. These positions, collectively called universalism or sometimes absolutism, hold that, in principle, acts that are called morally right or wrong are right or wrong independent of social or personal views. Certainly some choices merely involve personal taste: flavors of ice cream or hair lengths vary from time to time, place to place, and person to person. But these are matters of preference, not morality. Other evaluations appeal beyond the standards of social and personal taste to a more universal, an ultimate frame of reference. When these are concerned with acts or character traits—as opposed to, say, paintings or music—they are thought of as moral evaluations.

However, the nature of the universal standard is often disputed. For the theologically oriented, it may be a single divine standard as we see in the monotheistic religions. According to this view, calling it right to disconnect a respirator that is keeping a terminally ill, comatose patient alive is to say that God would approve of the act or that it is in accord with God's will. This position is sometimes called theological absolutism or theological universalism.

Still another view among universalists takes empirical observation as the model. The standard in this case is nature or external reality. The problem of knowing whether an act is right or wrong is then the problem of knowing what is in nature. Empirical absolutism, as the view is sometimes called, sees the problem of knowing right and wrong as analogous to knowing scientific facts.[6] While astronomers try to discern the real nature of the universe of stars and chemists the real nature of atoms as ordered in nature, ethics, according to this view, is an effort to discern rightness and wrongness as ordered in nature. The position sometimes takes the form of a natural law position. As with the physicist's law of gravity, moral laws are thought to be rooted in nature. Natural law positions may be secular or may have a theological foundation, such as in the ethics of Thomas Aquinas and traditional Catholic moral theology.

Still another form of universalism or absolutism rejects both the theological and the empirical models. It supposes that right and wrong are not empirically knowable, but are nonnatural properties known only by intuition. Thus, the position is sometimes called intuitionism or nonnaturalism.[7] Although for the intuitionist or nonnaturalist, right and wrong are not empirically knowable, they are still universal. All persons should in principle have the same intuitions about a particular act, provided they are intuiting properly. Still others, sometimes called rationalists, hold that reason can determine what is ethically required.[8]

There are other answers to the question of what makes right acts right. One view—in various forms called noncognitivism, emotivism, or prescriptivism—

which ascended to popularity during the mid–twentieth century, perceived ethical utterances as evincing feelings about a particular act.[9]

A full exploration of the answers to the question of the source, meaning, and justification of ethical claims—this most abstract of ethical questions—is not possible here.[10] Ultimately, however, if an ethical dispute growing out of a case is serious enough and cannot be resolved at any other level, this question must be faced. If one says that it is wrong to dispense abortifacients and another says that it is right to do so in the same circumstances, some way must be found of adjudicating the dispute between the two views. If the dispute is a moral one, the act cannot be both right and wrong at the same time. One must ask what it is that makes right acts right, how conflicts can be resolved, what the final authority is for morality, and whose judgment about what is right should prevail.

What Kinds of Acts Are Right?

A second fundamental question of ethics moves beyond determining what makes right acts right to ask: What kinds of acts are right? This is the realm of *normative ethics*. The main question at this level is whether there are any general principles or norms describing the characteristics that make actions right or wrong.

Consequentialism

Two major schools of thought dominate Western thought regarding general ethical principles. One position looks at the consequences of acts; the other, at what is taken to be inherently right or wrong. The first position claims that acts are right to the extent that they produce good consequences and wrong to the extent that they produce bad consequences. The two principles of consequentialist ethics are referred to as beneficence (the idea that actions are right insofar as they produce benefits) and nonmaleficence (the idea that actions are wrong insofar as they produce bad consequences). The key evaluative terms for this position, known in various forms as utilitarianism or consequentialism, are good and bad. The focus is on the consequences or ends of action. This is the position of John Stuart Mill and Jeremy Bentham as well as of Epicurus, Thomas Aquinas, and capitalist economics. Aquinas, for example, argued that the first principle of the natural law is that "good is to be done and promoted and evil is to be avoided."[11]

Since Aquinas stands at the center of the Roman Catholic natural law tradition, he illustrates that natural law thinking (which is one answer to the first question of what makes right acts right) is not incompatible with consequentialism. The two positions are answers to two different questions. While natural law thinkers are not always consequentialists, they can be.

Classical utilitarianism determines what kinds of acts are right by figuring the net of good consequences minus bad ones for each person affected and then adding up to find the total net good.[12] The certainty and duration of the benefits and harms are taken into account. This form of consequentialism is indifferent to who obtains the benefits and harms. Thus, if the total net benefits of providing expensive drug therapy for a relatively healthy but powerful figure are thought to be greater than those of providing the same to a sicker Medicare recipient, the healthy and powerful ought to be given the care without further ethical debate.

Traditional pharmacy ethics, like physician and nursing ethics, is oriented to benefiting patients. This tradition combines the utilitarian answer to the question of what kinds of acts are right with a particular answer to the question of to whom moral duty is owed. Loyalty is to the patient, and the goal is toward what will produce the most benefit and avoid the most harm to the patient.

The ethics of the pharmacy profession has traditionally held that the pharmacist's primary commitment is to the patient's care and safety. Some interpret this as giving first priority to protecting the patient from harm rather than to benefiting the patient. Like the principle of physician ethics, primum non nocere or "first of all do no harm," this view gives special weight to avoiding harm over and above the weight given to goods that can be produced.

Among some health professionals the principle of doing no harm is often interpreted conservatively. When a potentially risky intervention is contemplated, harm may be avoided by refusing to intervene. That way no harm is done (although the health care provider thereby avoids doing any good that the intervention could have brought). This form of consequentialism, which gives priority to avoiding harm, needs to be distinguished from classical utilitarianism, which counts goods and harms equally in calculating the net benefit of an action.

Problems arise from tension between classical utilitarianism (which counts benefits to all in society equally) and traditional, or Hippocratic, health care ethics. Hippocratic ethics, referring to the ethics of the Oath named after the father of Western medicine, focuses on the individual patient and sometimes gives special weight to avoiding harms through the prescriptive duty of advocacy. These issues are raised in the cases presented in Chapter 4.

Deontological or "Duty-Based" Ethics

Over against these positions that are oriented to consequences, the other major group of answers to the question of what kinds of acts are right asserts that rightness and wrongness are inherent in the act itself, independent of the consequences. These positions, collectively known as formalism or deontology, hold that right- and wrong-making characteristics may be independent of consequences, that morality is a matter of duty rather than of merely evaluating consequences. Hence this approach can be called "duty-based" ethics. Kant stated the position most starkly.[13] It is based on ethical principles that express these duties, the duty to respect autonomy or to avoid killing being possible examples.

Chapter 5 takes up problems of health care delivery and in doing so poses probably the most significant challenge to the consequentialist ethic. Today some of the most challenging ethical problems in health care arise in cases in which pharmacists have so many demands placed on them that they cannot do everything they would like for their patients. One approach is to simply determine which course of action will do the most good overall. That, however, could mean leaving some patients virtually without care. It seems unfair or unjust (even if it turns out to be efficient in maximizing the total good done). One principle that is sometimes thought to restrain the production of overall good is the principle of justice. Taken in the sense of fairness in distributing goods and harms, justice is held by many to be an ethical right-making characteristic even if the consequences are not the best.

The problem is whether it is morally preferable to have a higher net total of benefits in society even if unevenly distributed or to have a somewhat lower total good but to have that good more equally distributed. This issue will be the focus of the cases in Chapter 4. Utilitarians may acknowledge that the distribution of the good is relevant but only because the net benefits tend to be greater when benefits are distributed more evenly. The benefits may be larger because of decreasing marginal utility—that is, because the more benefits one possesses, the less valuable each marginal additional benefit is. They claim that the only reason to distribute goods, such as health care, more evenly is to maximize the total good. However, the formalist who holds that justice is a right-making characteristic independent of utility does not require an item-by-item calculation of benefits and harms before concluding that the unequal distribution of goods is prima facie wrong, that is, wrong with regard to fairness.

Another major challenge to consequentialism comes from the principle of autonomy. Classical utilitarianism demands noninterference with the autonomy of others in society only when this produces greater net benefits. By contrast, Kantian formalism leads to the moral demand that persons and their beliefs be respected even if doing so will not produce the most good. Conflicts between the health care provider's nonconsequentialist duties to respect the autonomy or self-determination of individual patients and the provider's consequentialist duties to produce benefit are discussed in Chapter 6.

Another ethical principle that many formalists hold to be independent of consequences is that of veracity or truth telling. As with the other principles, utilitarians argue that truth telling is an operational principle designed to guarantee maximum benefit. When truth telling does more harm than good, according to the utilitarians, there is no obligation to tell the truth. To them, telling the dying patient of his condition can be cruel and therefore wrong. In contrast, to one who holds that truth telling is a right-making ethical principle in itself, the problem of what the dying patient would be told is much more complex. Telling a lie is wrong in itself even if telling the lie does more good than telling the truth. This problem of what the patient should be told is the subject of Chapter 7.

Another principle that formalists may believe to be right-making independent of consequences is fidelity, especially the keeping of promises. Those who include the principle of fidelity in their normative ethics hold that people owe to others certain acts based on commitments they have made. Keeping these commitments is morally obligatory even if the consequences would be better if they were not kept. Kant and others have held that breaking a promise is wrong independent of the consequences. The utilitarian points out that breaking a promise often has bad consequences. For them, we usually should keep our promises, but only because of the bad consequences if we do not. The formalist, although granting this danger, argues that there is something more intrinsically wrong in breaking a promise and that to know this one need not even go on to look at the consequences. The formalist might, with the utilitarian, grant that to look at consequences may reveal even more reasons to oppose promise-breaking, but this is not necessary to know that promise-breaking is prima facie wrong.

The provider-patient relationship can be viewed essentially as one involving promises or contracts or, to use a term with fewer legalistic implications, covenants. The relationship is founded on implied and sometimes explicit promises. One of these promises is that information disclosed in the provider-patient relationship is confidential, that it will not be disclosed by the health care provider without the patient's permission. The duty of confidentiality in ethics is really a specification of the principle of promise-keeping in ethics in general. In Chapter 8, cases present the various problems growing out of the ethical principle of fidelity.

The cases of Chapter 9 introduce a final principle that can be included in a general ethical system: the avoidance of killing. All societies have some kind of prohibition on killing. The Buddhists make it one of their five basic precepts. Those in the Judeo-Christian tradition recognize it as one of the Ten Commandments. The moral foundation of the prohibition on killing is not always clear, however. For some people, who base their ethic on doing good and avoiding evil, prohibiting killing is simply a rule summarizing the obvious conclusion that it usually harms people to kill them. If that is the full foundation of the prohibition on killing, then killing is just an example of a way that one can do harm.

This presents a problem, however. Many people believe they are aware of special cases where killing someone may actually do good, on balance. It will stop a greater evil that the one killed would otherwise have committed, or it will, in health care, possibly relieve a terminally ill patient of otherwise intractable pain. Is killing a human being always morally a characteristic of actions that tends to make them wrong, or is it wrong only when more harm than good results from the killing? For those who hold that killing is always a wrong-making characteristic, avoiding killing takes on a life as an independent principle, much like veracity or autonomy or fidelity. The pharmacist is increasingly being asked to dispense prescriptions that could be used to terminate life. This practice is legal in Oregon as well as the Netherlands, and may arise outside the law in other jurisdictions. The cases of Chapter 9 explore these questions.

Other Issues of Normative Ethics

In health care ethics over the past 30 years, the major issue in normative ethics has been the debate over what are the principles of morally right action. The two consequence-oriented principles of benefiting the patient (beneficence) and protecting the patient from harm (nonmaleficence) have been contrasted with the duty-based principles, such as justice, respecting autonomy, avoiding killing, veracity, and fidelity. Sometimes ethical controversy involves other issues, however. Here it is important to get the terminology straight. Ethicists contrast principles, virtues, and values. When they speak precisely, these terms refer to different aspects of normative ethics.

Principles, as we have seen, are general criteria that make human actions morally right or wrong. They refer to the actions (or groups of actions) rather than to the character of the actors. Hence, a pharmacist with a despicable character could, theoretically, fulfill all the moral principles. He or she might do so even though it was done for selfish reasons or bad motives. Sometimes ethical evaluations address the character of the actor rather than the nature of the behavior. When we assess the character of an actor, we use the terms *virtue* and *vice*. In our everyday interactions with others, we make the distinction between character and actions. For example, when a generally unpleasant colleague does something nice, our reaction could easily be one of suspicion regarding this seemingly out-of-character action. Virtues are praiseworthy traits of character, and vices are blameworthy ones. Among the virtues often arising in health care ethics are compassion, humaneness, and caring. A pharmacist might fulfill the principle of veracity without showing any of these virtues (or violate the principle of veracity while being compassionate, humane, or caring). Principles refer to the actions; virtues, to the disposition or character of the actor. In this volume we will focus primarily on principles of right action, though sometimes we may want to assess the character of the pharmacist as well.

For normative ethics that are concerned about consequences, there is still another dimension of normative ethics. If producing good consequences or avoiding harmful ones is seen as important in ethics, then we need to ask what outcomes count as good or bad consequences. We will use the term *value* to refer to a good outcome and *intrinsic value* to refer to whatever counts as an outcome that is good in itself. Money is valued by most people but usually because it enables us to buy things we consider valuable. Money and similar goods can be thought of as *instrumentally valuable*. Those things that are good in themselves are *intrinsically valuable*. One branch of normative ethics is devoted to "value theory," that is, the theory of what is intrinsically valuable. Among the goods often seen as intrinsically valuable are knowledge, aesthetic beauty, and health. Health is, of course, particularly important to pharmacists and other health care professionals.

We will use the word *principle* to refer to general characteristics of actions that make them morally right (independent of the character of the actor) and *virtue* to refer to persistent dispositions or traits of people that are considered praiseworthy (independent of whether the behavior of those people always conforms to ethical principles). We will reserve the word *value* to refer to those things that are considered good or beneficial.

How Do Rules Apply to Specific Situations?

A third question that also is important in providing a full ethical evaluation of a pharmacist's conduct stems from the fact that each case raising an ethical problem is at least in some ways situationally unique. The ethical principles of beneficence (producing benefit), justice, autonomy, veracity, fidelity, and avoidance of killing are extremely broad. They constitute a small set of criteria that make up the most general right-making characteristics of actions or practices. The question is: how do the general principles apply to specific situations?

As a bridge to the specific case, an intermediate, more specific set of rules is often used. These intermediate rules probably cause more problems in ethics than any other component of ethical theory. At the same time, they probably are more helpful than anything else as guides to day-to-day ethical behavior.

The problems arise in part because of a misunderstanding of the nature and function of these rules. Rules may have two functions. They may simply serve as guidelines summarizing conclusions we tend to reach in moral problems of a certain kind. When rules have the function of simply summarizing experiences from similar situations of the past, they are called guiding rules or summary rules.

In contrast, rules may function to specify behavior that is required independent of individual judgment about a specific situation. The rules against abortion of a viable fetus or against killing a dying patient are examples of rules that are often directly linked to right-making characteristics. Sometimes this kind of rule is called a rule of practice. The rule specifies a practice that, in turn, is justified by the general principles. For example, a rule of the practice of pharmacy has been that the pharmacist should not cooperate in the active, intentional killing of patients by dispensing pharmaceuticals that are intended to end a patient's life. Even if the patient is terminally ill and suffering, intentional killing has been considered to be ethically unacceptable. According to this rules-of-practice view, it is unacceptable to overturn a general practice simply because the outcome in a particular case would be better.

The conflict between those who believe that the rules themselves should be the defining factor and those who consider the situation itself to be the most critical determinant of moral rightness led to a major ethical controversy in the mid–twentieth century. It is sometimes called the rules-situation debate.[14] At one extreme is the rigorist who insists that rules should never be violated. At the other is the antinomian (literally "against rules") who claims that rules never apply because every situation is unique. Probably both positions taken to the extreme lead to absurdity. Rigorists are immobilized when two of their rules conflict. Antinomians are immobilized when they treat a situation as so brand new that no moral help can be gained from past experience.

Between these two extremes are two more complex but more plausible views. A situationalist is one who considers every situation as unique and will not legalistically apply rules but is willing to be guided by the moral rules. Those rules are seen as summarizing past experience in similar situations, as guidelines, but not as rules to be followed blindly. A second intermediate position is closer to the rigorist end of the spectrum. Those endorsing what is called the "rules-of-practice" view take moral rules very seriously. They hold that normally the rules should just be applied rather than each case evaluated from scratch. Nevertheless, holders of the "rules-of-practice" position are willing in special situations to reassess the rules to see if the rules should be reformulated to reflect more accurately the requirements of the moral principles. Sometimes an analogy to the game of baseball is cited by defenders of the rules-of-practice position. On the one hand, they claim that, in baseball, the rules cannot be changed in the middle of the game—that it is inappropriate to propose in the late innings that it should take four strikes to make the batter out. On the other hand, also in baseball, there are special moments when those in charge might get together to reassess the rules, for example, at the annual meetings of the baseball team owners. So, likewise, defenders of the rules-of-practice view claim that at special moments in history moral rules may be reevaluated in order to formulate a more accurate specification of the general principles. Society has reassessed certain practices in pharmacy such that the moral rules have changed. Fifty years ago, pharmacists were not supposed to tell patients the name of the drugs they were taking because of concern that patients would misunderstand and suffer psychological harm. For example, taking a pharmaceutical that had many uses might lead a patient mistakenly to believe that he or she had some condition other than the one for which the drug was dispensed. Over the years the rule against disclosing the name of a drug has changed. The rules-of-practice view accepts these changes in the rules—perhaps expressed in a change in the code of ethics of the pharmaceutical association while it does not accept the notion that the pharmacist should decide in the individual case whether the rule applies. The situationalist is more willing to reassess the rules on a case-by-case basis.

This difference over how seriously rules should be taken cuts across the answers to the question of what kinds of action are right. One can be a utilitarian, who assesses the consequences case by case, or a *rule-utilitarian,* someone who believes in the rules-of-practice view, holding that rules should govern individual moral choices but that the rules should be chosen based on their expected consequences. Likewise, someone who is a *deontologist,* who believes there are certain inherent right-making characteristics of actions independent of the consequences, can either apply the general principles (such as autonomy or veracity) directly to individual situations or use them to generate a set of rules, which are then applied to individual cases. The former would be an *act-deontologist*; the latter, a *rule-deontologist.*

The rules-situation debate does not lend itself to special cases grouped together. The problem arises continually throughout the cases in this volume. The final question we address is what ought to be done in specific cases. This question requires special chapters with cases selected to examine the problems raised.

What Ought to Be Done in Specific Cases?

After the determination of the source and meaning of ethical judgments, what kinds of actions are right, and how rules apply to specific situations, there are still a large number of specific situations that make up the bulk of problems in pharmacy ethics. The question remains, what ought to be done in a specific case or kind of case? Pharmacists and other health care professionals, being particularly oriented to case problems, are given to organizing ethical problems around specific kinds of cases.

The first two parts of this volume emphasize the overarching problems of how to relate facts to values, of who ought to decide, of respecting autonomy, veracity, fidelity, of avoiding killing, and of delivering health care in a just manner. These are among the larger questions of biomedical ethics. Part three shifts to cases involving specific problem areas. Cases in Chapter 10 raise the problems of abortion, sterilization, and conception control. Chapter 11 moves to the related problems of genetic counseling and engineering and of intervention in the prenatal period. The next chapters take up in turn the problems of mental health and the control of human behavior; formularies and drug-distribution systems; human experimentation; consent and the right to refuse medical treatment; and finally, death and dying.

The answer to the question of what ought to be done in a specific case requires the integration of the answers to all of the other questions if a thorough analysis and justification is to be given. The first line of moral defense will probably be a set of moral rules and rights thought to apply to the case. In abortion, the right to control one's body and the right of the health care professional to practice his or her profession are pitted against the right to life. In human experimentation, the rules of informed consent pertain. Among the dying, rules concerning euthanasia conflict with the right to pursue happiness, and the right to refuse medical treatment conflicts with the rule that the health care provider ought to do everything possible to preserve life.

In many cases in which the tension between conflicting rules cannot be resolved, the analysis escalates from an issue of moral rules and rights to the higher, more abstract level of ethical principle. It must be determined, for example, whether informed consent is designed to maximize benefits to the experimental subject or to facilitate the subject's freedom of self-determination. It must also be explored whether harm to the patient justifies withholding information from the patient or whether the formalist truth-telling principle justifies disclosure.

The Levels of Ethical Analysis

Metaethics: The Source, Meaning, and Justification of Ethical Claims

Normative Ethics: Principles, Virtues, and Values

Rules and Rights

Specific Cases

Solving the problem of what ought to be done in a specific case also requires a great deal of information beyond what is moral. It requires considerable empirical data. Value-relevant biological and psychological facts have developed around many case problems in biomedical ethics. The predictive capacity of a flat electroencephalogram may be important for the definition of death. The legal facts are relevant for the refusal of treatment. Basic religious and philosophical beliefs of the patient may be critical for resolving some cases in health care ethics. It is impossible to present all of the relevant facts such as medical, genetic, legal, cultural practices, and psychological that are necessary for a complete analysis of any case, but it is possible to present the major facts required for understanding. Readers will have to supplement these facts for a fuller understanding of the cases, just as they will have to supplement their reading in ethical theory for a fuller understanding of the basic questions of ethics.

Notes

1. American Pharmaceutical Association. "Code of Ethics for Pharmacists." Washington, DC: American Pharmaceutical Association, 1995. This code was adopted October 27, 1994, and published the following year. The organization changed its name to the American Pharmacists Association in 2003 but retains this code of ethics.

2. Frankena, William. *Ethics.* Second Edition. Englewood Cliffs, NJ: Prentice-Hall, 1973, p. 62.

3. Beauchamp, Tom L., and James F. Childress, Editors. *Principles of Biomedical Ethics.* Third Edition. New York: Oxford University Press, 1989, p. 18.

4. Fried, Charles. *Right and Wrong.* Cambridge, MA: Harvard University Press, 1978, p. 12.

5. Beauchamp and Childress, *Principles of Biomedical Ethics,* Third Edition, pp. 20–21; Also see Rawls, John. *A Theory of Justice.* Cambridge, MA: Harvard University Press, 1971, pp. 131–136; and Baier, Kurt. *The Moral View.* New York: Random House, 1965, pp. 106–109.

6. Firth, Roderick. "Ethical Absolutism and the Ideal Observer Theory." *Philosophy and Phenomonological Research* 12 (1952): 317–345; Broad, C. D. "Some Reflections on Moral-Sense Theories in Ethics." *Proceedings, the Aristotelian Society* (1944–1945): 131–166.

7. Ross, W. D. *The Right and the Good.* Oxford: Oxford University Press, 1939.

8. Kant, Immanuel. *Groundwork of the Metaphysic of Morals.* H. J. Paton, Translator. New York: Harper and Row, 1964.

9. Ayer, A. J. *Language, Truth, and Logic.* London: Victor Gollancz Ltd., 1948; Stevenson, C. L. *Ethics and Language.* New Haven, CT: Yale University Press, 1944; Hare, R. M. *The Language of Morals.* Oxford: Clarendon, 1952.

10. For basic surveys of ethical theory see Frankena, *Ethics,* and Warnock, G. J. *Contemporary Moral Philosophy.* New York: St. Martin's, 1967. For more detailed introductions see Brandt, Richard B. *Ethical Theory: The Problems of Normative and Critical Ethics.* Englewood Cliffs, NJ: Prentice-Hall, 1959; Beauchamp, Tom L. *Philosophical Ethics: An Introduction to Moral Philosophy.* New York: McGraw-Hill Book Co., 1982; Feldman, Fred. *Introductory Ethics.* Englewood Cliffs, NJ: Prentice-Hall, 1978; and Taylor, Paul W. *Principles of Ethics: An Introduction.* Encino, CA: Dickenson Publishing Co., 1975. For works containing classical sources see Brandt, Richard B. *Value and Obligation: Systematic Readings in Ethics.* New York: Harcourt, Brace, & World, 1961; and Melden, A. I., Editor. *Ethical Theories: A Book of Readings.* Second Edition. Englewood Cliffs, NJ: Prentice-Hall, 1967.

11. Thomas Aquinas. *Summa theologica* I–II, A. 94, Art. 2. Fathers of the English Dominican Province, Editors. London: R & T Washbourne Ltd., 1915.

12. Bentham, Jeremy. "An Introduction to the Principles of Morals and Legislation." In Melden, *Ethical Theories,* pp. 367–390.

13. Kant, *Groundwork of the Metaphysic of Morals.*

14. Rawls, John. "Two Concepts of Rules." *Philosophical Review* 44 (1955): 3–32; Fletcher, Joseph. *Situation Ethics: The New Morality.* Philadelphia: Westminster, 1966; Ramsey, Paul. *Deeds and Rules in Christian Ethics.* New York: Charles Scribner's Sons, 1967; and Bayles, Michael D., Editor. *Contemporary Utilitarianism.* Garden City, NY: Doubleday, 1968.

Part I

Ethics and Values in Pharmacy

1

A Model for Ethical Problem Solving

After the determination of the source and meaning of ethical judgments, what kinds of actions are right, and how rules apply to specific situations—the topics of the introduction to this volume—the question remains of what ought to be done in a specific case or situation. Pharmacists and other health professionals often go through the process of determining the correct action in a specific case unconsciously. Furthermore, if asked, they would be hard pressed to articulate just what steps they went through to arrive at a sound and justifiable decision. There are many normative models for resolving ethical problems in the health science literature,[1] but all require critical thinking and should result in a choice that is morally justifiable. Decision-making, whether in ethics or any other area of life, is often thought of entirely in terms of its anatomy or structure and the relationships among the structures. To appreciate the complexity of ethical decision-making, one must also understand the functions of the parts of the decision-making process. The majority of the volume addresses the "function" of how general ethical principles apply to ethical problems in pharmacy. Here, a framework is offered that includes the principles and a step-wise process to systematically resolve ethical problems in particular cases.

The Five-Step Model

The five steps listed below provide the structure for the decision-making process, and they are linear, that is, they should be carried out in the order presented:

1. Respond to the "sense" or feeling that something is wrong.
2. Gather information/make an assessment.

3. Identify the ethical problem/consider a moral diagnosis.
4. Seek a resolution.
5. Work with others to determine a course of action.

The steps in the model outline a process, a way of making judgments about what should be done in a particular situation. Additional steps could be added, and much elaboration could be included within each step. But the basic framework is sufficient to focus moral judgments and simple enough to recall and apply in actual clinical practice.

Application of the Model

The five-step structure will be applied to Case 1-1 to illustrate the process of decision-making.

CASE 1-1   Reporting a Possibly Lethal Error: Who Needs to Know?

Roger Lucas, 70 years old, was admitted to the medical intensive care unit from the surgical floor of the hospital with what appeared to be a pulmonary embolism. Mr. Lucas had fractured his femur in a fall at the nursing home where he is a patient and was awaiting surgery the next morning when he developed dyspnea, tachypnea, and tachycardia.

At almost the same moment that Mr. Lucas arrived in the ICU, another patient, Ronald London, was admitted in the next room under equally emergent conditions. Mr. London was 60 years old and had a history of liver cirrhosis from alcohol abuse. Mr. London had ruptured esophageal varices. Helen Fowler, Pharm.D., was the pharmacy supervisor for the evening shift for the six intensive care units in the hospital. She and two other pharmacists worked frantically to fill all the orders for intravenous drugs and parenteral solutions that came from the intensive care units.

Later, after the rush had subsided, Dr. Fowler decided to conduct rounds and learned that Mr. London had died. The code team was still picking up their equipment when Dr. Fowler got to the unit. "That's a shame," Dr. Fowler said to the nurse who was straightening up the room and conducting postmortem care so that Mr. London's family could spend some time with him before his body was sent to the morgue. Then Dr. Fowler noticed the label on the IV bag in the trash, the one that had held the IV the nurse had just removed from Mr. London's arm. Dr. Fowler was shocked to see that the empty IV bag included heparin, not the octreotide he should have received. A hemorrhaging patient should never receive heparin.

Without saying anything to the nurse, Dr. Fowler stepped next door to see what solution was hanging in Mr. Lucas's room. Much to her dismay, Mr. Lucas was receiving octreotide when he should have been receiving heparin. And, the two names had been switched on the labels. In the rush and confusion surrounding the admissions and the critical nature of both patients, the IVs were inappropriately labeled. Apparently no one checked the bags for the name of the drug before hanging them since in each case the patient's name and room number were correct.

CASE 1-1   *Continued.*

Dr. Fowler knew that the risk of mortality is high with patients who have ruptured esophageal varices, so the mix-up with the heparin may not have had anything to do with Mr. London's death, but she knew that such a patient should not receive heparin.

Dr. Fowler believed the next step should be to stop the octreotide IV and notify the pharmacy to send up the right drug for Mr. Lucas. She thought she had to tell Dr. Janice Mann, the intensivist who was treating both patients, but dreaded doing so because Dr. Mann did not tolerate mistakes. But, Dr. Mann needed to know so that she could adjust Mr. Lucas's treatment. Then there was the issue of Mr. London's family. Dr. Fowler wasn't as sure that they needed to be told about the error.

Commentary

This case is complex but reveals potential ethical concerns. As the pharmacist involved in the case, Dr. Fowler will need to decide what she needs to do and why. The five-step model can help Dr. Fowler work toward a justifiable resolution.

1. Respond to the Sense That Something Is Wrong

The first step in the ethical decision-making process is to respond to the intuitive sense that something is wrong in a given situation. Unlike obvious signs and symptoms, such as a rise in partial thromboplastin time or a drop in hemoglobin level, there are no objective signs that one is involved in an ethical problem. It is obvious that urgent care areas, such as the emergency department and intensive care units, can be fraught with stress and emotion. Do these emotional signs indicate that an ethical problem is in progress? The answer, as is often the case in ethics, is yes and no. Just because people are emotionally upset with each other or under a lot of stress does not necessarily mean that an ethical problem is involved. However, heightened emotional sensitivity—along with ". . . stress and tension intrapersonally or interpersonally; and ineffective communication patterns such as avoidance, nagging, or silence"[2]—is often a warning sign that one is involved in an ethical problem.

In Mr. London's case, Dr. Fowler happened to notice the discarded IV bag that led to her discovery of a drug error that may or may not have contributed to Mr. London's death. Dr. Fowler also experiences a sense of dread when she thinks about reporting the error to the intensivist in charge of both patients. She can certainly expect some type of negative reaction from Dr. Mann based on past interpersonal interactions. She may also feel guilty about the error that has occurred. She expresses "dismay" when she sees the wrong drug being administered in Mr. Lucas' room. These negative emotions are indications that an ethical problem is present. This first step in the decision-making process merely requires one to respond to the feeling that something is wrong. One should then move on to the next step.

2. Gather Information

There is an old saw in ethics: "Good ethics begins with good facts." Clearly, to make an informed decision, one must have the facts. To organize the numerous facts in the situation in which Dr. Fowler is involved, one can classify them into clinical and situational information.

Clinical information deals with the relevant clinical data in the case in question. The following types of clinical questions are relevant when reviewing a case: What is the medical status of the patient or patients involved in the situation? Medical history? Diagnosis? Prognosis? What drugs are involved, and what are their actions, side effects, etc.? What is the patient's probable life expectancy and general condition if treatment is given? What is the patient's probable life expectancy and general condition if treatment is not given?

In Mr. London's case, the clinical information appeared to be unambiguous. His illness was acute and life-threatening. If not treated immediately with appropriate drug therapy and other life-saving measures, Mr. London would certainly die from hemorrhage and shock. Even if the treatment was effective in managing the bleeding, it would not resolve the underlying problem of cirrhosis. Additionally, the chance that treatment would be effective was small given the underlying condition. The administration of heparin to a patient who is already hemorrhaging would increase the risk of bleeding, but it may not have hastened Mr. London's death. As much as possible, it is important to clarify the relevant clinical information in the case before moving on to a more in-depth analysis of the moral relevance of these facts.

Situational information includes data regarding the values and perspectives of the principals involved; their authority; verbal and nonverbal communication, including language barriers; cultural and religious factors; setting and time constraints; and the relationships of those immediately involved in the case. In other words, even if the clinical "facts" of a case remain constant, changes in the situational or contextual factors, such as the values of a key principal in the case, could change the ethical focus or intensify the ethical conflict. Of all the situational data mentioned, the most important is the identification and understanding of the value judgments involved in a case. An extensive discussion of value judgments is in Chapter 2.

The main players in this case are the two patients, any family involved, Dr. Fowler, Dr. Mann, the pharmacist(s) who prepared the drugs, and members of the nursing staff responsible for hanging the IV medications. All the individuals involved in the case possess values about many things, including values about health, honesty, professional competence, and loyalty, to name a few. We know specifically that Dr. Mann ". . . did not tolerate mistakes." What does this mean in practical terms? Do individuals who make mistakes lose their jobs? The case also includes a situational factor that impinges on the case—urgency and time constraints. Two emergencies occurred almost simultaneously. If the two admissions to the intensive care unit had been spaced further apart, it is possible that the error would not have happened. We know that responsibility for the error-free care of Mr. London and Mr. Lucas rested with various members of the health care team. Each member's responsibilities are distinct yet overlap. As part of the information-gathering step it is important to sort out the various responsibilities, not for placing blame but for identifying moral accountability. For example, Dr. Fowler may not be the one who mislabeled the IV bags, but as evening supervisor she has overarching responsibility for all medications that leave the pharmacy. Second, she is the one who discovered the error. Knowledge of the error carries its own responsibility. These are only some of the facts affecting ethical decision-making in this case. Once all the facts are outlined, they can be examined to see whether the situation has the characteristics of an ethical problem.

3. Identify the Ethical Problem/Moral Diagnosis

As has been noted in the introduction, ethics deals with a wide range of imperatives and obligations regarding human dignity and conduct. The distinct characteristics of moral evaluation, also mentioned in the introduction, apply to this third step of the five-step model, that is, they must be ultimate, possess universality, and treat the good of everyone alike. Ethical principles are relevant sources of ethical guidance and can serve as guidelines to identify the types of ethical problems involved in a case. The values, rights, duties, or principles that are in conflict should be identified. The ethical principles most often involved in complex cases, such as Dr. Fowler's situation, are (1) patient and health professional autonomy, (2) beneficence and nonmaleficence, and (3) justice. In this volume, veracity, fidelity, and avoidance of killing are treated as possible principles as well. Separate chapters presented in Part II develop each of these principles.

At a minimum the principles in conflict in this case are nonmaleficence and veracity. Clearly an error has occurred. In the case of Mr. London, the degree of harm caused by the error is still in question. Even an autopsy might not be able to determine whether the error contributed to his death. All we know for certain is that the error deprived him of drug therapy that could have provided benefit. The error may have caused harm to Mr. Lucas as well. He too was deprived, at least for a while, of a treatment that could have helped him. Thus, harms have occurred that, at this point, are unknown to key players in the case. Nonmaleficence suggests that Dr. Fowler has a duty to protect the pharmacist involved from having to endure the unjustified wrath of Dr. Mann but also to prevent further harm to Mr. Lucas by making sure he begins to receive the right drug. Nonmaleficence would also suggest a duty to initiate procedures to make sure this kind of error does not occur again.

Also at stake is the principle of veracity, the moral notion that one is obligated to speak truthfully, especially when one's role in the situation makes it ethically impossible to keep silent. As far as we know to this point, only Dr. Fowler knows about the error. As soon as she calls attention to the error by stopping the octreotide IV and ordering the correct medication from the pharmacy, others will become aware of the error too. She believes she is obligated to tell the truth to Dr. Mann so that she can adjust Mr. Lucas's treatment. But there are others involved in the case who have a claim on knowing the truth, the other members of the health care team, such as the nurses and pharmacists, as well as Mr. London's family.

Dr. Fowler seems to feel quite certain that she has a duty to inform Dr. Mann but isn't as clear about her obligation to Mr. London's family. One could propose arguments for either telling or withholding the truth from the family. The harm to

Mr. London has already occurred and is irreversible. The principle of nonmaleficence, or of doing no harm, could lead Dr. Fowler to be concerned about causing unnecessary psychological stress on his family. Traditionally, the Hippocratic ethic permits, or even requires, health professionals to remain silent whenever information would be needlessly disturbing to patients or families. On the other hand, the family could benefit from knowing what happened. They could pursue legal action that would benefit them financially and may help them gain closure over the incident. Beneficence involves balancing the burdens and the benefits of an action, an analysis that can be extremely difficult.

The ethical principle of fidelity requires that people act out of loyalty to those with whom they stand in a special relationship, such as between health provider and patient. The requirements of fidelity when a provider interacts with family members are more complex, but a case could be made that, in this situation, Dr. Fowler owes it to Mr. London's family to let them know truthfully what happened. At this point, exploring various courses of action requires both determining which principles are involved and what their implications are. At that point, we can move to the fourth step in solving the problem at hand.

4. Seek a Resolution

Proposing more than one course of action and examining the ethical justification of various actions is, indeed, the working phase of decision-making. Many people try to avoid this step and, at the same time, to reduce the stress of the situation by settling for the first option that comes to mind or for what initially appears to be the safe choice.

Several courses of action are open to Dr. Fowler: (1) She could fully share information about the error with all those involved; (2) she could tell Dr. Mann about the error and other internal entities in the hospital but not inform Mr. London's family or Mr. Lucas's family; (3) she could keep the knowledge to herself and not tell anyone and try to correct the error without being caught or just let the wrong drug continue to infuse into Mr. Lucas; or (4) she could wait to tell Dr. Mann about the error with Mr. Lucas's medication until she can determine if it is having any side effects. These actions actually fall into the categories of telling, not telling, or waiting to tell, the last being a version of not telling. Because the error affected two patients, the range of possible actions doubles.

To determine which options are morally justifiable, one must project the probable consequences of each action and the underlying intention of the action as well as whether there are moral duties that prevail independent of the consequences. This process involves the application of the ethical principles presented earlier and the ethical theories described below. By following this process, one can reject some options immediately because they would result in harm or would conflict with another basic ethical principle.

Choosing the first option would be in compliance with deontological (or duty-based) ethical theories, which assert that the rightness of an act can be judged insofar as it fulfills some principle of duty, in this case particularly the duty of veracity. This option would be compatible with the respect, dignity, and equality that all human beings deserve. Telling the physician fulfills the principle of veracity vis-à-vis the physician but leaves open what that principle requires with regard to the family. The duty-based principles of veracity and fidelity require showing respect for others, especially when some special relation exists. Not telling the family members does not respect the dignity of the family members. The third option of withholding the truth about the error and not doing anything else would be hard to justify from the perspective of these duty-based principles. Furthermore, not telling and trying to correct the error without telling anyone about it is fraught with problems, not the least of which is the great possibility of getting caught in the act of a cover-up. The credibility of not only Dr. Fowler but of the entire pharmacy would be at stake should that happen. The fourth option delays the truth but holds open the possibility that it will be disclosed at a later time. This option seems to be based on the assumption that disclosure is warranted only if the consequences require it. This brings us to consideration of the consequence-oriented principles—beneficence and nonmaleficence.

Two major versions of consequence-oriented ethics were presented in the introduction: utilitarianism and Hippocratic ethics. Hippocratic ethics would focus on the principles of beneficence and nonmaleficence, but only insofar as the action has an impact on the patient. Mr. London is dead; he cannot be affected one way or the other. Mr. Lucas, conversely, is very likely to be affected. At least he needs to begin immediately receiving the right medication, but that may not require disclosure of the error. Then, too, disclosure may be distressing to him. A good case can be made that the error should be kept between Dr. Fowler and those who need to know in order to correct it.

Utilitarianism differs from Hippocratic ethics by not focusing on the principles of beneficence and nonmaleficence but on which consequences are relevant. Utilitarianism holds that the option that would bring about the greatest good for the greatest number should be chosen. If telling the truth would likely produce more benefits for all the affected parties than any other alternative, then it would be good and right. If not, it would be bad and wrong. To decide whether the various options are right or wrong one would have to consider the effects of each on everyone concerned. Utilitarianism would consider the effects not only on the two patients, Mr. Lucas and Mr. London, but also on the pharmacist who apparently made the error and the nurses who failed to check the medications and catch the error. It would consider the families involved. Most critically, it would consider the effects on future patients who might benefit if the error is reported and procedures are put in place to make sure it does not happen again.

We have at this point identified several possible courses of action and the implications of various ethical principles for each of those courses.

5. Work with Others to Choose a Course of Action

No one makes decisions alone in a health care setting. The same is true for ethical decisions. A better decision can be reached if the people who are legitimately involved have the opportunity to openly discuss their perceptions, values, and concerns. In a complex case such as this, Dr. Fowler should call on the input of colleagues in pharmacy, the physician, and the nursing staff. By discussing concerns together, they can reach a more comprehensive decision that is ethically justifiable.

It is apparent that the duty-based principles, such as autonomy, veracity, and fidelity, push very hard toward requiring disclosure of the error—at least to Dr. Mann and other hospital authorities and probably to the patients' families as well. On the other hand, the Hippocratic form of a consequence-based ethic provides the most plausible basis for supporting nondisclosure. Mr. London cannot be helped by the disclosure, and Mr. Lucas probably can be helped as much without it. A more social form of a consequence-based ethic, such as utilitarianism, leaves us in an ambiguous spot. Harms can come—to the families who will be placed in distress and certainly to the pharmacist who made the error. Significant benefits from disclosure also can be expected, perhaps to Mr. Lucas but definitely to future patients. It is possible that the family members might gain benefits as well.

Notes

1. Purtilo, Ruth. *Ethical Dimensions in the Health Professions*. Third Edition. Philadelphia: W. B. Saunders, 2005; Fletcher, John C., Editor. *Fletcher's Introduction to Clinical Ethics*. Second Edition. Frederick, MD: University Publishing Group, 2005; Haddad, A., and M. Kapp. *Ethical and Legal Problems in Home Health Care*. Norwalk, CT: Appleton and Lange, 2001; Rule, James T., and Robert M. Veatch. *Ethical Questions in Dentistry*. Second Edition. Chicago: Quintessence Books, 2004.

2. Salladay, Susan, and Amy Haddad. "Point-Counterpoint Technique in Assessing Hidden Agendas." *Dimensions of Critical Care Nursing* 5, no. 4 (1986): 238–243.

2

Values in Health and Illness

It might appear that ethical and other value problems arise infrequently for the pharmacist. Although the physician is increasingly seen as confronting such issues—in decisions about abortion, euthanasia, test-tube baby cases, and genetics, for example—the pharmacist's day may, to the layperson, seem less filled with such controversial issues. In fact, there are pharmaceutical dimensions to almost all of the dramatic ethical problems in health care. Abortion can involve decisions about the use of abortifacient agents; euthanasia, about the use of barbiturates and narcotic analgesics to hasten death; pharmaceutical agents are used in producing superovulation that precedes in vitro fertilizations; and genetic engineering includes many pharmaceutical applications in drug manufacturing and decisions about alternative therapies.

Thus almost every dramatic and controversial issue in health care ethics can pose problems directly related to pharmacy. Nevertheless, many of the day-to-day ethical dilemmas faced by the pharmacist arise not in the context of these dramatic, ethically exotic cases, but in much more normal, routine pharmacy practice. Every prescription raises issues about informed consent, assessment of risks and benefits, and the ethics of determining a fair price. Many patients will be faced with difficult choices about the wisdom of using drugs their physicians have prescribed. Other patients will turn directly to the pharmacist for medical advice, raising questions not only about the ethics of informing patients, but also about the moral limits on the pharmacist's role as health care practitioner.

Before turning to specific topics, such as the ethics of informed consent, pricing, and the dispensing of morally controversial medications, some preliminary work must be done. Having developed a five-step model for analyzing ethical cases, we now need to examine the ethical and other value judgments in pharmacy decisions (the focus of this chapter) and the problem of where moral judgments are grounded (the topic of the next chapter).

Identifying Value Judgments in Pharmacy

Normative judgments (or evaluative judgments) occur constantly in all health care decisions. It is impossible to get to a clinical conclusion—to prescribe a drug, use an over-the-counter medication, substitute a generic, check the accuracy of a dosage with the physician, include a medication in a formulary, or report a suspected drug abuser—without making a normative judgment. Whenever someone decides to act (or refrain from acting), some evaluation has taken place. A decision is made that a particular course is the *right* one. It is *better* than available alternatives. It is what one *ought* to do.

One key to learning to recognize that evaluative judgments have taken place is to watch for value terms. Words like *right, better,* and *ought* all signal a process of evaluation. It is the nature of a clinical science like pharmacy that these evaluations take place constantly.

Case 2-1 does not raise a dramatic or grave ethical issue. It may not raise any ethical issue at all. It does involve a number of evaluations, however. In deciding how the pharmacist should respond to the patient/customer in this case, one has to be able to identify what value judgments are being made. In reading through this case, note all the words signaling that an evaluation is taking place.

CASE 2-1   Over-the-Counter Diet Pills

Although it was still the middle of winter, Bess Williams noticed that the new swimsuits were on display in the department store window. As she admired the latest in swimwear, she made a firm resolution to lose weight. Ms. Williams had tried numerous diets over the years but always seemed to lose only a few pounds and then gain back even more. Also, she really hated exercise, so a quick-and-easy way to lose weight was what she had in mind. She stopped by the pharmacy she often patronized during her lunch hour. She found the "diet aids" section of the pharmacy and scanned the products until she found one she had seen advertised on the Internet. Ms. Williams remembered that the product, sold in several different forms, helps "curb your appetite" when you need it most and increases metabolism to "burn fat."

Since the drugstore wasn't busy, Steven Krause, Pharm.D., also the pharmacy owner, rang up Ms. Williams's purchases. Dr. Krause noticed the weight control pills and looked up to see if the buyer was truly overweight. He had noticed a seasonal increase in the sales of these pills following the holidays and leading into swimsuit season. Ms. Williams looked to be at least 50 pounds overweight for her height.

Ms. Williams asked Dr. Krause, "How do these diet pills work? I've just never had the willpower to stick to a diet, but I really want to lose weight this time."

Dr. Krause explained, "The main ingredients in these pills are herbs and other products. They contain chitosan, which binds to dietary fat and purportedly has an effect on

CASE 2-1   *Continued.*

reducing the absorption of fat. The formula also contains some bitter orange that will suppress your appetite to a certain degree. There is also guarana, and that has an effect similar to caffeine. These pills should be used on a short-term basis along with reduced caloric intake and exercise. The amount of weight reduction usually is small."

"You mean I have to be on a diet, too?" Ms. Williams groaned. Looking somewhat disappointed she said, "Oh well, it's worth a try. The worst thing that can happen is that I won't lose all the weight I want."

Dr. Krause replied, "Actually, other things could happen with these pills. Even though you don't need a prescription there are still some side effects you should know about. They have a stimulant effect, which can result in nervousness, restlessness, insomnia, dizziness, and headache. There is also the possibility of an increase in blood pressure and heart rate."

Ms. Williams was getting more and more discouraged. "I can't even drink coffee without getting all jumpy and irritable."

Ms. Williams stood in the checkout line with the diet pills in her hand, tapping them lightly on the counter as she decided what would be worse: being irritable and tired or not being able to wear a swimsuit again this summer.

Commentary

At first this case may appear to raise no evaluative issues at all. The customer wanted the diet pills, and the pharmacist was in a position to provide her with some information about them.

Searching for the value terms, however, reveals a number of judgments that are clearly in the realm of values. According to this pharmacist the pills *should* be used on a short-term basis along with reduced caloric intake. Two judgments are implied here. First, longer use would produce an unacceptable risk of bad results, in the pharmacist's judgment. But, second, it is acceptable to use them only in the short term. Both of these evaluations are controversial.

They rely in part on assessments of what the case refers to as *side effects.* The term is an interesting one. It is, in fact, a value judgment that certain effects are unintended and bad. (It would be quite odd to speak of a "good" side effect.) The pharmacist lists several such effects: nervousness, restlessness, insomnia, dizziness, headache, and possible increase in blood pressure and heart rate. The judgment that these are bad effects is relatively noncontroversial. It is a value judgment nonetheless. Moreover, these effects are worse for some people than for other people. Someone suffering from hypotension might be less concerned than a hypertensive.

We already see how such evaluations take the pharmacist beyond what pharmacological science can provide. The move becomes even more significant when the pharmacist and patient begin to compare the risks of these harmful side effects with the possible benefits of using the diet pills. In deciding to use any drug, the critical question is always how valuable the expected benefit is going to be. Normally that is not a medical issue. In this case, the critical question is how important it is to Ms. Williams to lose weight through the use of the drug. In order to answer that question we need to know not only how she values weight loss, but also how she compares the harms from the possible side effects with what she perceives as the disadvantages of other ways of losing weight (and of not losing weight at all). If every alternative is very unattractive, then (assuming continued use has at least some additional weight-loss effect) she might be willing to take on the risks of using the drug for a longer period. However, if losing weight is not as important, or if other methods are not terribly burdensome, then even short-term use of the substances commonly found in diet pills would make little sense. The evaluations are key, and it is hard to see how being trained as a pharmacist (or any other health professional) makes one an expert in making them.

What then is the pharmacist's role when educating patients about the so-called risks and benefits of pharmaceutical agents? Is it this pharmacist's duty to tell Ms. Williams what his personal opinions are about how one set of effects compares to another? Or is he simply charged to give her the facts? It seems strange that he would be expected to give her his personal value judgments. However, giving her just the facts would create serious problems as well. In the case of nonprescription products, such as herbs and vitamins, it may be very difficult for the pharmacist to know what the facts really are, since there is little convincing, scientific evidence about the benefit of any ingredient in weight-loss products. Also, stocking these products in the pharmacy implies a value of sorts, and that sends a message to patients when they look for assistance from the pharmacist. Moreover, in order to fully evaluate the risks, the pharmacist would have to know other important facts about the case, such as what products Ms. Williams had tried in the past and why she is worried about losing weight. Then, too, how can the pharmacist know exactly which medical facts to give her? Surely, more could be said about diet pills than is reasonable to tell to a patient. In addition, this particular patient may be unusually interested in certain relatively rare risks that would not be of concern to most.

Many interesting questions lie beneath the surface of this case, questions having relevance not only for over-the-counter medications, but also for value judgments made about the risks and benefits of medicinal agents as part of patient education. Learning to recognize value judgments is a crucial first step. Only after these issues are confronted can we turn to more directly ethical questions, such as whether patients should be permitted to take medicinal risks based on their own judgment and whether patients have the right to know about the risks and benefits in the first place.

Case 2-2 presents another opportunity to identify the evaluations taking place in a conversation between a pharmacist and a patient. In this case try to identify the value judgments made by the prescribing dentist, the pharmacist, and the patient.

CASE 2-2   Managing Dental Pain

Ian Jones, Pharm.D., could tell just by looking at Jerry Rudolph's face that he had just been to the dentist. Mr. Rudolph and Dr. Jones knew each other not only as pharmacist and patient, but as members of the same health club. Mr. Rudolph's speech was slightly slurred as he presented a prescription to Dr. Jones. Mr. Rudolph stated, "I just had a root canal, and my mouth is still numb. I can't talk very well yet. The dentist said the stuff he used to numb my mouth will last a long time, maybe up to 6 hours. What's the prescription for anyway? I wasn't paying much attention when I left the dentist's office."

Dr. Jones replied, "The prescription is for Tylenol #40, which is a combination of Tylenol and codeine, a narcotic analgesic. It's for pain relief."

Mr. Rudolph remarked, "I didn't ask for anything for pain. I'm not sure about taking strong pain medication when I really don't need it. Would aspirin or something else over-the-counter work just as well? Are there any side effects from codeine?"

Dr. Jones believes that pain and pain relief are completely subjective. Yet he doesn't like to encourage the use of narcotic analgesics until it is clear that the pain will not be relieved by nonopiate analgesics. He feels this is especially true in the case of dental patients who have received local anesthetic agents with a long duration of action. Should Dr. Jones encourage Mr. Rudolph to try aspirin, acetaminophen, or ibuprofen to relieve the pain?

Commentary

As in Case 2-1 there appear to be possible differences in value judgments about how to treat pain from a tooth extraction. Similar questions arise about what constitutes a side effect and how to determine just how bad the side effects could be. Mr. Rudolph seems to believe he will not need what he considers to be strong pain medication. Of course, the anesthetic has not worn off yet, but he may well know from past experience that he can tolerate the anticipated level of pain. The judgment that he will not *need* the codeine is actually a judgment that he prefers the risk of pain controlled only with nonnarcotic analgesics to pain controlled by a narcotic.

Dr. Jones apparently views these trade-offs differently. He believes he is in a position to know not only how much pain Mr. Rudolph is likely to experience, but also whether the risks of the narcotic would be justified in his case.

Attitudes about pain vary tremendously from one culture to another and from one individual to another. Some people are averse to using "strong," or narcotic, medication in part because of the psychological connotations of using narcotics. They may believe that the risk of addiction, no matter how small, is not worth it. They may also ground their judgments in even deeper cultural attitudes about the meaning of pain and its control. Moreover, in some cultures pain is perceived as affording some advantage, as a warning of an underlying problem or as a character-building experience in which the sufferer learns to cope. For other cultures and ethnic groups, pain is something to be expressed openly. This generates an attitude of sympathy while providing a rationale for explaining unusual behaviors related to pain.

In addition, there are those who hold the worldview that pain makes no sense (other than, perhaps, as a signal of a potential medical problem). According to this point of view, humans should have dominance over nature and make use of technology to suppress suffering. The dentist in this case seems to gravitate toward this view, while the patient is more cautious.

In effect, Dr. Jones is being asked to arbitrate a debate about which of these two worldviews is more appropriate for treating someone experiencing dental pain. Surely, there is no reason why the dentist's view is necessarily the more correct. Some would be inclined to say that these issues are simply matters of taste, that there is no "right" answer. In that case, the pharmacist is being asked as a friend to give counsel on a matter of personal preference, a role he might want to take on as a friend but surely not as a pharmacist. Even if we want to view the question of whether or not to fight pain aggressively as having a correct answer, it is not the sort of issue about which any medical professional—dentist, physician, or pharmacist—can really claim to have expertise. It is a question of aesthetics, of what kind of lifestyle is best. It may also be a question of what kind of lifestyle is ethical. This raises the question of the relationship between ethical judgments and other kinds of evaluative judgments, a question we address in the second half of this chapter.

CASE 2-3   Use of Generic Drugs

Sandra Kelly, Pharm.D., was impressed with the professionalism of her new employer, Mark Pierce, the pharmacist/owner of Midtown Pharmacy. Dr. Pierce took the time to counsel patients about the side effects of medications and often stepped out from behind the counter to assist a customer in selecting a nonprescription drug product. However, Dr. Kelly noted that Dr. Pierce seldom asked patients if they preferred generic or brand-name medications. Dr. Kelly had strong negative feelings about the bioequivalence of some generic drugs to innovator drugs, in particular, drugs with a narrow therapeutic index. Her suspicions had been fostered by several pharmacy school instructors who emphasized their personal biases against using generics for critical-dose drugs, such as immunosuppressive agents. One instructor went so far as to say, "A good pharmacist would not dispense generic drugs for critical-dose drugs."

Dr. Kelly asked Dr. Pierce why patients weren't routinely given the option to choose between generic and brand-name drugs. Dr. Pierce stated, "There is a sign on the cash register in the pharmacy that tells patients to ask about generic drugs. If they don't request one, I'm not going to encourage the patient to choose a brand-name product. We make a larger profit on generics, so I prefer dispensing them whenever I can." In addition to her general concerns about the effectiveness of generics, Dr. Kelly is uncomfortable with the specific practice of not giving patients a real choice. The sign on the cash register is not very large. Should she comply with the pharmacy's informal policy that encourages the use of generics, or should she let patients know they have a choice?

Commentary

Once again the problems of this case may appear to raise questions of medical science. Dr. Kelly and her instructors in pharmacy school have been impressed by the pharmacological data reportedly showing inconsistent bioequivalence of generic drugs as compared with name-brand medications. Furthermore, Dr. Kelly's instructors went so far as to make a value judgment on the quality of the pharmacist, suggesting that a bad pharmacist dispenses generics for critical-dose drugs. However, even if one assumes that there is less consistency in generic compounds as well as a greater risk of getting an ineffective dose, it does not automatically follow that the patient should prefer the brand name compound.

If through careful consideration of the pertinent research on the efficacy of generic drugs Dr. Kelly concludes that one can buy greater reliability by paying a higher price, she still must consider whether it is wise to spend more money for the extra margin of advantage from the brand name drug. The answer will depend on how one perceives the value of the extra benefit from a brand-name drug as compared with all the other things one might do with the extra money.

Choosing how to spend one's money is clearly not a question of medical science. It is a question of values. Different patients are likely to make different value judgments. If a patient is quite wealthy and has a high degree of concern about the effectiveness and safety of the drug being taken, it would certainly be understandable for that patient to spend the extra money to achieve an additional level of safety. This would to some degree depend on how important the hoped-for benefits would be. It may be more reasonable to take some risk with a generic drug for a headache than for the control of seizure activity.

However, those for whom the "alternative costs" of brand-name medications are high—those with less disposable income who are less concerned about the effectiveness of the medication—probably would prefer the generic. The value trade-off is in large part not medical. If one assumes that the generic drug is supposed to have met some minimal standards in the manufacturing process, the risk may be less than Dr. Kelly fears.

But Dr. Pierce seems to be engaging in evaluative judgments as well. He simply may not share Dr. Kelly's concern about the risks of filling prescriptions with generic drugs. His may simply be a different value judgment. There is a complicating factor, however. Dr. Pierce admits that the profit on the generic is greater. Insofar as the patient is maneuvered into the drug preferred by the pharmacist for reasons of personal profit, the case begins to raise ethical as well as nonethical questions. When the right of the patient to be informed and to choose among alternatives is violated by the pharmacist, the problem is no longer simply one of nonmoral value preferences. It is to cases that will help distinguish between ethical and nonethical evaluations that we now turn.

Separating Ethical and Other Evaluations

We have seen that evaluative judgments arise constantly in the practice of pharmacy, not just in the ethically dramatic cases, but also in making routine judgments about whether an effect is good or bad, whose good or bad it is, and whether the risk is worth taking given the alternatives available. Not all evaluations are *ethical* judgments, however. This section examines the relationship between ethical and other kinds of evaluations.

In order for an evaluation to be an ethical evaluation, certain criteria must be met. First, the judgment must be about a human action, or character, or about norms generally governing actions or character. When we say a painting is good, we do not make an ethical judgment; we make an aesthetic one. When we say a person is good, however, we can mean many things. If we say he or she is a good runner, we probably mean the person is technically proficient; we are not making a moral judgment. When we say a person is good, however, we may mean that that person is morally good.

In that case, we are judging the person's character or conduct. Moreover, we are judging it by what we take to be a certain standard, an ultimate or final standard from which no further appeal is possible. By contrast, a person may be good according to the standards of the local community or the culture. Or the person may be good according to a certain legal standard. In these cases we might agree that the person is approved of by the local community or culture or law but still ask meaningfully whether the person or the person's actions are ethical. An ethical evaluation is made according to the ultimate standard. For religious people that standard is most likely the will of God. For secular people it may be reason or natural law or some similar nonsacred standard.

The following cases provide an opportunity to try to separate ethical judgments from other kinds of evaluations. In reading them, try to identify the issues you consider to be ethical and those you think involve nonethical evaluations.

CASE 2-4   Nonprescription Access to Legend Drugs

Charles Vickers looked through his suitcase one last time before admitting he had left his prescription bottle of Bactrim DS (Sulfamethoxazole/Trimethoprim 800/160 mg) at home more than 1,000 miles away. Mr. Vickers was enjoying the first day of a 3-week vacation in the mountains. For the past 7 days, Mr. Vickers had been taking Bactrim DS twice daily for a painful urinary tract infection. His physician emphasized the necessity of taking the medication faithfully and completing the course of therapy, so Mr. Vickers left to find a pharmacy in a nearby town.

Mr. Vickers explained to the local pharmacist, Pat Martin, Pharm.D., that he had left his prescription medication at home. He gave Dr. Martin the name of his physician back home and the name and daily dosage of the drug. Dr. Martin was able to access Mr. Vickers's drug profile through the pharmacy's computer because Mr. Vickers was a member of a drug-card benefit plan. Since the prescription was for a single course of antibacterial therapy, there were no refills. Dr. Martin then called the physician and found out he was out of town and would return in 4 days. Dr. Martin relayed this information to Mr. Vickers. "Couldn't you just give me the rest of the prescription and then talk to the doctor when he returns? I'm heading up into the high country to fish. I just think I should finish my medicine because I sure don't want to be that uncomfortable again," Mr. Vickers stated.

Dr. Martin knows that state law prohibits a pharmacist from refilling a prescription without authorization. She could dispense the minimum amount necessary of a maintenance medication, but combination antibacterials don't really fall into the "maintenance" category. On the other hand, Bactrim DS is not the type of drug that has a serious potential for abuse. Besides, the adverse effects of the drug are minimal. Dr. Martin knows there are risks from stopping antibacterial therapy midcourse. It is really up to her to decide whether she will give a complete course of antibacterial therapy to Mr. Vickers since he has never had a prescription filled at her pharmacy and she doesn't really know him. Would it be that wrong to give him the rest of his prescription, to get him through his fishing trip?

Commentary

Many value judgments take place as this scene unfolds. Try to identify them. Look first for the judgments about the pharmacological effects of the medication. Mr. Vickers considers the Bactrim DS to have been successful; he is satisfied with the results. He believes he has benefited from the treatment and doesn't want to be uncomfortable again. Dr. Martin also makes evaluative judgments. She no doubt would like to help Mr. Vickers but feels an obligation to obey the law. She also believes, though, that the potential side effects are "minimal," and she knows there are risks in stopping an antibacterial therapy midcourse. Both judgments require evaluating not only the likelihood of certain risks occurring, but also how serious the risks are. In addition, the use of Bactrim DS has its own underlying value judgments. There are other drugs that could be used to treat the urinary tract infection, drugs with different risk-benefit profiles. Mr. Vickers, though, together with his physician, viewed the risks and benefits of Bactrim DS as appropriate. These are medical value judgments, but they are value judgments nonetheless.

There are also nonmedical value judgments. Mr. Vickers could have chosen other approaches to his problem. He must have decided that the problem was not serious enough to force him to return home or to seek out help from a local physician. Dr. Martin could have pursued Mr. Vickers's physician or someone covering for him. The value of the vacation in the mountains entered into the judgment as well.

Pat Martin, the pharmacist, believes that continuing the Bactrim DS will provide further benefit. She evaluates the side effects as minimal and considers the drug to have a low potential for abuse. Deciding that the side effects are minimal requires an evaluation of them. So does labeling something "abuse." None of these judgments by patient, physician, and pharmacist can rest on science though, to be sure, many of them are evaluations of scientific facts. Determining what the predicted side effects are is pharmacology. Deciding that they are bad and how bad they are is not.

These are evaluative judgments, but thus far we have encountered no judgments that could be considered "moral" per se. Likewise, some legal judgments were made by the pharmacist. Dr. Martin knows you cannot refill a prescription without an authorization. Even if there is an exception to the law in the case of the partial filling of a maintenance medication, that does not apply in this case. More importantly, the law does not settle the *ethical* question. When asking about the morality of dispensing without a prescription we are appealing to a different standard. We are asking whether such an action would violate some ultimate standard of right and wrong, not just the codified law of the land. In distinguishing between the moral and the legal we could have in mind that in some cases it could be moral to violate the law. If, for example, the pharmacist perceived that dispensing a legend drug such as Bactrim DS without a prescription was the only way to safely save a patient's life, we might think it would be moral to do so, even if it was illegal. If the pharmacist chose to break the law after careful moral deliberation in such a case, we might say that the pharmacist conscientiously violated the law.

We might also have in mind that sometimes we offer moral evaluations of existing law not for the purpose of considering whether to conscientiously violate it, but rather to determine whether it is a good law. Sometimes it is important to separate morality and law in order to purposely make legal certain actions that are believed to be immoral. (Some people take this view about abortion, for example.) In other cases, however, if we determined that an action, though illegal, was morally justified, we could use that conclusion to urge a change in the law. We might even insist that the law be obeyed as long as it exists while simultaneously working to change it.

When we ask whether Dr. Martin would be wrong to dispense the Bactrim DS, we seem to be asking if it would be immoral as well as illegal. Dr. Martin might conclude, for instance, that Mr. Vickers is a reasonably competent adult who should have the (moral) right to be self-determining regarding the risks he takes with his own body. If so, she might conclude that morality requires that he have access to drugs, even legend drugs, provided that the risk is only to himself. One who believes strongly in the priority of the moral principle of autonomy might reach that conclusion. A libertarian (one who gives absolute priority to autonomy) would reach that conclusion regardless of whether Mr. Vickers understood the actual risks and benefits of the drug. Others, utilitarians, for example, would give moral priority to making sure that the greatest good resulted. Even they, however, might support access to legend drugs, at least when the risks are small and the patient seems to understand them, especially, as in this case, when the risk of harm from not getting the drug also is real. Both of these reasons for supporting access are moral in character. They appeal to standards that can be taken by their proponents to be ultimate standards of action.

However, Dr. Martin may have moral reasons for refusing access. First, she is probably convinced that dispensing the drug without authorization is illegal. Since the time of Socrates, people have believed that if one agrees to live in a society one also agrees, or promises, to abide by its laws. We can be said to have a moral obligation to keep such commitments, even if we think the law is foolish, even if we think the law is immoral.

A second moral reason why Dr. Martin might oppose giving Bactrim DS to Mr. Vickers is that in calculating the consequences she could adopt the position that they should be assessed not on the individual case alone, but also by taking into account what would happen if everyone were to follow a similar rule. This position, based on what is known as *rule utilitarianism,* would ask that we consider whether society would work better if a rule was in place that allowed pharmacists to dispense legend drugs without a prescription whenever they thought the consequences would be positive and the risks minimal. If we worry about individual errors in judgment, we might believe that overall it would be better for us to obey a flat rule against dispensing without authorization, granting only the limited exception for maintenance drugs.

Whichever conclusion we reach, we should recognize that in this case, real moral issues are at stake. For those who favor dispensing, there are appeals to autonomy and to consequences. For those who oppose dispensing, there are appeals to the keeping of promises and to the consequences of alternative rules. Whichever conclusion is reached, we should recognize these appeals as moral.

CASE 2-5   What Should Be Behind the Counter?

Jose Emilio, Pharm.D., was a relief pharmacist for several independent pharmacies. On a Sunday afternoon when Dr. Emilio was the only pharmacist on duty, a patient asked him to help her find the Robitussin. Dr. Emilio took the patient to the allergy and cough-and-cold remedy section of the store. He wanted to make sure that she used the Robitussin with dextromethorphan; however, he could not find any products with dextromethorphan on the shelf. Dr. Emilio went back to the pharmacy office to call the owner, Allen Ryan, Pharm.D., to find out where the dextromethorphan products were located.

Dr. Ryan told Dr. Emilio, "I decided to place all products with dextromethorphan behind the counter because I do not feel that patients should be able to have easy access to such a potentially harmful medication without careful counseling. Make sure you tell that customer about the potential risks. Also make sure that she really needs the drug before you give it to her, and only sell her one bottle."

Dr. Emilio was confused and somewhat angry as he hung up the phone. Dextromethorphan had been approved for over-the-counter use. Dr. Emilio did not feel it was necessary to counsel a customer on a drug that had been judged safe for consumer usage. Also, he wasn't sure that Dr. Ryan had the legal right to control the use of an over-the-counter product merely because of personal concerns. Dr. Emilio handed the customer the bottle of Robitussin and stated, "I guess they just haven't had time to restock the shelves."

Commentary

While in the previous case there was a dispute about providing nonprescription access to a legend drug, here we have a similar dispute over access to an over-the-counter medication. Underlying the disagreement between Dr. Emilio and Dr. Ryan are evaluations about the risks and benefits of dextromethorphan. After all, for years it was thought to be risky enough that it was available only by prescription.

At this point, however, the social judgment has been made that, regardless of the potential for misuse, it should be available without prescription. Dr. Ryan is nevertheless worried that someone might be injured by taking the drug without adequate counseling. He is driven by the classical medical ethical principle of patient benefit. If asked, he surely would say he is trying to make access difficult for the patient's own good (as well as the good of others who could be injured if the patient does not understand the risks).

Dr. Emilio also is concerned about the patient but appears to be more concerned about the right of the patient to make a choice free of external constraints. He is expressing what in ethics is often referred to as the principle of autonomy, which holds that a competent adult patient has a right to develop and act on a life plan free from outside interference. Antipaternalists hold that such a right exists even if the individual could be hurt by acting on the choice.

In Chapter 6 we shall look at cases posing the conflict between autonomy and beneficence, between self-determination and patient benefit. We should note that the disagreement here seems to be different from that in the earlier cases, such as the choice between generic and brand-name drugs or between two analgesics. In those cases, the ultimate choice appeared to rest solely on personal preference. It would be hard to argue that one choice or the other was wrong in any ultimate moral sense.

In this case, however, participants in the dispute seem to be pursuing a moral controversy, not merely a matter of taste. One signal is the emergence of the language of rights and duties. In this case, Dr. Emilio appears to think patients' rights are violated if they do not have access; a higher issue is at stake (even if, as in this case, the stakes are not terribly high). Likewise, Dr. Ryan might believe that as a professional pharmacist he has a duty to protect the welfare of his patients. That duty is grounded beyond mere desire or preference. It is perceived as coming from outside the individual. Therefore, it is thought not to be a matter of personal preference but an obligation. Understanding the source of that duty—whether it comes from the profession, from the physician or health care institution, or from some greater religious or philosophical source—is the problem addressed by the cases in Chapter 3.

3

What Is the Source of Moral Judgments?

Once ethical and other evaluative judgments are identified, the next question is where one should look to determine what is moral. Health professionals view the problem of what is moral as a matter of "professional ethics." Pharmacists might turn to the code of ethics of the profession. For American pharmacists this might be the current Code of Ethics for Pharmacists of the American Pharmacists Association (APhA) (presented in the appendix of this volume). Someone might wonder, however, whether a pharmacist's conduct is always correct just because it conforms to the APhA Code of Ethics for Pharmacists.

The problem could be particularly acute when a pharmacist is in disagreement with a physician over what is ethical. It seems strange that a physician would want to yield to the APhA as an authority in such a disagreement. The physician might believe that the physician's personal moral judgment or the judgment of the physician's professional group (such as the American Medical Association) is the proper standard for assessing whether the physician's prescription or course of action is morally correct.

A pharmacist working in a hospital may have to contend with the ethical code not only of the physician, but also of the hospital. The hospital may have a locally generated code of conduct or may be subject to ethical positions taken by its sponsor or of the American Hospital Association. Should the pharmacist consider the hospital's ethical position to be the source of authority for determining what is ethical pharmacist conduct?

If the hospital is supported by a religious organization, the hospital's ethical code may be derived from the theological ethical commitments of the sponsoring religious group. For Catholic hospitals in the United States, for instance, this would be the Ethical and Religious Directives for Catholic Health Care Services.[1]

The pharmacist also may be aligned with a religious tradition, which may or may not be the same as that of the sponsoring hospital. Should a religious tradition be treated as an authoritative source for knowing what is ethical? If so, should it be the hospital's tradition or the pharmacist's? And how should either of these relate to the professional code of the pharmacist?

Finally, the pharmacist likely will confront ethical dilemmas involving a particular patient who also has moral standards that he or she feels should be the foundation of moral judgments involving his or her medication. Is the patient's ethical stance a defensible basis for grounding the ethical positions taken by a pharmacist? In this chapter cases are presented that provide an opportunity to examine alternative ways of grounding moral judgments. In each case, the important problem is not figuring out the right thing to do but, rather, determining the source of moral authority and upon what authority the pharmacist's behavior should be shaped.

Grounding Ethics in the Professional Code

A pharmacist confronting an ethical problem that poses a significant difficulty may want to turn to the professional code of ethics to determine what it says regarding the issue at hand. Often the professional code will provide insight based on years of collective experience of the members of the professional group.

Sometimes the apparent answer from the code seems so appropriate that no further consideration is necessary. In other cases, though, it may not be obvious to the individual pharmacist that the profession's collective wisdom is morally definitive. One problem arises because the professional group's code can change over the years. The APhA code, for example, was originally written in 1852[2] but was revised in 1922[3] and again in 1952[4] and 1969. Modest changes were made in 1975, 1981, and 1985.[5] Finally, in 1994 a completely revised code was adopted.[6] Each time the code changed did the ethically correct behavior for pharmacists really change or only what the APhA members believed was the correct behavior?

What about pharmacists who are not members of the APhA? Does its code determine what is ethically correct for those who are not members or only for those who are members? Can what is ethically correct for pharmacists change depending on whether they are members of their professional association? And what about pharmacists in other nations? Does the American professional code or the other nation's professional code determine what is right for these pharmacists? It seems odd that what is right for pharmacists should depend on the country in which they practice and when they practice. The following two cases ask what role the professional code should play in determining what is ethically correct conduct for pharmacists.

CASE 3-1   What Is "In the Best Interest of the Patient"?

Eighteen months ago, John Wilson was in an automobile accident that resulted in head trauma. After an acute hospitalization, Mr. Wilson responded fairly well to an extensive rehabilitation program. The only residual damage from the injury was grand mal seizure activity, which was adequately, though not completely, controlled with phenytoin sodium and valproic acid. Mr. Wilson wanted to return to work with the private roofing contractor with whom he had been employed for 10 years. Mr. Wilson spoke with the owner of the roofing company, Mark Adamson, about returning to work.

"Are you up to it, John?" Mark asked.

"Sure, sure," Mr. Wilson replied, "I'm just like new."

Later that week, Mr. Wilson returned to his neighborhood pharmacy for a refill on his anticonvulsant medications. In the course of filling the prescriptions, Mr. Wilson told the pharmacist that he had returned to work at the roofing company. The pharmacist, Ralph Jenkins, Pharm.D., was more than surprised because he knew that Mr. Wilson was not completely seizure free on his present medication regimen. Dr. Jenkins asked Mr. Wilson if he had told his employer about the possibility of seizure activity. "No way," Mr. Wilson replied, "I know when I'm going to have a seizure because I get this funny taste in my mouth and then I get dizzy. If that happens, I'll go find a safe place to lie down."

Dr. Jenkins is troubled by Mr. Wilson's response. He knows that the APhA Code of Ethics states that "a pharmacist promotes the good of every patient in a caring, compassionate, and confidential manner." Dr. Jenkins feels it would be in Mr. Wilson's best interest to warn Mr. Wilson's employer about the potential for grand mal seizure activity, yet he doesn't want to hurt Mr. Wilson's reputation or ability to work. Dr. Jenkins shudders to think what might happen if Mr. Wilson had a convulsion while working on a roof. Further, Dr. Jenkins is certain that Mr. Wilson's employer would be held at least partially responsible should Mr. Wilson sustain an injury. The Code of Ethics seems unclear about the ethically correct course of action in this type of situation.

Commentary

Until its most recent revision, the APhA code permitted violations of confidentiality when the pharmacist was convinced, as is Dr. Jenkins, that the patient's interest would be better served by disclosure; it may even have demanded disclosure in such situations. The earlier version of the Code of Ethics said that the pharmacist's first consideration should be the health and safety of patients. It is not implausible that disclosure would help protect the health and safety of Mr. Wilson. The present version of the APhA code is less clear about how Dr. Jenkins should respond. Its second principle is "A pharmacist promotes the good of every patient in a caring, compassionate, and confidential manner." The pharmacist is not only supposed to promote the good of the patient but, also, to do so in a confidential manner. Dr. Jenkins's problem is determining if he should break a confidence in order to promote his patient's good. Here we see that the professional code changes from time to time and sometimes is ambiguous.

As we shall see in Chapter 8 when we look in more detail at cases of confidentiality, other professional codes, including that of the American Medical Association, insist in such cases that, even if the patient's interest would be better served by breaking confidence, the confidence should still be kept, unless that patient gives permission to disclose.

The problem raised here is whether the professional association code is necessarily always the definitive authority for determining what is ethical for pharmacists. It seems to make sense to consult the code in difficult cases, but is that because the code *defines* what is right for pharmacists or because the code simply summarizes the judgment of the pharmacist's colleagues who have faced somewhat similar situations?

It could be that what is the right behavior for a pharmacist is whatever the code says. If the code literally defines what is ethical for members of the profession, then it is logically impossible for it to be wrong. Moreover, whenever the code is changed, then what is right for pharmacists changes. The alternative is that the foundation for ethics in pharmacy is something more basic than the current professional agreement. For example, for those standing in a religious tradition, what is ethically right and wrong might be determined by the approval or the will of the deity. For some secular thinkers what is right is determined by reason, by the moral laws of nature, or by other fundamental standards. The idea is that the standard for ethics is the ultimate appeal one can make, the point beyond which no further appeal is possible.

Some people have given up hope of recognizing the will of a deity, the moral laws of nature, or what reason requires. They may be convinced that the standard of ethics is a societal one. In that view, an act is right if one's society says it is. That, of course, leaves open the possibility that for other people in other societies, some other behavior would be ethical (because in their society some other behavior is approved). Still, there is possibly a difference between what society says a pharmacist should do regarding a problem, like breaking a confidence, and what the profession says a pharmacist should do.

Dr. Jenkins's problem is whether he is prepared to treat the professional association's statement of what is ethical regarding breaking a confidence as a standard beyond which there is no conceivable appeal. Is he prepared to say that whatever the APhA says ethically settles the matter? Or does he believe that the real standard of ethics lies elsewhere: in the will of God, in reason, in the laws of nature, in the broader society's judgment, or perhaps his own judgment? Where should Dr. Jenkins turn to find the ultimate standard for moral matters? A similar question arises in the following case.

CASE 3-2   Professional and Public Views on Closing a Pharmacy

Sidney Kalman had worked as a pharmacist-in-charge at the pharmacy of the Grand Union grocery store in Paramus, New Jersey, since September 1970. In early June of 1978, his supervisor, Stanley Brumer, informed him that, although the rest of the store would be open, the pharmacy section would be closed for the July Fourth holiday. Since the pharmacy section was not separated by a partition and was not capable of being secured, this disturbed Mr. Kalman. In fact, because of the inability to secure the prescription section, the entire store was licensed as a pharmacy.

When Mr. Kalman protested, the supervisor told him that the Board of Pharmacy had given its permission to close the pharmacy section, but Mr. Kalman, suspecting this was not true, phoned the Board and confirmed that the pharmacy was indeed required to be open if the rest of the store was. The pharmacy was kept open July Fourth with another pharmacist on duty.

CASE 3-2 *Continued.*

Upon reporting to work on July 5, Mr. Kalman was informed that his employment at Grand Union was terminated. Mr. Kalman eventually sued his former employer claiming he was discharged "solely for attempting to vindicate a state regulation and his own code of professional ethics." Mr. Kalman was what is called an "at will" employee, that is, one without a formal contract. In general an employer can dismiss such employees at will except when doing so violates public policy. Firings on blatant racial grounds or for refusal to grant sexual favors to a supervisor are examples of firings that have been held to violate public policy.

A lower court granted a dismissal of Mr. Kalman's case on the grounds that neither the state regulation nor the code of professional ethics was a clear expression of public policy that would prohibit firing of Mr. Kalman. The case was then appealed, at which time the higher court had to determine whether the mandates of state regulation and the professional code of ethics provided such clear expressions.

The appeals court first held that the state rules regulating the practice of pharmacy did impose a duty on the pharmacist to report the violation of the Pharmacy Act. It then turned to the question of whether the APhA Code of Ethics could also be a "source" of public policy. The question at this point is whether Mr. Kalman, in deciding whether to report the decision to open the store on the Fourth of July without opening the pharmacy section, should be guided by the APhA Code as well as by the rules of the Board of Pharmacy and, if so, whether the state should recognize such guidance.[7]

Commentary

The problem facing Mr. Kalman involves a complex combination of moral, legal, and public policy questions. For our purposes, it is important to focus on the moral ones. It seems sensible to say that the rule or regulation requiring Mr. Kalman to report the violation constitutes clear public policy. What, however, is the relation between the APhA Code of Ethics and the moral and legal dimensions of this case?

Professional organizations, such as the APhA, are not public agencies. They are private professional groups. They are not, in any way, under public control. In this sense, they are quite different from public agencies. By contrast, the Board of Pharmacy is a public agency normally appointed by and formally accountable to public officials. It would appropriately have authority to establish public policy not normally granted to private groups, even professional groups.

A public body, such as a state board of pharmacy, could adopt as its public policy a rule that whatever the professional group declares is ethical is automatically public policy as well. If it did, it would still have to determine whether it is endorsing the state association, the national association, or some international professional body's code of ethics. The underlying question, however, is whether it makes sense for the public to permit private professional groups to shape public policy, regardless of which group is selected. There is always the possibility that the public's view of what the policy should be will be different from the profession's view. In the event of a dispute between the public and the professional perception of public policy, it would seem strange to hear the public insist that the professional formulation should automatically prevail.

Even if the APhA was recognized as a legitimate source of public policy, the question remains of the relation between what is public policy and what is ethics. Since the courts were only dealing with the matter of what was the source of public policy, the question of what is ethical may not have been directly relevant. It is conceivable that opening the store without a pharmacist present was permitted by public policy but was still unethical. What should Mr. Kalman do in this case?

It is possible that Mr. Kalman would conclude that he should engage in civil disobedience, to violate public policy in order to do what is ethical. That is a major decision, however, one that should not be undertaken lightly. In this case, since public policy seems to concur with Mr. Kalman's ethical judgment, the problem probably would not arise.

This leaves us with the question, however, of how Mr. Kalman should judge what is ethical in such cases. If ethics sometimes requires civil disobedience, this implies that what is ethical is not determined solely by public policy of the society. However, it is not clear that the codes of the profession automatically determine what is ethical any more than they determine what is public policy. If the profession *determined* what was ethical for professionals, then the profession could never be wrong, yet many people would acknowledge that the profession is occasionally wrong. Perhaps the profession is no more an appropriate source of the ethics of professional conduct than it is a source of public policy. We are left with the question of whether the society, the courts, or Mr. Kalman should view the professional codes as a "source" of either public policy or of ethics. Does it make sense for Mr. Kalman to claim in defense of his behavior regarding the Fourth of July incident, that he was grounding his sense of obligation in the code of the profession of pharmacy?

Grounding Ethics in the Physician's Orders

In some situations a pharmacist is presented with ethical decisions that seem to be grounded not so much in either public policy or professional codes, but in the beliefs of practicing physicians. Of course, in reaching his or her moral conclusion, the physician may have to decide how important the professional code is, but by the time the physician has decided on a course of action, the pharmacist may be presented only with the doctor's order. The following two cases raise the question of whether the pharmacist should treat the physician's instruction as a grounding of moral positions taken in the practice of pharmacy.

CASE 3-3   Whether to Dispense a Potentially Lethal Drug

Jane Travis, Pharm.D., worked closely with the local hospice program. She was very familiar with pain-management protocols for terminally ill patients. Most of the patients were maintained at home on ambulatory infusion pumps that delivered continuous or bolus doses of morphine. As the patients developed tolerance to the morphine, the dosage was adjusted accordingly. Dr. Travis understood that opiate doses were determined by balancing analgesic effectiveness and side effects. She followed the National Cancer Institute recommendations that, at lower doses of opioids, for patients with uncontrolled

CASE 3-3   *Continued.*

pain, daily doses usually should increase by 25–50%, whereas for patients already on high-dose formulations, daily doses usually should increase by 20–30% from the previous dose.[8] Therefore, Dr. Travis was surprised when she received a phone order from Dr. John Crampton, who was caring for Mrs. Reynolds, a terminally ill hospice patient. Mrs. Reynolds had been receiving 100 mg/hour intravenous morphine and oral amitriptyline hydrochloride 20 mg/qd. Dr. Crampton increased the morphine dose to 275 mg/hour infusion. Dr. Travis had participated in hospice rounds earlier that morning and learned that although Mrs. Reynolds's blood pressure and heart rate were low, she was receiving adequate pain control at the 100 mg/hour rate.

Dr. Travis shared this information with Dr. Crampton and questioned his rationale for increasing the morphine so drastically. Dr. Crampton stated, "I have known the Reynolds family for a long time. Rebecca Reynolds has been slowly dying for 6 months, and the family is exhausted. Rebecca has no quality of life to speak of and certainly is ready to die. I have given this a lot of thought and feel it is the humane and moral thing to do. I take full responsibility for this decision." Dr. Travis was not comforted by Dr. Crampton's willingness to take responsibility for this decision. She wondered about her personal responsibility regarding dispensing a drug in a dosage that, regardless of Dr. Crampton's justifications, was patently lethal.

CASE 3-4   Respecting the Wishes of the Terminally Ill

Linda Marley, Pharm.D., worked in the intensive care area of a large, university hospital. Dr. Marley had been involved in the care of Oscar Donham, a 71-year-old patient who two months earlier had suffered a massive cerebral vascular accident (CVA). Mr. Donham had been a patient in the hospital several times before. He had a history of coronary insufficiency and two previous myocardial infarctions. During one of his stays in the coronary care unit, he told Dr. Marley, in the presence of his wife, that he did not want any aggressive treatment if he was "really out of it for good." Mr. Donham stated, "Look, I know what it feels like to have those paddles on your chest when they try to 'jump start you.' I just want to be made comfortable and left alone."

During this last hospitalization after the CVA, Mr. Donham was completely unresponsive. He had developed stasis pneumonia for which the causative agent was methicillin-resistant *Staphylococcus aureus*. To make matters worse, he also had *Pseudomonas* sepsis. Dr. Marley had prepared a plethora of parenteral antibiotics for Mr. Donham, all of which had proven ineffective. Dr. Marley was more convinced than ever that the patient was terminally ill and would refuse further treatment if he were able to communicate his wishes.

With that in mind, Dr. Marley decided that she could not prepare the new orders for vancomycin hydrochloride and ceftazidime until she spoke to the physician who wrote the order, Dr. Jason Scott. Dr. Marley approached Dr. Scott and told him about her past interactions with the patient. Dr. Marley stated, "Mr. Donham was very clear about what he wanted regarding aggressive treatment. I don't think he would consent to receiving these antibiotics." Dr. Scott responded testily, "Who are we to decide when treatment should stop? Everyone deserves all the treatment we have to offer until it doesn't work. We have a professional duty to do all we can to preserve life." Dr. Marley retorted,

CASE 3-4 *Continued.*

"I think that our duty as health care professionals is to respect the decisions of competent adults." Dr. Scott said, "Well, it appears that we disagree. Since I'm writing the medical orders on this case, I expect that those orders will be filled as written." As Dr. Scott turned to leave, Dr. Marley again reflected on her last conversation with the patient during which he stated, "I just want to be left alone and made comfortable." Even though Dr. Scott seemed to think the matter was settled, Dr. Marley did not agree.

Commentary

These two cases each leave the pharmacist having to evaluate the moral judgments of physicians. Jane Travis is being asked to participate in an act that the physician, Dr. Crampton, knows or should know would kill the patient, Mrs. Reynolds. Dr. Crampton conveys that he has reflected carefully on the matter and has concluded that the dose is ethical.

If this dosage was believed by Dr. Crampton to be a lethal one, then, as we shall see in the cases in Chapter 9, he would be engaged in what is called "direct killing." The intent would be to kill. That is often thought to be ethically different from giving a high dose of a narcotic knowing there is a *risk* of death but sincerely intending only to relieve pain.

Whether one accepts this ethical distinction, it is important to realize that it is a matter of moral controversy. It is also illegal to give a dose intended to kill, even though it is legal to risk death with a dose intended to relieve pain. We saw, however, in the previous case that it is possible for an action to be both ethical and illegal. The law does not necessarily determine what is ethical.

Should Dr. Travis operate on the assumption that jumping to 275 mg is ethical just because Dr. Crampton is convinced that it is? Surely sometimes physicians can be ethically mistaken. Somehow, Dr. Travis has to decide whether this is such a case. That dispensing the morphine at this dose level might also be illegal should give Dr. Travis extra reason to reflect carefully on Dr. Crampton's action. Many people hold that even though some actions that are illegal might still be ethical, other things being equal, the fact that an act involves breaking the law is one reason to consider the act unethical. We have, in some implied way, made a commitment to live by the law when we accept the privileges of citizenship.

Dr. Travis not only has to come to an independent judgment about the ethics of dispensing morphine at this dose level, she also has at least one reason to conclude it is unethical. Even if she ends up agreeing that it would be morally justified to give a lethal dose to Mrs. Reynolds in a world where it was not illegal to do so, she might nonetheless feel that it is immoral to break the law. She could end up concluding that it is morally wrong to give the drug in a jurisdiction where it is illegal. The core problem raised here is whether Dr. Travis should be inclined to think that dispensing the drug is the moral thing to do because Dr. Crampton has come to that conclusion.

Pharmacist Linda Marley faces a similar predicament. She has good reason to believe that the CVA patient, Mr. Donham, reached a decision that he would not want his pneumonia or sepsis treated, yet Dr. Scott has concluded that ethically the antibiotic must be given. Dr. Scott appeals to what he believes is the professional duty to do all that can be done to preserve life.

Dr. Scott has a problem here. In fact, no code of ethics for physicians has ever required that physicians do whatever is necessary to preserve life. To the contrary, the current American Medical Association code requires that the refusal of treatment by competent, terminally ill patients must be respected (even though we raised the question in the previous cases of whether conduct is ethical for a health professional just because it conforms to the professional code).[9]

By contrast, the current APhA code does not specifically require the pharmacist to honor a patient's wishes to refuse treatment. However, the Code of Ethics for Pharmacists does state that a pharmacist "promotes the right of self-determination and recognizes individual self-worth by encouraging patients to participate in decisions about their health."[9] We thus have the intriguing situation in which physician and pharmacist disagree while the physician is taking a position that seems to contravene his professional code and the pharmacist finds her professional code silent on the subject of the refusal of life-sustaining treatment. If the codes are definitive for determining behavior of the members of each profession, then presumably both would have grounds for changing their positions. Should Dr. Marley treat either the opinions of the professional groups or the opinion of Dr. Scott as morally definitive?

Grounding Ethics in Hospital Policy

If the pharmacist cannot automatically ground ethical judgments in a physician's moral views, societal opinion, or professional beliefs about what is ethically correct, can the institution in which a pharmacist works provide that grounding? Many pharmacists work in hospitals or other health care institutions that may have codes of ethics of their own. They may come from the large public or private organizations that sponsor the hospital, or they may be in a local institution that, through its board of trustees or its medical board, may have formally adopted a statement or code of conduct about what is believed to be ethical. To what extent should the pharmacist working within such institutions feel bound by such statements? To what extent is the institution the "source" of the pharmacist's ethical obligation?

CASE 3-5　A Medication Error on the Oncology Unit: Who Has the Final
　　　　　Word?

Since Edward Strunk, Pharm.D., was a new clinical pharmacist on the oncology unit, this was literally the first time he had ever discovered a medication error. At first he wasn't sure what to do. Dr. Strunk was in the process of reviewing the medical records of the patients on his unit and updating orders when he noted the error. It appeared that the physician had written an order for "L-PAM 2 mg." Lorazepam, an antianxiety agent, was mistakenly dispensed instead of melphalan, an antineoplastic agent. The patient had received lorazepam for 6 days instead of the melphalan. "L-PAM" was the formal and correct abbreviation for melphalan, but lorazepam was often incorrectly abbreviated as "L-Pam" as well, which caused considerable confusion and in this case a medication error by the pharmacist who originally filled the prescription.

CASE 3-5 *Continued.*

The physician had renewed the order for "L-PAM 2 mg." After confirming with the physician that a mistake had been made, Dr. Strunk dispensed the correct medication. He also reviewed the medical record to see if the patient had suffered any ill effects from the lorazepam. It did not appear that the patient had suffered any adverse drug reactions. Yet Dr. Strunk wondered how one could measure the harm that was done by not receiving the appropriate antineoplastic drug, especially since the patient was diagnosed with ovarian cancer?

Dr. Strunk decided to approach his supervisor with his discovery. The clinical supervisor told Dr. Strunk that it was hospital policy to complete a medication error report but not to inform patients of errors such as this on the grounds that it would only upset the patients and undermine their confidence in the hospital and their caregivers. The supervisor claimed that the risk-management committee reasoned that it was morally unacceptable to disturb patients if they had not been injured. In this particular case, no one would ever know that an error was made, as the melphalan and lorazepam look remarkably similar, and the nurses recorded that "L-PAM 2 mg" was given to the patient. Dr. Strunk was troubled that the patient was unaware of the mistake and felt that she had a right to be informed. He was also not certain that the hospital's policy was ethically sound.

Commentary

In this case, the hospital's moral policy seems controversial. One could easily suggest that it is grounded in self-interest, since the hospital could be in serious legal trouble if the patient learned of the error. Assume, however, for purposes of discussion that Dr. Strunk is convinced that the hospital's policy is, in fact, believed by administrators and the risk-management committee to have a moral, rather than a self-serving purpose—that they really believe it would be unethical to upset patients. This, after all, is a long-standing interpretation of the Hippocratic Oath's imperative to do whatever is believed to benefit that patient (see the appendix to this volume).

If the hospital's position is intended to have a moral purpose, then there is a real conflict between the holders of two ethical perspectives. The cases in Chapter 15 will explore in further detail the different ethical positions regarding disclosure of controversial, potentially upsetting, information. Here the issue is whether a pharmacist should treat the hospital as the legitimate source of morality. Presumably when Dr. Strunk accepted employment at the hospital he made at least an implied commitment to abide by its rules. To what extent does that commitment imply agreeing to accept hospital policy as a source of moral authority?

It some ways the problem is similar to the pharmacist in Case 3-2 who has to factor into his reasoning his moral obligation to obey the law. In this case, however, Mr. Strunk has real reason to believe that the hospital's policy is unacceptable. Can he acknowledge his general obligation to conform to hospital policy and, at the same time, still claim that there is a source of moral obligation beyond the hospital where he works?

Grounding Ethics in the Patient's Values

The patient is another possible source of the ethical and other evaluations that are incorporated into the pharmacist's practice. It is sometimes believed that, since there are so many different ethical positions possible on controversial issues, every person should have the right to choose his or her own ethics. A slightly different view, referred to by philosophers as *personal relativism,* is that to say something is ethical literally means nothing more than that it is the position approved by the speaker. According to this view, if one believes an action is morally right, it literally is right; that is the final standard. However, someone else may have a quite different perspective. For the other person, the same action could, for him or her, be wrong. There is no further appeal beyond the individual. The following case poses the problem of whether the pharmacist should treat the patient as the source of moral standards.

CASE 3-6   Is the Patient Always Right?

Laura Chen submitted a claim under her major medical insurance for several prescriptions, one for clomiphene, which she was taking as a fertility medicine since she had polycystic ovarian syndrome and was having difficulty conceiving. She was surprised that she received a denial for the cost of the clomiphene. The insurance company explained in its denial letter that her employer's benefit package did not cover the cost of fertility drugs. Ms. Chen checked with the personnel office at work and discovered that her employer chose not to cover this type of drug for treatment of fertility problems in order to keep the cost of health insurance down for all of its employees. Ms. Chen's employer did not view infertility as a health problem and did not feel obligated to pay for fertility drugs for employees.

This infuriated Ms. Chen, and she shared her feelings with Albert George, her community pharmacist. She explained to Dr. George that this was an unfair policy on the part of her employer. Why should her employer have the right to decide which drugs should be paid for? Ms. Chen had given this perceived injustice a lot of thought and had come up with a solution for which she needed Dr. George's assistance. At the counseling counter, Ms. Chen asked Dr. George to prepare a dishonest claim for another drug, any drug, so long as the cost was similar to the cost of the clomiphene and it was a drug covered by her benefit plan. Ms. Chen reasoned that she could then get the money she rightly deserved to cover the cost of the medication. Dr. George knew that Ms. Chen was asking him to commit fraud. He also knew that the insurance company would probably not check up on this small deception. Dr. George wasn't certain that Ms. Chen had been wrongly treated. However, Dr. George was certain that fraud was ethically wrong. What should he do?

Commentary

The question raised by Ms. Chen's request deals with the substantive questions of the ethics of dishonest insurance claims as well as the ethics of treatment for infertility. These will be explored further in the cases in Chapters 7 and 11, respectively. Here the problem needing attention is where Dr. George should turn to find the source of his moral obligation in this case.

The patient is making a moral claim. She feels she has been wronged by her employer's policy of excluding infertility treatment from health insurance. One might look at the case first from Ms. Chen's point of view. She might believe that her own feelings are the ultimate foundation of her moral judgment, or more likely, she may believe that she is appealing to some external source for deciding what is ethical—to a religious view, to reason, or to some moral "law."

Dr. George has similar options for places to turn. He might see the source of ethics in his own judgment, in his religious view of the world, in reason. He might also turn, as we have seen in previous cases, to the code of ethics of his profession. (The standards of a physician or a hospital do not seem relevant in this case.) The question is what role, if any, should Ms. Chen's conviction that the deceptive insurance claim is morally justified play in Dr. George's moral reflection?

A patient's views about certain medical treatments, such as chemotherapy for terminally ill patients, are important in deciding what is appropriate for the patient. A pharmacist might say that the right therapy depends on the patient's ethical judgment in these cases. Patient autonomy is an important part of contemporary ethics. Yet, in this case, not only the patient's life is being affected. Deciding what is right may not depend exclusively on the feelings of the patient.

Even in the case of chemotherapy for a terminal illness, the pharmacist might distinguish between what the patient wants and what is morally right. That reveals that the real grounding of the ethical judgment is not simply the patient's feelings or wishes. A pharmacist might say that even though a patient has made the morally wrong choice about the chemotherapy, he or she has a right to be wrong. In the insurance fraud situation, however, Dr. George may not only want to make an independent assessment of what is right, he might also insist that he cannot be involved in an action that violates what is right simply because Ms. Chen is satisfied it is moral.

Grounding Ethics in Religious or Philosophical Perspectives

Pharmacists sometimes find that they or the people with whom they interact claim they are grounding their ethical positions not in professional codes, public policy, or the opinions of physicians, hospitals, or patients, but see them as coming from certain religious or philosophical perspectives. The problem can be especially acute when, as in the following case, the pharmacist senses that his or her own religious or philosophical perspective may conflict with the professional code.

CASE 3-7   Oral Contraceptives: The Pharmacist's Refusal to Dispense

---

Phil Schwartz, Pharm.D., had always been a little uneasy about the distribution of standard birth control pills. But now that he had finished rabbinical study, he was certain that it was wrong to dispense oral contraceptives. Dr. Schwartz works in a chain pharmacy that sells oral contraceptives. He is sometimes the only pharmacist on duty. He has discussed his unwillingness to dispense oral contraceptives with the pharmacist-owner. Dr. Schwartz argued, "You must concede that most women who take the pills are not told about

CASE 3-7 *Continued.*

the possibility that the pills cause the woman's body to reject a fertilized egg. I refuse to distribute oral contraceptives. I believe I have the right to refuse to participate in a practice that I feel compromises my moral integrity and violates my understanding of rabbinical law."

The pharmacist-owner responded, "I respect your right, but what about the rights of the patients that come into this pharmacy expecting to get a legally valid, therapeutically sound prescription filled? The Code of Ethics states that ' ... A pharmacist places the well-being of the patient at the center of professional practice.'[10] Therefore, I believe that patients have the right to have access to appropriately prescribed medications regardless of your personal beliefs. Furthermore, you may have the law to contend with as well since the state is considering a law requiring pharmacists to fill all prescriptions." What should Dr. Schwartz do when he is the only pharmacist on duty?

Commentary

Dr. Schwartz perceives correctly that oral contraceptives in some cases may function to block implantation of a fertilized ovum and that some Jews (as well as Catholics and members of other religious groups) find them morally objectionable for this reason. As with the other cases in this chapter, the pharmacist is caught between two possible sources for his moral position.

There is something special in this case, however. In the other cases it seems hard to defend the claim that a behavior is right simply because it is in accord with the code of ethics of the professional group, is a matter of public policy, or is the opinion of a physician, hospital, or patient. However, one might imagine that a believer in a particular religious or philosophical tradition might claim that he or she knows a behavior is right because it is held to be so by the tradition of which he or she is a member.

Actually, most believers in such traditions do not literally hold that a behavior is ethically right simply because their group says so. Rather they hold that their group has a legitimate claim to being able to know what is right—what is God's will, what is in the moral law, and so forth.

Thus being a Jew includes being committed to the view that the Torah and the Talmud provide a way of knowing what is morally right and that the interpreters of that tradition are authoritative in such matters. Likewise, Catholics, while respecting moral conscience, give prominent place to the teaching authority of the Roman Catholic Church. Protestants affirm that the Bible is the source of moral knowledge. Even those who subscribe to secular philosophical movements do so, in part, because they accept the movement's claims about how moral positions can be known. To stand within one of these traditions is precisely to affirm its views about the source or grounding of morality. It is hard to imagine that Dr. Schwartz could say, "I am a Jew; in fact, I have undertaken rabbinical study, but do not consider the teachings of the tradition morally significant."

Could one imagine him saying, "I am a pharmacist and a member of my professional organization yet do not consider its moral positions definitive"? The problem presented in this case from the point of view of Dr. Schwartz is determining the grounding or foundation of ethical judgments and which sources should be relied upon for guidance.

It is the nature of religious and philosophical systems that they claim to provide a systematic framework of moral insight for knowing what is morally right. This is not to say that those who do not subscribe to these frameworks believe they make legitimate claims to this status, but from the perspective of an adherent, by definition, those claims are accepted. Should Dr. Schwartz give similar status to the claims of his profession or of any other groups of which he might be a member? If his religious group gets this special claim, what does this mean for the pharmacist-owner, who appears to have reached a different moral conclusion? What about the conflict between refusing to dispense a medication on religious grounds and state law that explicitly requires pharmacists to fill all prescriptions? Several states have enacted laws regarding pharmacists who refuse to dispense oral contraception and emergency contraception. Some laws allow pharmacists to refuse to dispense on religious grounds, while others specifically require pharmacists to fill valid prescriptions.[11] Should the owner in this case appeal to the professional code as having, for him, similar moral authority? What does this mean for potential patients who, perhaps based on their religious convictions, have concluded that oral contraceptives are acceptable or even morally necessary?

Notes

1. Committee on Doctrine of the National Conference of Catholic Bishops. *Ethical and Religious Directives for Catholic Health Care Services*. Fourth Edition. Washington, DC: United States Conference of Catholic Bishops Publishing Services, 2001.

2. "Code of Ethics of the American Pharmaceutical Association." *Proceedings of the National Pharmaceutical Convention, Held at Philadelphia, October 6th, 1852*. Second Edition. Philadelphia: Merrihew & Son, 1865, pp. 24–26.

3. American Pharmaceutical Association. "Code of Ethics of the American Pharmaceutical Association (Adopted August 17, 1922)." *Journal of the American Pharmaceutical Association* 11, no. 9 (1922): 728–729.

4. American Pharmaceutical Association. "Code of Ethics of the American Pharmaceutical Association, 1952." *Journal of the American Pharmaceutical Association* 13 (1952):721–723.

5. The texts of these and previous editions of the APhA codes appear in Buerki, Robert A., and Louis D. Vottero. *Ethical Responsibility in Pharmacy Practice*. Second Edition. Madison, WI: American Institute of the History of Pharmacy, 2002.

6. American Pharmaceutical Association. "Code of Ethics for Pharmacists." Washington, DC: American Pharmaceutical Association, 1995.

7. *Kalman v. Grand Union Co.* 183 N.J. Super. Ct. 153, 443 A.2d 728 (1982).

8. National Cancer Institute. "Basic Principles of Cancer Pain Management." National Cancer Institute Website, www.cancer.gov/cancertopics/pdq/supportivecarepain/HealthProfessional/page3#Section_121 (retrieved March 6, 2006).

9. American Medical Association. Council on Ethical and Judicial Affairs. *Code of Medical Ethics: Current Opinions with Annotations, 2004–2005 Edition*. Chicago: American Medical Association, 2004, p. 70.

10. American Pharmaceutical Association. "Code of Ethics for Pharmacists." 1995.

11. Feder, J. *Federal and State Laws regarding Pharmacists Who Refuse to Dispense Contraceptives*. Congressional Research Service Report for Congress RS22293. October 7, 2005. Available from http://digital.library.unt.edu/govdocs/crs/data/2005/upl-meta-crs-7544/RS22293_20050ct07.pdf (retrieved March 4, 2006).

Part II

Ethical Principles in Pharmacy Ethics

4

Benefiting the Patient and Others
The Duty to Do Good and Avoid Harm

One way to approach ethical decision-making in pharmacy is to examine principles that describe general characteristics of actions that tend to make them morally
right. In the introduction, the principles of beneficence (doing good), nonmaleficence (avoiding harm), fidelity, autonomy, veracity, avoiding killing, and justice are
mentioned. Ethical problems in pharmacy practice often involve conflicts between
these principles. In other cases the moral problem arises over the interpretation of
one of these principles.

The idea that it is ethically right to do good, especially good for the patient, is
one of the most obvious in health care ethics. The Hippocratic Oath has the physician pledge to "benefit the patient according to [the physician's] ability and judgment." The 1994 APhA Code of Ethics says that "A pharmacist promotes the good
of every patient in a caring, compassionate, and confidential manner." These are all
versions of the principle of doing good for the patient. While this seems so obvious
as to be platitudinous, in fact, many serious moral problems arise over the interpretation of this principle.

First, even if it is agreed that the benefits and harms that ought to be the focus
of the pharmacist's concern are the patient's, there is still considerable room for
controversy. The first group of cases provides an opportunity to sort out exactly
what it means to both benefit the patient and protect the patient from harm.

Equally controversial is the question of whether the pharmacist should limit his
or her concern to benefits and harms that accrue to the patient alone. For example,
what if protecting the patient will come at considerable risk of harm to society in
general or to specific identifiable people who are not patients? What if the interests
of the profession of pharmacy conflict with those of the patient? Or what if doing

what is necessary to help the patient conflicts with the interests of the pharmacist's family? Is it obvious that the pharmacist should always place the patient's interest above those of his or her family? These are the problems of the cases in this chapter.

Benefiting the Patient

Assume for the time being that it is agreed that an important moral principle is that the pharmacist should act so as to benefit the patient. Even limiting our concern to this apparently simple principle turns out to raise serious problems of interpretation. For example, many ethical systems take as their goal producing good results for people. The first case in this section forces the pharmacist to decide what should happen when nonhealth benefits might outweigh the health risks of a medication. Later cases exam the relationship between producing good and avoiding harm for the patient and between determining the good produced by various rules rather than the good in individual cases.

Health in Conflict with Other Goods

Health professionals are normally committed to restoring, maintaining, or improving the health of patients. Health is viewed by virtually everyone as a good, as something intrinsically desirable. Yet there are many other goods that rational people desire as well. These include knowledge, aesthetic beauty, psychological and material well-being. Often, unfortunately, these various goods that people want to pursue compete for scarce resources, including time, money, and energy. Deciding what mix of goods is the proper one is a complex and highly individual decision. Normally, however, rational people would not choose to give absolute priority to one of these goods over another. Just as people constantly sacrifice their future material well-being for pleasures of the moment, so they also make some compromise with their health for other goods they consider important. The reasonable goal is not maximum well-being in any one sphere (including health), but maximum well-being across all kinds of possible goods.

This poses a problem for health professionals. They are experts, at most, in the good of health. Normally, they cannot claim to be an expert in how to help people with their finances, art appreciation, or social well-being. At most they can advise how to maximize health. The current Code of Ethics for Pharmacists commits the pharmacist simply to the "good" of the patient; it does not limit the focus to health and safety, as was the case in the 1981 version of the APhA Code. However, health professionals will not normally be in a position to advise about what really benefits patients, only, at most, about what serves their health. But rational people would not normally want to maximize their health; they would want to maximize their overall well-being. Thus if pharmacists are committed first of all to the health and safety of patients, their patients should normally have a different objective, whereas if the pharmacist is committed to the overall well-being or "good" of the patient, he or she is going beyond his or her sphere of expertise. The following two cases illustrate this problem.

CASE 4-1   A Matter of Priorities: A Patient Who Chooses to Reduce
            Antihypertensive Medication

Mary Phillips, Pharm.D., prided herself on her ability to keep in touch with her patients. Dr. Phillips had known Cora Jackson for many years. Mrs. Jackson picked up the prescriptions for herself and her husband Jake on a regular basis. Dr. Phillips noticed that this past month Mrs. Jackson asked for the refill only of her husband's antihypertensive drug, furosemide. Dr. Phillips asked Mrs. Jackson if her prescription for torsemide had been discontinued or changed by Mrs. Jackson's physician. The patient replied, "Oh no, I haven't been to see Dr. Williams. We, that is Jake and I, just decided to cut some corners. You know how expensive these drugs are, especially mine. So we decided to just get one blood pressure prescription filled, and we'd share. Jake's was less expensive, and one pill is as good as another. I just split the pills in half. We don't have enough money to get both prescriptions filled and still pay the heating bills."

Dr. Phillips knew that her own heating bills had risen substantially in the subzero weather. She also knew that Mr. and Mrs. Jackson were literally on a fixed income. Dr. Phillips felt that she should try and persuade Mrs. Jackson to give higher priority to health. As a pharmacist, she also knew that splitting her husband's pills in half was not appropriate and would probably do less good than not taking any medication at all. Yet, Dr. Phillips recognized that the health and comfort of Mr. and Mrs. Jackson depended on adequate heating.

CASE 4-2   Aesthetics Versus Health

This was the fourth customer in as many days who had asked Ron Bettis, Pharm.D., about retinoic acid, a derivative of Vitamin A. David Levy had been a customer of Dr. Bettis's pharmacy since moving into the office building across the street. Mr. Levy, in his late forties, was very concerned about his personal appearance. He confided in Dr. Bettis, "I have several friends who have gotten a prescription for Retin-A, and their skin looks wonderful. All the wrinkles just disappeared. They look 10 years younger. I was wondering about getting some of the stuff myself. What do you think?"

Dr. Bettis knows that retinoic acid is supposed to be used for the treatment of acne vulgaris, principally grades I–III, not for removing wrinkles. Mr. Levy obviously does not have acne vulgaris. He would be using the drug for purely cosmetic reasons. Additionally, retinoic acid is not curative, and relapses generally occur within 3–6 weeks after the drug is discontinued. Therefore, once Mr. Levy started to use the drug, he would in a sense be committed to it and the expense that would entail on a long-term basis. Mr. Levy would also expose himself to the possibility of side effects, such as dry skin and increased sensitivity to the sun, wind, and cold. Dr. Bettis is not sure how to weigh the nonhealth benefits—a youthful complexion—against the overall benefit to the patient.

Commentary

These two cases reveal how complicated it is for the pharmacist to try to promote the well-being of patients. In the case of Mr. and Mrs. Jackson, the couple who shared antihypertensive medication, it is not even clear exactly what the effects of splitting tablets are on their hypertension. At one point Dr. Phillips says that taking half the medication is probably worse than not taking any at all. That may be true, but there may be a linear dose/response relationship such that, if one cannot receive the full prescribed dose, getting half the dose could actually provide a significant fraction of the benefit. In fact, it could lower their blood pressures from critical to tolerable (if not ideal) levels. However, other arrangements could be far better. A less expensive medication, though not as effective as the full dose of the prescribed medication, might provide more effective treatment than the half dose. If Mr. and Mrs. Jackson have blood pressure problems with different degrees of severity, as it appears they do based on the two medications in question, it might not be proper for them simply to split the dose. Perhaps they should divide it differently. There might even be some way that Medicare or some other third-party payer could cover additional costs. It seems clear that Dr. Phillips needs to point out the complexities of simply splitting doses without the involvement of the physician.

It seems wrong, however, to assume that the correct course for Mr. and Mrs. Jackson, all things considered, is to allocate their limited resources so that they get the ideal blood pressure medication at the ideal dose while they suffer serious inadequacies in other areas of their lives. Physicians often assume that their responsibility is to prescribe the best possible medication, not taking into account the impact on other areas of the patient's life. In this case, it is not even clear whether putting the money toward medication rather than heating maximizes the patients' health. Dr. Phillips recognizes that their health depends on adequate heating. It could be that complicated tradeoffs between short-term and long-term health would lead to different mixes of investments in their health. It is also possible that different health goals—preservation of life, relief of suffering, and maintenance of mental well-being—require different arrangements. Even if it is only the health of the patient that is at stake, there may not be any single, definitive arrangement that is ideal. Even if Dr. Phillips is committed to the health of her patients, it is not clear what she should recommend.

Dr. Phillips acknowledges, however, that it is not only health, but also comfort that concerns Mr. and Mrs. Phillips. This raises the question of whether there is any degree of comfort that would justify any compromise with health. Anyone who decides not to exercise to maximum health advantage has probably concluded that there is. Thus before Dr. Phillips intervenes she needs to reflect on how important comfort ought to be in her patients' lives and whether any compromise with blood pressure medication is justified by concern over warmth.

Ron Bettis's patient who asks about retinoic acid raises a similar question. Here a pharmacist is concerned about the use of a pharmaceutical with some modest risk of side effects when the only benefits are cosmetic. Is there any way that removing wrinkles could be considered a health benefit? Only if one takes an extremely broad definition of health as including the psychological well-being of the patient. When the APhA Code of Ethics said that the well-being of the patient should be the center of professional practice, is this what it had in mind?

More likely, this is a case in which the patient, if asked, would have to acknowledge that he is contemplating a modest risk to health for a nonhealth benefit perceived to be important. Is it Dr. Bettis's task to try to figure out what would be beneficial overall for Mr. Levy, taking into account both the risks of pharmacological side effects and the benefits of a youthful complexion, or should he stick to the pharmacological assessment leaving to others the tradeoff of the health and nonhealth benefits?

Relating Benefits and Harms

After the problem of relating health benefits to overall benefits is solved, a second question needs to be addressed if the pharmacist is to figure out what it means to do what will benefit the patient. Often the intervention that offers the greatest prospect for benefit is also most risky; it offers not only the greatest good, but also the greatest risk for harm. How is the pharmacist to relate the benefits and harms in attempting to determine what will produce the most good?

One possibility is to approach the problem arithmetically. The benefits could be viewed as "pluses" and the harms as "minuses" on a common scale. According to this view, the harms are subtracted from the goods to determine what course will result in the most "net" good. This is the position of many utilitarian philosophers. It is sometimes identified with the great nineteenth-century British utilitarian Jeremy Bentham.[1] In carrying out such mental calculations, one has to factor in the probability of each envisioned benefit or harm. Some of these benefits, such as expected numbers of years of life added by an intervention, and harms are rather easily quantifiable. Others, such as pain and suffering or the benefit of getting to see a loved one, can, at best be approximated. Policy analysts have developed sophisticated strategies for estimating such benefits and harms. For example, the quality adjusted life year (QALY) method is designed to take into account not only number of years of life, but also the quality of the years.[2]

It is not obvious morally that it is correct to pursue the course of action that is expected to produce the greatest net good. Many believe there are moral constraints on such actions based on other moral principles, principles to be explored in cases in later chapters. But even for those who limit their ethics to beneficence and nonmaleficence, to doing good and avoiding evil, there are problems. For example, one might try to maximize the benefit/harm ratio rather than maximize the net goods. This approaches the problem of relating benefits and harms geometrically rather than arithmetically. If one imagines two courses, the second of which has twice the expected benefit and twice the expected harm, according to the ratios method there is no difference between the two, but according to the method of subtracting harms from benefits, the option with twice the benefits and twice the harms would produce a net gain that is twice as large as the alternative. According to the arithmetic method, one is always obliged to choose the high-gain/high-risk option, whereas according to the ratios approach, the two options would be treated as equally attractive.

Still another way of relating benefits to harms is to give nonmaleficence, the duty to avoid causing harm, moral priority over beneficence. According to this view, the duty to not harm is more stringent than the duty to help. One is morally free to try to help only when one is sure that harm will not be done. In contrast to the approaches that calculate net good done or ratios, giving priority to avoiding harm gives a preference to the more cautious course. In fact, if carried to an extreme, it would always lead to doing nothing. In that case, at least one will have avoided harming (even though one would also have missed opportunities to do good and to prevent harm). The following case provides an opportunity to compare different ways of weighing benefits and harms of alternative courses of action.

CASE 4-3   The Benefits and Harms of High-Risk Chemotherapy

Joe Cavanaugh, a 58-year-old professor of economics, was diagnosed with chronic myelogenous leukemia (CML) several months ago. Though this particular type of leukemia is somewhat less responsive to chemotherapy, Dr. Cavanaugh responded well to a course of busulfan and hydroxyurea, which he took orally shortly after his diagnosis. Dr. Cavanaugh's last blood count indicated that his white blood count was greatly reduced. During the course of his chemotherapy, Dr. Cavanaugh had become close to Heather Eyberg, Pharm.D., the clinical pharmacist in the cancer treatment center.

After a follow-up visit with the oncologist, Dr. Cavanaugh stopped by Dr. Eyberg's office. Dr. Cavanaugh said, "The doctor has suggested several possibilities regarding my treatment. I trust you, and I would appreciate your opinion on my options. The doctor said that now that I have finished taking the oral chemotherapy I could start interferon alpha, or if I want to be "cured," I should think about a stem cell transplant. The type of leukemia I have can rapidly change from this chronic phase into acute leukemia. If that happens, it is unlikely that anything would help, and I wouldn't have long to live. The doctor wants me to think about a stem cell transplant. The doctor said I could remain in this latent phase for years but that there's no way of knowing. Or I could have high-dose chemotherapy and stem cell transplant. What do you think?"

Dr. Eyberg respects Dr. Cavanaugh and his capacity to understand the risks and benefits involved regarding stem cell transplantation. She knows that allogenic hematopoietic stem cell transplantation (HSCT) is the only therapy proven to cure CML. If Dr. Cavanaugh has a sibling that is a match and has the HSCT within the first year of his diagnosis, he has a better five-year survival rate than do those who undergo HSCT after the first year of diagnosis. The two options presented to Dr. Cavanaugh are essentially: watch, wait, take the interferon alpha, and hope that the disease never progresses to the blastic phase or take a chance on HSCT now. The risks of HSCT are substantial. The possibility of infection and other complications is very high. It is not inconceivable that Dr. Cavanaugh could die from the HSCT itself.

Since Dr. Eyberg is part of the cancer treatment team, she is unsure of where her moral commitment should lie. Should she counsel Dr. Cavanaugh to choose the least harmful course of therapy? The conservative route would probably be to watch and wait and take the interferon alpha. Yet, if the disease progresses to acute leukemia, there is little anyone could do to help Dr. Cavanaugh. However, Dr. Cavanaugh could be in the percentage of patients who never progress to this fatal phase of the disease. Even if he eventually did change to the blastic phase, Dr. Cavanaugh might have many good years with his wife and children until then.

Dr. Eyberg could also counsel Dr. Cavanaugh to choose that option which maximizes the benefit for him. It is hard in this situation to determine which course of action will do the most good in the long run. Clearly, HSCT holds greater risk in the short run but in the long run offers the potential for a cure of Dr. Cavanaugh's leukemia.

Finally, Dr. Eyberg is troubled by the memory of another patient with a similar diagnosis who recently chose the option of HSCT and did not survive the procedure. Given all of these considerations, Dr. Eyberg is not sure where to begin.

Commentary

The issue in this case is whether there is a *moral* reason to prefer one course or the other. If, for example, there was a moral priority to avoid harm, even to oneself, then the correct moral advice would be to take the "safer" course and avoid the transplant. No one would then engage in a risky action that could be directly responsible for harming Dr. Cavanaugh, even causing his death.

A second approach is to attempt to calculate the *net* benefit from the alternative courses. Sometimes this is hard to do; often one can only estimate. She or Dr. Cavanaugh might feel that the chance of doing harm is greater with the transplant but that the risk of harm is offset by the potential increase in benefit. In that case, the extra quantity of expected good equals the extra expected harm. If one subtracts harm from good in the two cases, the results would be the same. If one is a Benthamite utilitarian, then one is *morally* obliged to choose the course that would produce a greater net good. If the net is the same, there is no moral reason to prefer one course over the other.

This suggests a third approach. It could be that in comparing benefits and harms, the correct approach is to compare ratios of benefits and harms and choose the course that has the greatest ratio of benefit to harm. If the ratios were essentially the same, then one would be morally indifferent between the two choices. It would be a matter of taste. If Dr. Cavanaugh could see no difference, he would have to flip a coin or choose arbitrarily. In order for Dr. Eyberg to know how to advise Dr. Cavanaugh, she needs to know what the correct approach is to relating the benefits and the harms envisioned from the two courses of action.

Benefits of Rules and Benefits in Specific Cases

Even if the pharmacist solves the problem of relating benefits to harms as well as the problem of relating health to nonhealth benefits, there is still another difficulty in figuring out what will benefit the patient. Some people who calculate consequences do so with reference to the specific case considered in isolation. They look only at the effects of alternative actions in the specific case. Others are equally focused on consequences, but they are interested in the potential consequences of alternative rules. Those people, referred to in the introduction as "rule utilitarians," hold that one should look at the potential consequences of alternative rules and choose the rule that would produce consequences as good as or better than any alternative. Then, once the rule is adopted, morality requires that it be followed without reassessment in specific cases. Only at the stage of adopting rules do consequences count, according to this view. Rule utilitarians oppose case-by-case calculations either for pragmatic reasons—because they think there is too much room for error in the heat of a crisis and because such calculations are too time consuming—or for theoretical reasons—because morality is simply a matter of playing by the rules once they have been adopted. The following case illustrates how these two approaches to calculating consequences impact on a pharmacist's moral choices.

CASE 4-4   When the Exception Breaks the Rule: Charitable Use of Outdated
Drugs

Boris Petrov is a physician who immigrated to the United States from the former Soviet Union. Dr. Petrov is scheduled to depart on a mission to his homeland with Project Assist. Medications are in very short supply, and Dr. Petrov would like to take some with him.

Dr. Petrov asks Harold Hawkins, director of pharmacy at the local hospital, if he will donate any expired or soon-to-expire products to Project Assist. Dr. Petrov explains that he believes that any medications, even those that are not fully potent, could be used. Pharmacist Hawkins reminds Dr. Petrov that hospital procedures may prevent the pharmacy from donating medications. For example, current hospital policy is to return all eligible medications for partial credit and to incinerate all others. Pharmacist Hawkins explains that the FDA also prohibits the distribution of expired medications. Nevertheless, pharmacist Hawkins also believes that the soon-to-expire medications he has should be given to Dr. Petrov.

Should pharmacist Hawkins follow his conscience and give the soon-to-expire drugs to Dr. Petrov, even if that means he has to get around the hospital's policy?

This case first appeared as "Distributing Soon-to-expire Medications to the Commonwealth of Independent States." *American Journal of Hospital Pharmacy* 49 (November 1992): 2773–2777. It is reprinted with the permission of the *Journal*.

[handwritten annotation: rule-utilitarian approach — would follow the rules that already exist — act in accordance w/ FDA & hospital policy]

Commentary

Here the pharmacist, Harold Hawkins, is intent on doing what is best. He decides that providing the outdated drugs in these circumstances would produce better consequences than the alternative course, even though both law and hospital policy seem to prohibit their use. Surely, the writers of the hospital policy and the state law had nothing like this situation in mind when they required returns or incineration. Mr. Hawkins could make a plausible case that in this specific case dispensing the outdated medication would result in more good than any alternative course of action.

The real issue needing attention at this time is whether it is morally acceptable for Harold Hawkins to consider the benefits and harms of this specific act in isolation. If he gives Dr. Petrov the medications, he seems to be operating on a rule that the prohibition on dispensing outdated drugs can be overridden by a pharmacist whenever the pharmacist judges that doing so will produce more benefit than not dispensing it. Should the FDA or the hospital change the rule so that it would authorize any pharmacist to use his or her own judgment about the wisdom of making an exception? That would expose patients to risks that some pharmacists might miscalculate or take advantage of the exception even when it would be better not to dispense.

Mr. Hawkins might conclude that, on balance, even though he was convinced that in this case it would be better all around to give Dr. Petrov the outdated drugs, the practice of permitting pharmacists to overturn such rules whenever they thought the consequences justified doing so would have such a bad result that it is better to affirm the rule, "don't dispense outdated drugs." If he took that position, he would be a rule utilitarian.

While this might sound legalistic, it need not be viewed as a totally exception-less position. For instance, a pharmacist on an isolated island whose only dose of a drug needed for a clear life-saving intervention was outdated might decide that the rule about dispensing outdated drugs would have to give way, even if it would not when less was at stake. The exception clause might require that the consequences of not dispensing the outdated drug would have to be overwhelming in order to justify making an exception.

The problem facing Mr. Hawkins is one of deciding whether he will calculate the consequences looking only at the specific case or whether he calculates consequences of alternative rules and chooses the rule that has the best consequences.

Benefiting Society and Individuals Who Are Not Patients

The focus of benefit in the cases presented thus far in this chapter is the patient. Occasionally benefits to others emerged in the cases, but it was usually in a very marginal way. In other situations the pharmacist appears caught between doing what will benefit the patient and doing something else that will have much greater benefit on other parties.

According to the classical Hippocratic ethic, the health professional was, in such cases, to choose to benefit the patient. The APhA Code of Ethics for Pharmacists uses the language of overall good, referring to the "good of every patient."

As early as the nineteenth century, the writers of the professional codes began to realize that sometimes the moral obligation of the health professional extended beyond the individual patient. The emergence of public health in the nineteenth century made code writers realize that sometimes the health professional has to consider the welfare of the population as a whole. More recently pharmacists have recognized ethical tensions created by their obligation to others, such as the family of patients, the profession as a whole, or to their own families. These cases raise this conflict between benefits to the patient and to others.

Benefits to Society

During the past century health professionals have gradually reached the conclusion that they bear responsibilities not only to individual patients, but also to the community. The 1922 version of the APhA code captures this movement. According to it, the "Pharmacist should be willing to join any constructive effort to promote the public welfare and he should regulate his public and private conduct and deeds so as to entitle him to the respect and confidence of the community in which he practices."[3] The current Code of Ethics for Pharmacists also includes reference to the larger community that pharmacists serve by asserting that the "primary obligation of a pharmacist is to individual patients. However, the obligations of a pharmacist may at times extend beyond the individual to the community and society. In these situations, a pharmacist recognizes the responsibilities that accompany these obligations and acts accordingly."[4] Many other codes of the health professions have incorporated similar notions of the pharmacist's duty to the community (as opposed to just the individual patient).

The ethically difficult issue is what should happen when the pharmacist's opportunity to serve the public comes at the expense of the individual patient. Pharmacists are variously asked to participate in medical research for the purpose of creating generalizable knowledge, in public health campaigns, and in cost-containment efforts. None of these is ethically possible on strictly Hippocratic (individual patient welfare) grounds. The next case forces a pharmacist to choose between serving a community of patients and an individual patient.

beneficence and non-maleficence

CASE 4-5 The Benefit of Cost Savings in a Health Maintenance Organization

---

William Edwards was 39 years of age when, during a routine physical exam, his physician discovered that he had paroxysmal supraventricular tachycardia (PSVT). The cardiologist first prescribed quinidine, but it failed to control the arrhythmia.

Disopyramide was successful in controlling it, but Mr. Edwards complained of severe blurred vision and dry mouth. When the dosage was reduced, the side effects disappeared but the arrhythmia returned. At this point the cardiologist decided to combine the disopyramide with propranolol, a common beta-blocker known to be effective in certain arrhythmias. This controlled the problem, without side effects.

Mr. Edwards continued with this medication regimen for 2 years until moving to a new town, where he joined a health maintenance organization (HMO). He immediately consulted Dr. Sam Forester, the HMO cardiologist.

Dr. Forester agreed that medication was needed, but he was concerned about disopyramide, since some problems had been reported in some patients. Moreover, Mr. Edwards and his original physician had never tried the obvious approach of using propranolol alone.

Both Dr. Forester and Mr. Edwards concluded that there were also risks in shifting to the single drug. Although it was generally safer than disopyramide and probably should have been tried first, there was a small chance of a fatal arrhythmia if the propranolol by itself were not effective. Moreover, while disopyramide presents some risk of side effects, most of those occur during the first month a patient is on the medication. Since Mr. Edwards had been on it for over 2 years, his risks were minimal. On balance both agreed that the status quo was slightly better for the patient, so Dr. Forester wrote prescriptions for disopyramide and propranolol and told Mr. Edwards to present them at the HMO's pharmacy.

John Williams, Pharm.D., was the pharmacist on duty. When he entered the prescriptions in the computer, he noticed the financial ledger for Mr. Edwards's care, which included the cost of the medications, which were paid for in full by the HMO. The yearly cost of the disopyramide was $1,500; the propranolol cost $700.

Later he happened to meet Dr. Forester in the physician's lounge. Dr. Forester shared with him what he thought was an interesting problem in comparing risks and benefits of the alternative medical regimens, explaining that he felt that even though he would normally use the propranolol first, in this case the combination seemed slightly better for the patient.

At this point Dr. Williams recalled the prices he had seen in the computer. He realized that even a significant increase in the propranolol dosage, something that would involve little risk, would still reduce the HMO's medication bill considerably. He wondered whether he should point this out to Dr. Forester, potentially saving the HMO considerable money.

Should Dr. Williams suggest to Dr. Forester that he consider a change in medication based on the cost saving for the HMO, or ought Dr. Williams's duty be to work solely on the basis of the welfare of the patient?

Commentary

The pharmacist, Dr. Williams, confronts an interesting problem of whether his moral obligation is to benefit the patient even if it will cost the HMO a considerable amount to do so or whether he should compromise the patient's interest in a case where a slight sacrifice of the patient will provide significant benefit for the group. Here the group could simply be the HMO management or owners who will pocket the savings. Even then Dr. Williams might consider himself their employee with an obligation to serve their interests, at least when he can do so without seriously compromising the patient. It may also be that the institution has a pool of funds dedicated to patient care so that the savings for this patient will ultimately benefit the community of patients. If the savings were for Medicare or some other public insurance fund, that would be the case.

The unusual facts of this case make it such that considerable savings would result from a very small compromise of the patient's interest. In fact, if the propranolol were expected to be equally beneficial while much cheaper, Dr. Williams's ethical problem would essentially disappear. No conflict would exist between the specific patient and others in the HMO group. Dr. Williams might have a diplomatic problem in dealing with Dr. Forester, or an emotional problem worrying about that interaction, but it seems clear that if the less expensive drug is just as good as the expensive one, then the less expensive one should be used.

In this case, however, a drug that is a little more than twice as expensive is expected to be a bit better. (Of course expectations can be wrong, but the only way medical decisions can ever be made is on the basis of the best estimate of outcomes.) If the disopyramide is expected to offer a slightly better outcome (or a slightly better chance of the same outcome), then, by definition, it is in the patient's interest to get it. Yet from the point of view of the system, it makes no sense to spend twice as much to get only a small margin of extra benefit. If patients (including the patient needing the disopyramide) could decide on a policy objectively without knowing whether they would need the drug, they would surely insist that some limits be placed on buying very small margins of benefit when they come at a high price.

The real question in this case, however, is whether the pharmacist should take the perspective of the group or whether he should be an advocate for the interests of the specific patient. One possibility is to expect clinical professionals to become advocates for their patients, relying on others, administrators perhaps, to set limits on inefficient uses of resources.

The other possibility is that in some limited way clinicians should include the interests of others as well as the patient whose interests are served with the expensive drug. The problem with that approach, however, is how can the pharmacist start to consider the interests of others without ending up completely subordinating the patient whenever the aggregate interests of the community outweigh those of patient? One possible way out of this serious difficulty is to permit the interests of others to come into play only when some specific principle other than beneficence requires it. In discussing Dr. Williams's predicament, focus on the specific reasons that would justify considering the interests of those other than the specific patient in a morally acceptable way.

Benefits to Specific Nonpatients

A variant on the problem in the previous case arises when the pharmacist can promote the interests of those other than the patient and those others are specific, identifiable nonpatients. The other person might be someone at risk from the patient by a threat of violence or an exposure to acquired immunodeficiency syndrome (AIDS). It might also involve the interests of members of the patient's family as in the following case.

CASE 4-6   The Interests of the Patient Versus His Family: Burdens on
            the Caregiver

Patrick Ross managed his diabetes fairly well over the years since his diagnosis, but he still ended up with many of the problems associated with long-term diabetes, including retinopathy, cardiovascular decompensation, and peripheral neuropathy. He has been in and out of the hospital for congestive heart failure (CHF) over the past few months. Although he was treated daily with digoxin, hydralazine, furosemide, and captopril, the CHF was refractory to therapy. Hence, the frequent hospitalizations. Mr. Ross was not a good candidate for a heart transplant because of his age and multiple health problems. The only treatment that might prevent complete heart failure was dobutamine hydrochloride infusions. Mr. Ross specifically requested that this therapy be provided at home if at all possible. Although the current CHF guidelines did not recommend dobutatime infusions at home, the physicians finally agreed.

Mrs. Ross asked Nanci Borger, Pharm.D., the clinical pharmacist on Mr. Ross's case, if she could talk to her about the proposed drug therapy. Mrs. Ross said, "I have a real dilemma. I love my husband, but I am literally at the end of my rope physically and emotionally. He is always very nice when he is in the hospital, but I can tell you he is a different man at home. I am literally on call 24 hours a day. I have to monitor his insulin and all of his other medications. I have to help feed him some of the time and help him walk and get to the toilet. We do get a little help from home care, but not nearly enough, and we just can't afford more. He needs to go to a nursing home or stay here if he is going to take this new drug. I just can't bear the additional responsibility. He won't listen to me. Can you convince him?"

Dr. Borger knows that this is the last thing Mr. Ross would want. He has been in a nursing home before and told Dr. Borger that he would rather die than go back there again. Dr. Borger also knows that it is likely that the intravenous medications would be paid for in full if Mr. Ross stayed in the step-down unit of the hospital.

If Mrs. Ross is truly as exhausted as she maintains, it might not be safe for Mr. Ross to receive the intermittent ambulatory dobutamine hydrochloride therapy at home, since she would have to monitor at least some of the infusion, take his pulse and blood pressure, and watch for side effects. The dobutamine would no doubt improve his quality of life with minimal complications. However, the factor of where he should receive the therapy as it relates to the cost to his wife, his sole caregiver, is considerable in this case. Dr. Borger thought that the benefits of the proposed treatment probably outweighed the additional burden to Mrs. Ross. Yet, she could not deny the real hardship that would befall Mrs. Ross with this additional therapy. She wasn't sure if she should take the welfare of Mr. Ross's wife into account when she weighed the benefit of treatment for Mr. Ross.

Commentary

If Dr. Borger's duty is to serve the interests of her patient, as the Hippocratic ethical tradition suggests, then her focus should be on Mr. Ross's welfare. In this case it might be argued that it is in Mr. Ross's interest to consider the welfare of his wife. But what should Dr. Borger do in a case where Mr. Ross does not express an interest in the impact on his wife, or where he is so ill that he is unable to express his views about his wife's welfare? Is it ethically acceptable for Dr. Borger to extend her perspective beyond the patient himself to those he probably cares about—or should care about? Is the wife's interest any more legitimately on Dr. Borger's agenda than that of any other person? If the clinician can take into account the interest of a spouse, even when it conflicts with the patient's interest, does the same reasoning lead to subordination of the patient to the aggregate interests of the members of the society?

Benefits to the Profession

One of the possible groups other than patients that could command the attention of the pharmacist is the profession of pharmacy. Its members perceive that they have an obligation to the professional group. It commands loyalty that requires certain sacrifices on the part of the individual. This is sometimes thought to include an obligation to conform to the moral standards of the profession, a problem addressed in the cases of the previous chapter. It also is sometimes believed to include a duty to promote the good of the profession. Since pharmacists are traditionally thought to have a duty to promote the good of the patient, this raises an interesting problem when the good of the profession conflicts with the good of the patient. The following case poses the problem dramatically.

CASE 4-7   For the Welfare of the Profession: Should Pharmacists Strike?

The clinical pharmacists at University Hospital were showing all the signs of professional burnout—irritability, fatigue, and impatience. Due to institutionwide budget cuts and an overly cost-conscious chief executive officer (CEO), the out-patient pharmacy had not been able to fill any of the vacancies created by retirement and resignations. Therefore, the pharmacists who were left were required to fill more and more prescriptions with less and less staff. The pharmacists met to discuss their dilemma.

One of the clinical pharmacists, Michelle Newman, Pharm.D., stated, "I have copies of several studies that I retrieved from the professional literature that correlate the number of prescriptions filled per hour with drug errors. We are well over the safe limit of the number of prescriptions we should be filling per hour. Additionally, I don't think any of us can continue to take this much stress. I think we have to take a stand on the number of prescriptions we can safely and sanely fill. If we have to, I think we should go on strike." After considerable discussion, the other pharmacists concurred with Dr. Newman.

All of the pharmacists in the department signed the draft of their demands and presented them to the director of the pharmacy department, Charlotte Collis, Pharm.D. Dr. Collis was quite concerned about her staff's plans to strike if their demands were not met.

CASE 4-7   *Continued.*

She knew that this type of action would certainly get the attention of the CEO. She had been trying for months to get permission to hire additional staff but had been turned down. The out-patient clinic could not survive long without pharmacy services. Most of the patients that used the clinic were completely dependent on obtaining their drugs from the out-patient pharmacy, as there were no other community pharmacies in the vicinity that would take Medicaid patients. A strike might or might not be effective in changing the CEO's mind. One thing was certain, the strike had the potential of exposing a substantial number of patients to inconvenience and perhaps even considerable risk. Although Dr. Collis did not think a strike would last long, even temporarily withholding services did not seem right to her. However, she was acutely aware of the physical and emotional toll that this pace was taking on her staff.

Commentary

This case presents what appears to be a conflict between the welfare of patients and the interests of the profession. The conflict Charlotte Collis faces appears to be a conflict between the interests of patients in getting their prescriptions filled and the interests of her professional colleagues in having tolerable working conditions. In fact she will have to do considerable work to sort out whose interests are in conflict here. The most obvious patient-welfare issue is the interest of the relatively small group of patients who may need to get prescriptions filled in the hospital pharmacy during the strike. Other patient interests are at stake as well, however.

We might also ask if there are ways in which patients' interests would be served by the strike. In the longer run, the pharmacists could argue that they are really pursuing patients' interests by striking. After all, if the errors increase, it is the patients who could be injured. Hence, in some ways this is a case of pitting one group of patients against another.

From another perspective, however, it might be that the interests of the profession and its members are in conflict with those of patients. On the one hand, the profession has traditionally claimed that its first interest is the well-being of patients. If that is so, then striking might simultaneously be a professional obligation as well as in the interest of those patients who will eventually benefit from the strike. On the other hand, the strike can be seen as serving the interests of the pharmacists, whose working conditions would eventually be made better (at the expense of those patients who will not be able to get the pharmacists' services during the strike). It appears that the interests of the employees, then, does conflict with the interests of at least some patients.

This raises the question of whether the interests of the profession should be taken to mean the sum of the personal interests of all members of the profession. Is it possible that there is something called a professional interest beyond this interest of individual pharmacists? For instance, if pharmacists were objecting to a hospital productivity policy that risked the quality of the pharmacist's service in order to save money, would that count as a true professional interest that differs from the self-interest of pharmacists?

If so, would that be legitimately on the pharmacist's agenda if this professional interest conflicted with those of the patient?

Benefits to the Pharmacist and the Pharmacist's Family

There is one final group of interests that could conflict with those of the patient: those of the pharmacist and his or her family. In the traditional Hippocratic health professional ethic, the only welfare that counted was that of the patient. There was never a formal recognition that the interests of the health professional could ever legitimately compete with those of the patient. Of course, health professionals have always recognized some limits to serving the patient. The following case explores those limits.

CASE 4-8 Choosing Between Patients and Pharmacist's Family

It was 2:45 A.M. Thursday morning when the phone rang for the third time. Tom Skinner, Pharm.D., groggily answered the phone. Dr. Skinner was one of two pharmacists who owned and operated Home Care Infusion Services, a home-infusion company. Since the company was small and working to establish a reputation in the community, Dr. Skinner and his business partner were doing their utmost to provide quality and conscientious service to their patients. This included the availability of pharmacy support on a 24-hour basis. Therefore, Dr. Skinner and his partner had to share the responsibility for being on call 24 hours a day.

This particular call was from Mrs. Mangiamele. Home Care Infusion Services provided equipment, solutions, and support to Mr. Mangiamele, who was on home total parenteral nutrition (TPN) for short-term bowel rest. Mrs. Mangiamele said that she hated to bother Mr. Skinner but that the spike had accidentally come out of the bag of TPN solution, and it had all run out. Mrs. Mangiamele knew how to change the bag, but there were no more bags of TPN solution in the house. Dr. Skinner had planned to deliver 7 days' worth of solution later Thursday morning.

Dr. Skinner thought sleepily about his options. He could get up now and go into the office and deliver the new bags of TPN to the Mangiamele's house. Or, he could tell Mrs. Mangiamele to hang a bag of 5% Lactated Ringer's solution, which she did have, and run it slowly to gradually bring Mr. Mangiamele's blood glucose level down. The latter option would allow Dr. Skinner to get a full night's sleep, which he desperately needed. Dr. Skinner had been on call for the last 4 nights because his partner had been sick.

Further, Dr. Skinner wanted to be at his best tomorrow morning because he and his wife were scheduled to meet with his daughter's teacher. Apparently, his daughter's work had declined over the past several months, and the teacher felt it was imperative to meet with both parents. Dr. Skinner had already rescheduled this meeting twice with his wife and the teacher and just could not do so again. Dr. Skinner felt he had been devoting more and more of his time to his patients and was neglecting his family.

Dr. Skinner realizes that if he waits until later in the day, it will pose little to no serious risk to Mr. Mangiamele. By this time, Mr. Mangiamele had probably received at least half of his TPN and, therefore, missing the rest of the TPN for this one night would not result in any great harm. Yet Dr. Skinner worries about the reputation of his fledgling business. Dr. Skinner wonders where the limits are to his commitment to his patients.

Commentary

Dr. Skinner is challenged to find out whether he literally believes that the pharmacist always works for the well-being of the patient. If his only concern is his patient's welfare, it is hard to see what else he could do but deliver the new solution in the middle of the night. Presumably if that were his only concern, he would keep answering calls in the middle of the night until he became so starved for sleep that his patients' interests were jeopardized. Yet no pharmacist really would do this.

Dr. Skinner also lives other roles in life. He is husband, father, neighbor, and citizen. He has made commitments in these other roles to work for the welfare of others in his life. A utilitarian would resolve such conflicts by asking which course would do the most good taking into account the effects of all parties—his patient, his children, and everyone else. Is this the way Dr. Skinner should decide whether to deliver the TPN solution in the night?

Suppose that Dr. Skinner realizes that there are occasions in which he could do more good overall if he simply ignored his patients and did something good for a stranger. According to utilitarian reasoning, he should abandon his patient in such cases. What is the difference between Dr. Skinner's duty to his children, his patient, and strangers? One possibility is that these conflicts cannot be resolved ethically solely by looking at which course will do the most good. Perhaps one has to take into account other moral obligations grounded in principles other than beneficence and nonmaleficence, principles calling for distributing goods justly, respecting autonomy, telling the truth, keeping commitments, and avoiding taking human life as well as the amount of good that is done. In the next five chapters we shall examine how these moral principles are factored into moral decisions confronting pharmacists.

Notes

1. Bentham, Jeremy. "An Introduction to the Principles of Morals and Legislation." In *Ethical Theories: A Book of Readings*. A. I. Melden, Editor. Englewood Cliffs, NJ: Prentice-Hall, 1967, pp. 367–390.

2. Weinstein, Milton C., and William B. Stason. "Foundations of Cost-Effectiveness Analysis for Health and Medical Practices." *New England Journal of Medicine* 296 (1977): 716–721; Kaplan, R. M., and J. W. Bush. "Health-Related Quality of Life Measurement for Evaluation Research and Policy Analysis." *Health Psychology* 11 (1982): 61–80; Mehrez, Abraham, and Amiram Gafni. "Quality-Adjusted Life Years, Utility Theory, and Healthy-Years Equivalents." *Medical Decision Making* 9 (1989): 142–149.

3. "Code of Ethics of the American Pharmaceutical Association (Adopted August 17, 1922)" *Journal of the American Pharmaceutical Association* 11 (1922): 728–729.

4. American Pharmaceutical Association. "Code of Ethics for Pharmacists." Washington, DC: American Pharmaceutical Association, 1995.

5

Justice

The Allocation of Health Resources

The principles of beneficence and nonmaleficence—of doing good and avoiding harm—were the focus of the previous chapter. One of the problems raised was the conflict between the welfare of the patient and the welfare of other parties. The utilitarian solution to this problem is to strive to maximize the total amount of good that is done, regardless of the beneficiary. We saw that sometimes the utilitarian approach conflicted with the Hippocratic ethic, which requires the health professional to focus exclusively on the welfare of the patient.

Pharmacists often find themselves in situations in which the interests of their patients are in conflict. The pharmacist must choose between patients or between a patient and those who are not patients. Whether to provide medications for those who cannot pay the full costs and shift the costs onto those who can is one example. The Hippocratic mandate to serve the interests of the patient (in the singular) does not help. However, it seems ethically crass simply to count up the total amounts of good and harm and choose the course that maximizes total social outcome regardless of the impact on the individuals affected. That could lead, for instance, to refusing to provide services to those who are not useful to society or to those who can benefit only modestly from the pharmacist's services.

The problems of allocating scarce resources arise in pharmacy in planning health care system formularies and in the operation of drug-distribution systems. Cases involving these programs are presented in Chapter 13. Before turning to these applications, however, we need to set out the ethical principles that are involved. Some ethical theories introduce a new ethical principle to deal with this problem—the principle of justice. While beneficence and nonmaleficence are devoted, respectively, simply to producing as much good and preventing as much harm as possible, justice is concerned with how the goods and harms are distributed. Justice is concerned with the equity or fairness of the patterns of the benefits and harms.[1]

Among those who hold there is a principle of justice that is concerned about the ways goods and harms are distributed, there are many schools of thought regarding what counts as a just or equitable distribution. The just distribution might focus on the effort of the various parties (even if sometimes those exerting great effort do not produce beneficial outcomes). Others, especially in health care, look at the needs of the parties. In health care, those who are in the greatest need (the sickest) may not be the most efficient to treat. In such cases, a choice must be made between using health care services in the way that will do the most good (sometimes treating healthier, more stable patients) and treating those with the greatest need. Any ethical principle that focuses on maximizing the good done for patients would tolerate—indeed require—that those with the greatest need be sacrificed. However, a principle of justice that focuses on need would accept the inefficiencies of an allocation of health resources that concentrates on the neediest. The cases in this chapter look at various problems of health resource allocation and the conflict between maximizing efficiency, called for by the principles of beneficence and nonmaleficence, and distributing resources equitably, called for by the principle of justice.

Justice Among Patients

Some pharmacists accept the traditional Hippocratic ethic that limits the focus of the pharmacist's ethical responsibility to the welfare of the patient. They hold that it is simply outside the moral scope of the pharmacist's role to worry about saving society money, catching welfare cheaters, or serving other societal interests.

Even the Hippocratic pharmacist sometimes still must allocate resources. He or she may face a direct conflict between the interests of different patients. The next two cases raise such conflicts.

CASE 5-1   The Hypochondriac and the Patient in Crisis: Whose Needs Take
          Priority?

Marian Jorgensen was a familiar patient at the outpatient pharmacy at University Hospital. Ms. Jorgensen sustained a work-related back and wrist injury 2 years ago. Ever since the injury, she had spent a great deal of time in the outpatient clinic for one sort of ailment or another. As far as the medical staff could determine, there was nothing specifically wrong with Ms. Jorgensen. Yet, she persisted in seeking relief for various vague complaints. The medical staff had informally labeled her a hypochondriac and malingerer. Her physicians responded to her complaints by ordering a medication for relief of each new symptom.

Ms. Jorgensen handed her newest stack of prescriptions to Randall Citron, Pharm. D., who worked the day shift in the outpatient pharmacy. Dr. Citron was familiar with Ms. Jorgensen and knew that she liked to spend considerable time talking with the pharmacist about her medications and other health-related concerns. Dr. Citron decided to fill Ms. Jorgensen's prescriptions at the end of the shift so that he could spend uninterrupted time

CASE 5-1   *Continued.*

with her. Dr. Citron told Ms. Jorgensen, "Its going to take longer to fill these. Could you come back later, say around 3:30 P.M.? I promise you, we'll have time to talk."

After Dr. Citron finally finished out the shift and his co-workers had left for the day, he called Ms. Jorgensen to the window. At the same moment, Ms. Riley rushed up to the pharmacy window with her infant daughter. Ms. Riley stated, "I need to talk to a pharmacist. The doctor gave me all these prescriptions for my baby. She's very sick. I need to start these medicines as soon as possible. The doctor told me some of the medicines have to be measured very carefully, but I don't remember everything the doctor told me."

Dr. Citron attempted to hand Ms. Jorgensen her prescriptions so that he could turn his attention to Ms. Riley. But Ms. Jorgensen would not be brushed aside so easily. Ms. Jorgensen said, "Hey! Wait a minute! You promised to spend time answering my questions. I made an extra trip back here today like you asked. I'm a sick woman. I deserve some attention too." Dr. Citron feels that his time would be better spent with Ms. Riley. Ms. Riley has an extremely ill child and is obviously in distress. Ms. Jorgensen always complains vigorously about her physical condition but does not appear to be ill. Yet, Ms. Jorgensen has a legitimate claim to his time, even though it sometimes feels like a waste of time to hear her repeat her litany of aches and pains. Dr. Citron pondered what to do next as both women stared tensely at him.

Commentary

This is a problem from which Randall Citron cannot escape, even if his approach is purely Hippocratic. He may insist that his only concern is to benefit his patient, but here two patients are in need of his attention. He cannot give his sole attention to both at the same time.

First, consider what Dr. Citron would do if he were acting only on the basis of the more social version of an ethic of beneficence and nonmaleficence, if his only goal was to do as much good as possible considering the sum of the effects. He would have to calculate the benefits and harms, much as was done in the cases presented in Chapter 4. What are the relevant effects of giving attention to each of these patients? Is there any case to be made for Ms. Jorgensen, any effects that could possibly lead to the conclusion that dealing with her first would produce more net benefit overall? Does one factor in the psychological effects of her having been put off? Does one consider that she will feel annoyed, angry, or upset, or are these psychological dimensions irrelevant?

Now consider what else Dr. Citron might take into account other than the sum of the benefits and harms. He seems to believe that more good would come from dealing with Ms. Riley first. But it is also true that Ms. Riley's child seems sicker. Is it the fact that the child is sicker that is important, or the fact that he believes more good will come from turning to Ms. Riley first? Imagine that Dr. Citron knows that even though Ms. Riley's child is very sick, the delay will not be of any consequence. If delaying Ms. Jorgensen would be very upsetting to her while delaying Ms. Riley would be less upsetting, then more good might come from turning to the better-off patient first. Which is morally critical: doing as much good as possible or treating the sicker patient first?

There are other factors to consider here. What should Dr. Citron make of the fact that Ms. Jorgensen had been waiting longer? Does the idea of first come/first served apply here, and if so, why? What should Dr. Citron make of the fact that he has previously given Ms. Jorgensen a great deal of his time? Does Ms. Riley have a claim to equal time? Finally, what should Dr. Citron make of the fact that he had promised Ms. Jorgensen that he would see her at a certain time? Does that promise give her a special priority?

CASE 5-2   The Obligations of Pharmaceutical Manufacturers

It was reported on April 18, 1991, that a male infant was born at Schneider Children's Hospital in New Hyde Park, New York, with an extremely rare condition—congenital adrenal hypoplasia—that resulted in an inability to produce the corticosteroid cortisone. The infant required intramuscular injections of cortisone acetate until he was old enough to take the medication orally. Unfortunately, the medical and pharmacy staff could not locate a supply of the intramuscular preparation of cortisone acetate. Dr. Paula Kreitezer, a physician in pediatric endocrinology at Schneider's, worked with the infant's parents and the pharmacists at the hospital to locate a pharmaceutical manufacturer who made the intramuscular preparation of cortisone acetate. Although there were numerous pharmaceutical manufacturers in the *American Hospital Formulary Service Drug Information Book* who listed intramuscular cortisone acetate, none of them had the drug in production. When Dr. Kreitezer contacted Merck Sharp and Dohme (MSD) she learned that they had stopped production of the intramuscular preparation of the drug a few months prior to her request. There had been little request for the intramuscular preparation of the drug. Additionally, the drug did not fall into the "orphan drug" category even though the disease was rare. The dilemma revolved around the type of preparation of the drug, since more than one manufacturer produced an oral version. MSD responded to Dr. Kreitezer's request and found a supply of the drug that they sent to Schneider's for the infant. MSD also reinstituted production of the intramuscular preparation of cortisone acetate for this infant and others like him with adrenal hypoplasia even though it occurs rarely. The infant has now matured to an age where he is able to take the oral preparation and no longer requires the intramuscular injections.

Source: Paula Kreitezer. "Pediatric Endocrinology." New Hyde Park, NY: Schneider Children's Hospital.

Commentary

If the manufacturer believed in pure, free-market principles, presumably it could offer to manufacture the injectable cortisone for the small number of patients who needed it and charge whatever it liked. The price presumably would be beyond what many parents could afford. The question here is whether a manufacturer has a moral duty to resume production and, if so, how the costs should be borne.

Assuming that this patient (or his family) cannot bear the cost alone, the only possibilities would be to insist either that insurance pay the full costs or that the manufacturer absorb the costs, shifting those costs onto other pharmaceuticals that are more profitable.

Imagine, for purposes of discussion, that the insurer bears these costs. The funds will come from a pool of money available to pay for the care of the subscribers. Should insurers be responsible for bearing the high cost of producing a specialized drug of this kind? Suppose that the same funds could be spent on other patients in the insurance plan, for example, on immunizations, well-baby clinics, and the like and that such an expenditure will predictably do more good in aggregate than for this one patient. Even though the other children are much better off than this child, more good would be done spending the insurance funds on them. If so, is it ethical to divert the insurance funds to the less efficient care of the child who is much sicker?

Alternatively, the manufacturer could be expected to eat the costs of the production of the intramuscular preparation. In effect, that means shifting the costs to other products, which, in turn, means getting healthier people who have less need to pay for the costs of production of the orphan drug. Leaving aside the market considerations (the cost shifting might make the price of the other products less marketable), is it ethical for the manufacturer to expect other, healthier customers to absorb the costs of the drug for this one sick baby? Either way the intramuscular preparation is funded, some group of healthier people is going to end up paying the costs of the sick person's care. If the costs of manufacture are great enough, it is likely that more good (in aggregate) could be done if the money were spent in some other, more efficient way. If so, does the fact that this child is terribly sick give him a claim of justice to have the resources used for his benefit?

Justice Between Patients and Others

In both of the previous cases, patients were competing among themselves for scarce resources—a pharmacist's time in the first case, the funds to support health care in the second. Sometimes, however, a patient is competing with others who are not patients. A pharmacist must choose between the patient and others. Of course, in purely Hippocratic ethics, the patient is the only interest that is morally relevant. Neither other patients nor those who are not patients count morally. Either way, the pharmacist has a duty to totally ignore the interests of others. The following cases make clear that sometimes this is hard to do.

CASE 5-3   The Distraught Husband: Balancing the Needs of Patients and
            Others

Gwen Yee, Pharm.D., had worked with Mr. and Mrs. Estee since Mrs. Estee had been diagnosed with ovarian cancer last year. Dr. Yee knew that Mrs. Estee's prognosis was poor. Mrs. Estee's present hospitalization was for surgical correction of radiation-induced abdominal adhesions. Dr. Yee had arranged to meet with Mrs. Estee preoperatively to teach her about the patient-controlled analgesia (PCA) she would be using after surgery. Mrs. Estee had confided in Dr. Yee in the past that above all else she was fearful of pain and wanted everything done to keep her as pain free as possible.

When Dr. Yee walked into Mrs. Estee's room with the PCA pump, she noted that Mr. Estee was there as well. As Dr. Yee started to teach Mrs. Estee about the pump, she could tell that Mr. Estee looked strained and distraught. Dr. Yee asked Mr. Estee, "How are you?" Mr. Estee could barely contain the emotion in his voice, but only replied, "Fine. Just tired."

CASE 5-3   *Continued.*

Dr. Yee knew that Mr. Estee had been a stoic source of support for his wife throughout her illness, yet he now looked as if he could use some support. Mrs. Estee seemed unaware of her husband's status and was completely absorbed with questions about the PCA pump. Even though Dr. Yee felt that her patient was her first priority, she could not seem to concentrate on teaching Mrs. Estee when her husband appeared to be in so much need.

Commentary

Dr. Yee has entered into an ongoing clinician-patient relationship and, according to traditional Hippocratic ethics, has a duty to do what she can to benefit her patient. She definitely has a service she can offer. Yet she is distracted by someone else, someone she also could benefit, perhaps even more than Mrs. Estee. Even though no ongoing clinician-patient relationship exists, and though it might take considerable time to make the proper connections for Mr. Estee, Dr. Yee appears to believe she can help him as well. To what extent, if any, does Dr. Yee have a moral obligation to benefit this man who is not her patient? How should she decide to allocate her time?

One approach would be to decide how she could do the most good choosing among Mrs. Estee, Mr. Estee, and others (whether they are patients or not). That is what utilitarian ethics would require. Another approach would be to ask which people are worse off and concentrate her efforts on helping them. It is possible in this case that Mrs. Estee is worse off but that Mr. Estee could be helped more. She, after all, has cancer; he is under stress that might be amenable to intervention, but by comparison, he is in relatively good shape.

Finally, what difference, if any, does it make that one of these is a patient while the other is not? Is the difference morally relevant for Dr. Yee in deciding how to spend her time?

CASE 5-4   Compromising the Welfare of Others: The Patient Cheating
             Medicaid

Celestine Morano, Pharm.D., had suspected for some time that Shara Walsh was abusing Medicaid by obtaining prescriptions from the various community ambulatory clinics. Dr. Morano confirmed her suspicions when Ms. Walsh handed her 2 prescriptions, 1 for a barbiturate and 1 for an analgesic, for the second time in 3 weeks. The prescriptions were legitimate. However, Dr. Morano learned by calling various colleagues in pharmacies near the other general assistance program clinics that Ms. Walsh had used her Medicaid card to fill 25 prescriptions for analgesics and sedatives within the last 2 months.

Dr. Morano suspected that Ms. Walsh was selling the drugs. Regardless, Dr. Morano knew Ms. Walsh was abusing Medicaid and should be reported. But Dr. Morano also knew that Ms. Walsh had three children, all under the age of 10. Dr. Morano worried that if she reported Ms. Walsh to the Medicaid authorities, Ms. Walsh's children also would lose their Medicaid benefits. Dr. Morano had filled only a few prescriptions for the Walsh children, but the image of them standing in line behind their mother in the pharmacy remained in Dr. Morano's mind as she decided how to proceed.

Commentary

Ms. Walsh, and especially her children, seem to be in special need. They might easily qualify as being among the more poorly off members of society. Assuming Celestine Morano considers both Ms. Walsh and the children to be her patients, she might also assume she has a special duty to benefit them. Some would argue that it is her obligation to serve as an agent for society, protecting society against Medicaid abuse; others, however, might claim that it is her special obligation to serve the interests of her patients and leave it to others to worry about the broader social dimensions of this case.

From a purely Hippocratic perspective of having the pharmacist do what will benefit the patient, a case can be made for ignoring the broader social dimensions. From the perspective of justice the analysis of the case seems more complex. First, it is not really clear whether Ms. Walsh and her children are really worse off than the others who are being injured by her behavior. Is she taking Medicaid funds that would go to persons in even greater need? If so, then justice would require that Celestine Morano focus her attention on the others.

There is another dimension involving justice in this case. So far we have focused only on how poorly off various parties are. But what should be made of the fact that Ms. Walsh is engaging in a behavior that is cheating the system, a behavior that is illegal as well as unethical? Suppose she was not obtaining illicit drugs and presumably selling them in an illegal manner but only cheating on her Medicaid claim. Suppose, for example, that Celestine Morano knew that Ms. Walsh, though poverty stricken, was not eligible for Medicaid, that she was continuing to use a Medicaid card even though she was no longer eligible. If she had a desperate need for medications for her children, would a pharmacist be justified in ignoring the Medicaid ineligibility? Is the goal to benefit the patient, to help the person who is worse off, or to make sure that cheating the system is prevented so that Medicaid resources can be stretched as far as they can?

Justice in Public Policy

The questions of justice in the allocation of resources arise not only in clinical situations, but also in matters of policy. A key difference is that the pharmacist facing policy decisions does not have a specific patient or patients in mind whose interests can be served. If a specific patient's case is debated, it is as an example of a more general policy question in which the interests of a group are at stake, as the HMO subscribers in the following case, or in a community whose interests must be treated fairly. The pharmacist in such cases is not acting as an agent for the specific patient so much as for the entire group.

CASE 5-5   Maximizing Benefits in a Health Maintenance Organization

---

Howard Andrews, Pharm.D., was the chair of the drug utilization and review committee of Better Care, Inc., a small health maintenance organization (HMO) in the northwest. The committee monitored all of the medication profiles of the HMO enrollees to ascertain the efficacy and cost of medication regimes. Better Care itself was not in very good financial health because its members were mostly adults in their 50s through 60s with the usual chronic illnesses and acute hospitalizations common to these age groups. There were very

CASE 5-5   *Continued.*

few healthy, child-bearing-age families enrolled in the HMO to offset the expenditures of the older, high-use enrollees. Therefore, the drug utilization and review committee members were formally charged to do all they could to keep drug costs down.

Dr. Andrews was reviewing patient records for medication orders before the next committee meeting when he came across a diagnosis he had never seen before: severe cold agglutinin disease. The patient in question was Derek Grosklaus, a 62-year-old man who had been diagnosed with the condition the previous year. The patient's physician recently ordered recombinant interferon alpha-2b at a dose of 3 million units/m^2 of body surface subcutaneously 5 times a week. Dr. Andrews decided to speak to the physician, Dr. Ellen Joseph, about the diagnosis and the treatment.

Dr. Joseph stated, "Cold agglutinin disease is a rare condition in which an antibody reaction destroys red blood cells when blood vessels are exposed to low temperatures. Mr. Grosklaus had to wear heavily insulated gloves to reach into the refrigerator or to go outdoors without experiencing painful ischemia and hematuria. I read about the treatment with alpha-interferon and decided to try it on Mr. Grosklaus." Dr. Andrews knew that alpha-interferon was very expensive. A modest estimate would place the cost of Mr. Grosklaus's medication at approximately $5,000 per month. Dr. Joseph estimated that Mr. Grosklaus would need the medication for at least a year. Although the medication held a small chance of success for Mr. Grosklaus, it also held a steep price tag. Dr. Andrews believed that his responsibility was to focus on the needs of the entire membership rather than on the needs of the few. After all, Dr. Andrews reasoned, this was not a life-threatening illness if certain restrictions and precautions were observed, and the cost to the membership as a whole would be quite high. Though Dr. Andrews was sympathetic to Mr. Grosklaus's predicament, he was not certain that the drug utilization and review committee would justify the expenditure for the alpha-interferon.

CASE 5-6   Erectile Dysfunction Therapy: Who Should Pay?

The discussion about pharmacotherapy for erectile dysfunction with the Pharmacy & Therapeutics Committee (P & T) was inevitable. Marietta Sowers, Pharm.D., could not remember more media hype about any class of drugs in recent history. The HMO for whom Dr. Sowers worked had numerous male members who were over the age of 65 in the Medicare side of the HMO and many more men in their late 40s and early 50s in the regular HMO as well, all potential candidates for PDE-5 inhibitors, a relatively new class of vasoactive drugs such as sildenafil, tadalafil and vardenafil. The HMO had to decide whether it would cover the cost of these drugs.

Dr. Sowers began describing the usual elements of a new drug review. She stated, "Although sildenafil was the first of the PDE-5 inhibitor drugs to hit the market, the others soon followed. Their biochemical potency and selectivity are relatively similar. The other thing they all have in common is that they are expensive, about $10 per tablet. Also, there are serious risks. Sexual activity carries an increased risk of cardiovascular events. The incidence of erectile dysfunction is about 5% at age 40 but increases to 18% in men 50–59 years of age, and it also affects diabetics. The possible patient demand for these drugs is enormous due in large part to media attention and direct-to-consumer advertising."

CASE 5-6   *Continued.*

Emil Zanders, M.D., spoke next, "I know that the cost is a factor here, but what if instead this was a drug that could temporarily cure paralysis in spinal cord injury patients, even if only for a few hours? Wouldn't the brief restoration of function be worth the cost?"

Dr. Sowers interjected, "That's just the point. Let's say there was such a drug to cure paralysis. The number of paralyzed individuals in society is small. The number of adult males who might benefit from these pharmacological agents is substantial. Furthermore, we have to consider the off-label use of these drugs. There is nothing to prevent physicians from prescribing these for patients who don't really suffer from erectile dysfunction. In a word, it is a potential bank breaker."

"So what are you saying?" Dr. Zanders asked. "The future holds many new drugs like this, ones that will enhance lifestyle but not cure a disease. Is there a medical need for these drugs? If so, I think we're obligated to cover them."

"But how do we define medical need?" Dr. Sowers queried. "And how do we factor in the cost of these drugs compared to other products that do provide a cure or amelioration of symptoms? Maybe these are the sorts of products that people should pay for out-of-pocket or at least share more in the form of a higher co-payment. If we decide to cover the cost for lifestyle-enhancing drugs, I hope we realize that we are establishing a policy for many other products that are likely to follow," Dr. Sowers finished.

Commentary

The medications in these cases pose an intriguing question. They have the chance of benefiting the patient but at an enormous cost. This is quite a different problem from that faced by a utilization review committee after a physician has prescribed a drug that the committee knows cannot offer any benefit whatsoever. If the drug can offer no known benefit, there is no ethical problem in eliminating it. (There may, of course, be an interpersonal relations problem if the physician is offended by the committee's action.)

In these cases, however, there is a real chance of benefit. It is the cost in relation to the benefit that raises the question. In Case 5-5, the cost is projected to be about $60,000 per year; the benefit is avoiding the wearing of insulated gloves. Dr. Andrews, the pharmacist who chairs the drug utilization and review committee, knows that that same $60,000 spent in many other ways would offer more benefit to the patients of Better Care, Inc.

The first issue to settle is whether it is the clinician's duty to do what is best for the individual patient. If it is, then it seems clear that the clinician in Case 5-5 should prescribe the interferon. It almost certainly offers more benefit than harm, taking into account the degree and probability of benefits and harms envisioned. Yet, even if the clinician has a duty to try to do what is best for his patient, it is irrational for a health care system to let him get away with it. There will always be some interventions that offer vanishingly small net benefit and yet are very expensive. Some of those should be foregone in favor of other treatments that offer more chance of benefit for the same cost or offer more of a chance to benefit those who have stronger claims. Even if Dr. Joseph has a duty to recommend the interferon, somebody in the HMO has to decide whether this treatment has a high enough priority.

There are basically two criteria Dr. Andrews and his committee could use. First, they could ask whether spending $60,000 on this one case does as much good in total as would every other possible use of those funds. They would have to imagine every way $60,000 could be spent that is not presently funded and authorize the interferon only if Mr. Grosklaus's treatment offers the best chance of net benefit. That is the approach of the utilitarian.

Alternatively, they could ask who has the greatest claim of justice to the resources. If justice is interpreted as distributing resources according to medical need, then they would have to determine whether someone suffering from severe cold agglutinin disease is worse off than any other patient who could be treated with the resources. Justice would support a practice of using resources to benefit the worst-off patients, even if doing so is not as efficient at maximizing the net benefit produced. This suggests that if severe cold agglutinin disease were a terrible condition, if it were like acute heart failure, for example, then it would command resources, even if using the resources that way is inefficient.

There is, of course, another possibility. The committee could disapprove of the alpha-interferon without using the funds for any other group of more needy or more efficiently treated patients. They could simply let the funds accumulate as increased profits. Ethically, how would such a decision be assessed? Some would argue that this is a fair margin of profit for an HMO or other health facility. One could think of the funds in an HMO or insurance plan as being divided into two pools, one that should be reserved for patient services to be allocated on the basis of the claims of equity and efficiency and a second that is a fair margin of profit for a profit-making HMO or operating reserve for future development in the event the HMO is not-for-profit.

Case 5-6, which raises the issue of whether an HMO should fund PDE-5 inhibitors, poses this problem in a slightly different context. As in Case 5-5, the P & T committee must decide whether to fund a potentially expensive treatment. It must realize that excluding coverage could save considerable money, either to save funds for other patient services or to increase HMO net profits.

If the committee views the funds as committed to patient services, it must decide whether to spend the limited funds available on pharmacotherapy for erectile dysfunction or some other treatment, perhaps for some other group of patients. Moreover, it must choose whether to decide based on maximizing benefits to the subscriber population or whether to give priority to the worst-off patients. Either moral criterion will pose some difficult problems. If it chooses the criterion of maximizing benefits to the subscriber population, it will need to know such things as how much benefit comes from treating erectile dysfunction compared with other potential uses of the funds. If it chooses the criterion of serving the worst-off patients, it will need to know how poorly such patients are doing compared to other patients with other needs. Attempting to compare the burden of Mr. Grosklaus, the man in Case 5-5 with severe cold agglutinin disease, with patients in Case 5-6 with erectile dysfunction, could be enormously difficult. That would be true whether we want to know how much good is done or which patients are worse off without treatment. These are the sorts of problems discussed in the previous chapter.

One creative possibility might be to view these problems as issues to be resolved by some representative group of subscribers. A patient representative board could be asked to decide whether to use utility or justice (doing the most good for subscribers or serving the worst-off subscribers). Such a group could be asked to decide the proportion of funds dedicated to subscriber services that should be used for each purpose. In making such decisions a board (or the P & T committee) would have to decide whether it is morally relevant if a condition merely improves lifestyle rather than curing a disease. It would have to decide if it makes any difference whether a condition is rare, such as the agglutinin disease, or more common, such as erectile dysfunction. At least such a patient board might be asked to decide whether the goal should be to maximize the amount of good done (even if the patients who benefit are relatively well-off to begin with) or to help those who are worse off (even if the benefit is more marginal).

Case 5-6 can also be looked at as a problem for public policy. Until the creation of the prescription benefit (Medicare Part D), Medicare funded only a select number of medications, e.g., pain medications for symptom management for hospice beneficiaries, and did not fund any medications for ambulatory patients, so it avoided having to decide which medications have the strongest claim for support. Now, however, with Part D, it is not be able to escape these choices as easily. Still, some drugs offering potential benefits will be excluded under all plans. Medicaid also funds prescription drugs. Moreover, it has mandated that PDE-5 inhibitors be funded. This means that Medicaid program administrators must make the same judgments that challenged the P & T committee in Case 5-6. It has to decide whether to strive to maximize the total good it can do with its funds (the principle of utility) or to benefit the worst-off patients (the principle of justice). It then has to decide how much benefit comes from a drug like tadalafil compared to other drugs and other treatments it might cover. It also has to decide whether patients with erectile dysfunction are among the worst off. Are these questions that the general public should be answering or those on P & T committees?

Justice and Other Ethical Principles

We have, throughout this chapter, been examining how the principle of justice relates to the principles of beneficence and nonmaleficence. Nonutilitarians hold that right-making characteristics of actions other than the net amount of good produced are morally relevant. Justice, that is, some morally right pattern of the distribution of benefits and burdens, is just one such principle of rightness. In later chapters other principles that are sometimes identified as right-making characteristics will be discussed. These include respect for autonomy, truth telling, fidelity to promises, and the duty to avoid killing. We shall see that sometimes these come into conflict. When they do, a comprehensive ethic will have to have some method for resolving the conflict. One approach is to view the various principles (the right-making characteristics) as elements that identify characteristics that will tend to make actions right. Then considering only the single dimension, the action can be said to be right. It would be right if there were no conflicting considerations pulling it in the other direction. If ethical principles are used to identify these right-making elements, they are sometimes called prima facie principles. They identify characteristics that would make an action right, other things being equal. In the following case, we can identify what justice requires, but we might also have to take into account that certain commitments have been made that would pull the pharmacist in a different direction. Here is an example of a conflict between the principles of justice and fidelity.

CASE 5-7   Justice Versus Fidelity

Douglas Winters, Pharm.D., was the owner of Central City Infusion Care. He prided himself on the personal attention he gave to each new patient. Dr. Winters had hired two other pharmacists, but he still liked to perform the initial visit in the home with new patients.

The Rhodes family was one of the first cases that Central City Infusion Care agreed to take on during its first year of operation. The Rhodes' daughter, Emily, had malabsorption syndrome and required total parenteral nutrition (TPN) via a central line. Dr. Winters had scheduled a family conference with Mr. and Mrs. Rhodes, the nutritionist, the nursing agency staff, and the pediatrician to discuss Emily's current status, changes in her TPN, and a new infusion pump. Dr. Winters worked with the nursing agency for several days to plan the conference. It had taken a great deal of effort to coordinate everyone's schedule. Dr. Winters promised Mr. and Mrs. Rhodes that he would personally attend the meeting to discuss the pros and cons of the new infusion pump.

At 4:30 P.M. Dr. Winters received a phone call from the discharge planner at Morning Valley Hospital regarding a referral for home TPN. The new referral, a 28-year-old man with Crohn's disease, was being discharged the following day and needed an assessment visit that evening. Dr. Winters knew that if he turned down the opportunity to do the assessment visit the discharge planner would call another infusion company. Unfortunately, the only other company in the area was new. Dr. Winters was convinced that it really was not competent to handle the case. According to the discharge planner, this was a very difficult patient who needed special care. He could ask the discharge planner to delay the discharge until the next day, but that seemed unfair to the patient. He did not want to send a substitute to either appointment because he felt his presence was necessary at both places.

Commentary

Dr. Winters's problem is that there is a head-on conflict between justice and fidelity to the promise he has made. The new patient with Crohn's disease is an emerging case. If he used as his only criterion the duty to benefit the patient with the greatest need, the Crohn's disease patient would undoubtedly have first claim on his time. If, however, he used as his only criterion the duty to keep commitments, then the Rhodes family would have first claim. Two characteristics of these situations seem morally relevant: the fact that one of the patients has greater need and the fact that the other patient has been promised a visit. Both justice and fidelity to promises are prima facie principles or right-making characteristics. We can say of the case that insofar as justice is concerned, the Crohn's disease patient has first claim, but we can also say that insofar as promising is concerned, the Rhodes family has first claim.

If we could agree that priority is always given either to justice or to fidelity to promises, the dilemma would be solved. Most people, however, believe it is impossible to assign such a priority to either justice or fidelity. If not, how should this dilemma be resolved?

Some might introduce beneficence and nonmaleficence at this point. If we could determine that much more (net) good would be done by seeing one patient or the other, that might resolve to conflict. Some ethical theories treat beneficence and nonmaleficence as prima facie principles just like justice and fidelity to promises.[2] Others believe that this gives too much weight to benefits and harms. It would mean that if there were enough social benefits just about anything could be justified no matter how much it violated the rights of individuals. They are not willing to treat beneficence and nonmaleficence as prima facie principles on a par with such considerations as justice and fidelity. They may, however, be willing to let beneficence and nonmaleficence come into play in a case where two prima facie principles are in a standoff.[3] In either case, consideration of outcomes would be considered a morally relevant factor in cases of conflict between two other principles. Whether that would resolve Dr. Winters's conflict depends on how one sees the outcomes in the two cases.

Notes

1. The most important twentieth-century work on the concept of justice is Rawls, John. *A Theory of Justice.* Cambridge, MA: Harvard University Press, 1971. He sees justice as providing a pattern of fair distribution and considers justice morally prior to maximizing utility. For a good summary of Rawls's work see Buchanan, Allen. "Justice: A Philosophical Review." In *Justice and Health Care.* Earl Shelp, Editor. Dordrecht, Holland: D. Reidel Publishing Co., 1981, pp. 3–21. The utilitarian perspective on distribution is still best represented by the classic work by John Stuart Mill,. "Utilitarianism." In *Ethical Theories: A Book of Readings.* A. I. Melden, Editor. Englewood Cliffs, NJ: Prentice-Hall, 1967, pp. 391–434. The most direct rejection of the idea that patterns of distribution are morally important appears in Nozick, Robert. *Anarchy, State, and Utopia.* New York: Basic Books, Inc., 1974. Other helpful basic sources on justice include Bedau, Hugo A., Editor. *Justice and Equality.* Englewood Cliffs, NJ: Prentice-Hall, 1971. Many sources discuss the principle of justice applied to health care. Helpful discussions include Shelp, *Justice and Health Care;* Daniels, Norman. *Just Health Care.* Cambridge: Cambridge University Press: 1985; and the President's Commission for the Study of Ethical Problems in Medicine and Biomedical and Behavioral Research. *Securing Access to Health Care.* Vol. 1. Washington, DC: U.S. Government Printing Office, 1983.

2. Beauchamp, Tom L., and James F. Childress, Editors. *Principles of Biomedical Ethics.* Fifth Edition. New York: Oxford University Press, 2001.

3. Veatch, Robert M. *A Theory of Medical Ethics.* New York: Basic Books, 1981.

6

Autonomy

In the previous chapter we saw that in social ethics the principles of beneficence and nonmaleficence (which taken together underpin the ethic maximizing aggregate total net benefits) may not be the only morally relevant considerations. The principle of justice affirms that certain patterns of distribution of the good, such as distribution based on medical need, also may be morally relevant. Justice as distribution is not the only moral consideration that can provide a check on the principles of beneficence and nonmaleficence. In this and the following chapters we shall explore several other moral principles—autonomy, veracity, fidelity, and avoidance of killing—principles that all, in one way or another, refer to right-making elements or actions or practices that do not focus on maximizing the net good produced.

Justice is concerned with the distribution of goods in morally preferred patterns. It, therefore, always involves more than one potential beneficiary. The remaining principles that we have yet to explore—autonomy, veracity, fidelity, and avoidance of killing—are relevant, however, even if there is only one person affected by our actions. Thus these principles are particularly important in traditional clinical health care ethics in which the professional is thought of as acting on one and only one patient. In fact, we increasingly recognize that even in these clinical situations many people are affected by the clinician's actions. There is not only one patient, but other patients whom the clinician could be treating. Family members of the patient, friends, and citizens as well as fellow health professionals may be affected by each treatment decision.

Nevertheless, many ethical decisions in health care can be analyzed as if there is only one party who is principally affected. When we contemplate violating a patient's autonomy, lying to a patient, breaking a promise to a patient, such as the promise of confidentiality, or acting in a way that will kill a patient, it is the patient's moral interests that primarily are affected. Other people's interests are much more indirect. Therefore, while remembering the important ethical issues raised by the principle of justice in the previous chapter, the cases in this and the following chapters in this part of the book will focus primarily on the more individual ethical concerns. These begin with the moral principle of autonomy.[1]

Autonomy is both a psychological and a moral term. Psychologically, autonomy is a term describing the mental state of persons who are free to choose their own life plans and act on those plans substantially independent of internal or external constraints. One leads the life of an autonomous person to the extent one is free to be "self-legislating." Autonomy means creating one's own legislation. As such it should be apparent that being autonomous is always a matter of degree. No one is "fully autonomous" in the sense of being totally free from internal and external constraints. Some people may be totally lacking in autonomy—infants and the comatose, are examples. Many people whom we call nonautonomous, however, possess some limited capacity to make their own choices. Small children, the mentally retarded, the mentally ill, and the senile all may be able to make limited choices based on their own beliefs and values and yet are hardly autonomous enough to be called self-determining in any meaningful way.

Thus being an autonomous person is a matter of degree. Those persons who have a sufficient degree of autonomy we treat as being essentially self-determining; we call them "substantially autonomous persons." For purposes of public policy, we assume that persons below the age of majority, usually 18, unless proven otherwise, are lacking sufficient autonomy for a range of publicly significant decisions. We admit that a particular 16-year-old may have both the internal knowledge and intellectual capacity and be sufficiently free from external constraints to be as autonomous as some adults. Occasionally courts will recognize such minors as "mature" for purposes of making medical decisions on their own. But the working presumption is that minors lack competence to make many substantially autonomous decisions.

By contrast, those who have reached the age of majority are presumed to be substantially autonomous unless there is adequate evidence to the contrary. One type of evidence comes from a judicial determination of lack of competence. There is a striking problem with adult patients who are clearly unconscious. By law they are presumed competent to make their own decisions, and they have not been declared incompetent through a formal proceeding, such as in a court, but, nevertheless, they are obviously not capable of making autonomous decisions. One approach is to require a clinician or a family member who believes another person is clearly incapacitated to take reasonable steps to inform the patient of that belief. Of course, if the patient is unconscious, no such action is necessary. But, if the patient is capable of disagreement and coherently expresses that disagreement, then the patient should be presumed to be competent until adjudicated otherwise. If he or she fails to disagree, then a presumption of lack of capacity to make substantially autonomous choices seems reasonable.[2]

This does not mean, however, that a health professional is automatically free to do what seems reasonable to those who are not substantially autonomous. In the case of children, we presume that only parents and those so designated by the courts are free to act as surrogate decision-makers. In the case of adults, even if the presumption of lack of autonomy is warranted, it is still necessary to determine who is authorized to speak for the individual. The health professional—pharmacist, physician, or other health worker—does not automatically have that authority. And even if one is believed to be substantially autonomous, it does not necessarily follow that he or she should be free to make all decisions about his or her actions. If one's actions are likely to harm others, we routinely accept the idea that they can be restrained. This might be supported on what can be called the harm-to-others principle. From the time of John Stuart Mill, this limit on action has been well recognized, even among defenders of human liberty.[3]

The principle of justice also might be a basis for constraining actions that affect others. That is, we may want to control people because of the effect of their actions on the distribution of goods as well as because of the total amount of harms one's actions will bring to others. Still others believe that it is acceptable to constrain people who we believe are substantially autonomous in order to produce a greater good for society. Constraining in order to produce good for others is, however, more controversial than constraining to protect others from harm or to promote justice. Finally, some people believe it is acceptable to constrain those who are substantially autonomous in order to produce good for those individuals themselves. This is what is called *paternalism*.

If a person's substantially autonomous actions have no appreciable effect on other people, it is an open question whether it is ethically right for others to constrain his or her behavior, that is, to act paternalistically. Even if their free choices affect only those making the choices, some people hold that it is morally appropriate to constrain those actions. This is where autonomy surfaces as a *moral* principle. The moral principle of autonomy holds that an action or practice is morally wrong insofar as it attempts to control the actions of substantially autonomous persons on the basis of a concern for their own welfare.

Classical Hippocratic ethics in the health care professions has been committed to the principle that the health care worker should do whatever is necessary to benefit the patient. This has been understood to include violating the autonomy of the patient. Pharmacists, in the name of Hippocratic paternalism, have refused to tell patients the names of drugs they are taking, filled prescriptions for placebos, refused to dispense drugs believed dangerous, and engaged in all manner of violations of the autonomous choices of patients. They have done so not out of a concern to protect the welfare of others or to promote justice, but rather out of concern that the patient would hurt himself or herself. Classical Hippocratic professional ethics contains no moral principle of autonomy.

By contrast, the moral principle of autonomy says that patients have a right to be self-determining insofar as their actions affect only themselves. The principle of autonomy poses increasingly difficult moral problems for pharmacists, first in determining whether patients really are sufficiently autonomous so that the principle of respect for autonomy applies; second, in deciding whether persons who are, in principle, sufficiently autonomous are being constrained by external forces that control their choices; and finally, in deciding whether it is morally appropriate to override autonomy in order to protect the patient's welfare. The following cases confront these issues.

Determining Whether a Patient Is Autonomous

Some persons may lack the capacity to make many substantially autonomous decisions. They may, through age or brain pathology, lack the neurological development to process information necessary for making choices. They may suffer from severe mental impairments, delusions, or errors in understanding.

In the easy cases this capacity is totally lacking. In these cases, such as in small children, we presume by public policy that autonomy is absent and designate someone as a surrogate, such as a parent or court-appointed guardian. In adults in whom autonomy appears to be totally lacking matters are more complex. First, the adult may have made choices while competent that are thought to be still relevant. Second, public policy does not automatically designate any adults incompetent (as with someone under the age of majority). It is here that we are still striving to develop legal and public policy mechanisms for transferring decision-making authority.[4] Presently no clear legal authority exists for health professionals, on their own, to declare incompetency and assume the role of surrogate decision-maker. Competence is a legal term that can only be determined by the courts.

Since adults are normally presumed competent until adjudicated otherwise, there is a real problem for adults in need of medical treatment who appear to lack the capacity for making autonomous choices and yet need medical treatment immediately. Legally, consent is presumed in cases of emergency.[5] That presumption is not valid, however, for situations that are not emergencies, such as planning to write a medical order not to resuscitate a patient in the case of a cardiac arrest. It is probably not valid either for emergencies in which the patient is coherent enough to demand not to be treated. As a society we are moving toward a consensus that in cases in which the patient is so lacking in capacity that he or she cannot respond coherently to a declaration of incompetency, the transfer of decision-making to the appropriate surrogate is acceptable, even without a formal court review. Still, that leaves open the question of who the appropriate surrogate should be. The pattern emerging seems to be that it is the legally designated next of kin rather than the health professional in charge.

In cases in which the patient can respond to a declaration of lack of capacity by the care provider, it is much less clear what should be done. If the patient acknowledges that he or she cannot make decisions and accepts the suggestion that the next of kin take on that role, it seems reasonable to proceed, but if the patient claims to be able to make his or her own decisions, no clear policy guides health professionals on what to do. If there is enough time, it probably is best to seek informal help from an ethics committee or a formal, legally binding review from a court. If there is not enough time, it is far less clear what should be done.

CASE 6-1   The Partially Competent Patient

Mario Gonzales, Pharm.D., a clinical preceptor in a rehabilitation hospital for a pharmacy school, was conducting clinical rounds with two of his doctor of pharmacy students. As they neared Room 459, Dr. Gonzales asked one of the students, Irene Sawyer, to present the medical history and medication profile of the patient in Room 459.

Ms. Sawyer began, "Mr. Larry Craig is a 22-year-old Caucasian male who was involved in a motor vehicle accident in which he was the unrestrained driver. Mr. Craig sustained multiple injuries, including bilateral arm and leg fractures and a closed-head injury. He has progressed through rehabilitation with some difficulty with agitation, persistent memory loss, short attention span, impaired awareness, and mild to moderate depression. He is presently taking lorazepam for the agitation, oxycodone for pain, donepezil for the memory problems, sertraline for depression and as adjunct to pain control.

"Although Mr. Craig has family in the community, he is going to be transferred to an assisted-living facility that specializes in fostering independent living in group-type houses on a large campus. He will live with seven other adults with similar disabilities. Since he regained consciousness after his accident, he has participated in decisions about his care, largely consenting to all procedures and treatments. He has not been formally declared incompetent. He did not have an advance directive or a durable power of attorney, and no one could recall Mr. Craig having expressed any relevant views about how patients in such a condition should be treated.

"Mr. Craig and his roommates are responsible for meal preparation and general housekeeping in addition to their jobs in a workshop on the campus. A social-service worker stops by on a weekly basis to oversee the residents' finances, but there is no on-site health care service, and daily supervision is not offered to the residents. Mr. Craig will have to administer his own medication."

Dr. Gonzales entered Mr. Craig's room with his students. Dr. Gonzales began by asking Mr. Craig if he knew where he was. Mr. Craig responded, "Some rehab place." Mr. Craig had to look at the calendar to recall the month and date. He appeared to be easily distracted and mildly agitated during Dr. Gonzales's attempts to review Mr. Craig's medications with him. When he asked Mr. Craig if he had any concerns or questions about managing all of the medications he would be taking, Mr. Craig responded, "I've got this all under control, Doc."

Dr. Gonzales was acutely aware of all the information Mr. Craig would have to assimilate in order to take his medications safely. At a minimum, Mr. Craig would have to remember when to take his medications and how to look for side effects from the drugs.

Dr. Gonzales observed as Ms. Sawyer explained the drug administration schedule to Mr. Craig. Ms. Sawyer had placed the medications in a weekly pill container so that it would be easier for Mr. Craig to remember when to take his medications. When Ms. Sawyer asked Mr. Craig if he was supposed to take his donepezil at the same time everyday, he appeared confused and responded, "I'm not sure." Even though Mr. Craig was competent enough to be responsible for the majority of his activities of daily living, Dr. Gonzales wondered if someone at the group home or a member of Mr. Craig's family should be involved in administering his medications instead of or in addition to Mr. Craig. Dr. Gonzales was somewhat worried that Mr. Craig might take too much pain medication or forget to take his medication at all. Dr. Gonzales was also concerned that the impaired self-awareness exhibited by Mr. Craig would cause him to overestimate his abilities to manage his medications.

CASE 6-2   Borderline Incompetence: HIV and Natural Remedies

Sophie DuBois was as regular as clockwork regarding when she came to the pharmacy clinic to pick up her maintenance drugs of didanoisine, zidovudine, and nelfinavir. Ms. DuBois had become HIV+ from using intravenous drugs. Not only had she managed to kick her heroin habit, but she was also involved in a nearby women's shelter for others in the same dire situation in which she had lived in the past. Garth Wardworth, Pharm. D., was surprised when Ms. DuBois placed several bottles of various vitamins and herbal remedies, including a garlic supplement, omega 3 oil, St. John's Wort, and Echinacea on the counter instead of her usual prescriptions.

"Where are your prescriptions?" Dr. Wardworth asked.

"Oh, I've got them right here in my pocket, but I'm not going to need them. I know the right thing to do now. Only natural products can go into my body. No more artificial chemicals for me. I've abused my body long enough," Ms. DuBois responded.

Dr. Wardworth immediately reacted to Ms. DuBois's statement by reciting all of the reasons she should continue with her triple combination antiretroviral therapy but to no avail. He emphasized that her decision need not be limited to either prescription drugs or natural products since she could take both at the same time. Still Ms. DuBois insisted that she did not want the prescriptions filled. She had been reading numerous articles and books on "alternative" healing and was convinced that this was the right decision for her. In addition, several of Ms. DuBois's friends who also were HIV+ were using these products and other complementary therapies too.

Dr. Wardworth was not only concerned about the decision Ms. DuBois was making, he also was worried about her ability to make such an important decision. Dr. Wardworth knew that many patients with AIDS had cranial and peripheral neuropathies, specifically human immunodeficiency virus (HIV) encephalopathy that affected memory, judgment, and thinking abilities. Since Ms. DuBois was a young HIV+ patient, she was more likely to develop AIDS dementia complex. Was this sudden change in her attitude toward her medications a sign of incapacity? Even though she didn't seem disoriented or confused, her decision to stop taking the medications that were most likely going to save her life struck Dr. Wardworth as irrational.

Commentary

Cases 6-1 and 6-2 both raise questions of the mental competence of patients to make crucial medical choices. Had Mr. Craig been more severely impaired, the ethical and clinical problem posed by this case would have disappeared. He would not have been living independently; he would have had a formal guardian designated, either a parent or some other named decision-maker. We would not have worried about whether to treat Mr. Craig as the one responsible for his own medical decisions. Likewise, if he were still a child, he would be treated as one needing parental permission for treatment. We would assume his lack of capacity to make medical decisions of this sort.

Mr. Craig, however, is an adult. He lives on his own. He has never been adjudicated to be mentally incompetent to make his own decisions. He has never had a guardian appointed. The working presumption is that he is competent to make his own medical choices.

Here, however, Dr. Gonzales has real doubts that, for this vital decision, Mr. Craig really possesses the requisite ability to consent to the treatment and follow the regimen adequately. Mr. Craig's limits are neurological. He clearly has an impairment in his judgment as a result of a closed-head injury. He needs to understand a drug regimen, the reasons why the regimen is important, the wide range of possible side effects, and what to do in case those effects occur. He needs to understand certain monitoring functions, such as watching for side effects from all of the medications he is taking.

Should side effects occur, as is quite possible, some choices will need to be made about whether to intervene to change the medication. Some effects, such as dizziness, headache, or orthostatic hypertension, could involve judgment calls about whether to report them to a health professional or try to tolerate them. If Mr. Craig is sufficiently autonomous, he should have the right and responsibility to make these decisions. If he is not, then, for his own protection, someone else should have that authority.

One strategy might be to ask Mr. Craig to voluntarily bring someone at his home or a family member into the decision-making process. Should he volunteer to do so, part of the problem will be solved. But if he values living independently, he may refuse to permit the involvement of others. More critically, even if he agrees to involving others, Dr. Gonzales and Ms. Sawyer need to decide whether to deal with Mr. Craig as a substantially autonomous adult (who is getting advice from others) or whether he, like a child, is consulted but not treated as the real decision-maker. The decision could have a significant impact on the respect and dignity accorded to Mr. Craig.

Ms. DuBois is in a similar situation. She is not obviously incompetent, yet Dr. Wardworth knows she has a condition that is known to affect mental function. Moreover, she is making a choice that, to him, seems unreasonable. The drugs the patient is taking are known to be effective in decreasing the advance of her disease. To him, her behavior seems "crazy."

Nevertheless, she has good reason to feel that placing what she thinks of as unnatural chemicals in her body can cause her harm. It has done so in the past. Furthermore, it is generally considered unacceptable to classify someone as incompetent simply because they seem to be making a bad choice. The seeming unreasonableness of her choice might well be reason for being alert to the possibility that the patient lacks adequate capacity to make autonomous choices, but the mere fact that people hold atypical values and make unusual choices because of them does not necessarily mean they lack capacity to choose based on their own idiosyncratic values.

If Dr. Wardworth is going to treat her as incompetent to consent or refuse consent for her prescribed medications, he needs to be able to show how she lacks capacity. If, for example, she could give no reason why she was afraid of the medication or why she believed the natural products were better, that might be reason to suspect a lack of capacity. The mere preference for natural products over potent medications, however, hardly seems to be evidence that she is not sufficiently autonomous to make her own choices. What would count as adequate reason for Dr. Wardworth to treat her as lacking sufficient capacity for autonomous choice in this important decision, and what should he do if she persists in claiming she has that capacity?

External Constraints on Autonomy

Persons may be substantially autonomous in the sense that they have the necessary neurological and mental capacity as well as adequate knowledge but nonetheless be constrained by external forces from making specific choices. Persons housed in special institutions, sometimes called "total" institutions, such as prisons, boarding schools, or the military, may be subject to substantial external control over their choices, including the threat of physical force.

One interesting problem in this area is whether a person's autonomy can be violated by the pressure of "irresistibly attractive offers." For example, if an imprisoned sexual offender is offered release if, and only if, he agrees to the implant of a long-acting hormone that is expected to control his sexual aggression, is such a person able to autonomously choose to accept or reject the offer? If not, is it because the offer is made while he is in prison, or is it because the option seems so attractive compared to the alternative? These, in fact, are the issues of a case presented in Chapter 12. Ethical problems of respect for autonomy can be created by external forces such as these. The following case illustrates the problem.

CASE 6-3   Can Prisoners Consent? External Factors That Infringe on
          Autonomy

The TriCounty Correctional Facility was an overcrowded state prison. The cells were originally designed to hold one inmate, but now each cell held two. There was barely enough room to walk down the center of the cell. The overcrowding had also limited the amount of time the inmates could spend in the "commons" area of the cell pods and outdoors. One of the inmates, Jared Almquist, was serving a 2-year sentence. Mr. Almquist was a slightly built 21-year-old who was serving his first prison term. One afternoon, Mr. Almquist was told to report to the health clinic of the prison. John Ressling, M.D., and Stuart Wise, R.Ph., two researchers from a local university, greeted Mr. Almquist. Dr. Ressling explained their reason for meeting with Mr. Almquist, "We are talking to all of the inmates who are between 21 and 30 years of age, are not on any medication, and have no preexisting conditions, such as diabetes or renal disease, and who are prehypertensive. You fall into this category, Mr. Almquist. Your blood pressure has been recorded around 125–130 systolic and 80–90 diastolic. Normally, standard treatment for borderline hypertension is modifications in lifestyle, such as changes in diet and activity. We want you to understand that you are not sick, but you have a common condition that frequently develops into a chronic disease. In fact, hypertension is a particularly serious problem in the black population. We are conducting a research study of a new medication that may help control your hypertension. The research is funded by Norton Pharmaceuticals and reviewed by our university institutional review board to assure that subjects are protected. If you decide not to participate in the study, you will still receive all the medical care that you might need while you are an inmate."

Mr. Wise added, "We would like to obtain your consent to participate in a clinical drug study to determine the effectiveness of early drug therapy in controlling the development of hypertension. We want to control all of the independent variables that we can, so the study participants will be housed in a separate unit from the other inmates. It will still be a controlled environment, but there will be one inmate per cell, and you will share

CASE 6-3 *Continued.*

a common room with a television and probably have much more privacy than you have now. The study participants will receive specially prepared low-sodium and low-fat diets and will have organized exercise sessions in the prison yard two times a day.

"If you give your consent to participate in the study, you will either be assigned to the experimental group, who will receive the medication, or the control group, who will not. In either case, you will still be housed in the study unit and participate in the diet and exercise program. All of this information is written out in greater detail on the consent forms that you will have to sign in order to be included in the study. Please read them and take them with you to review. You are free to withdraw your consent and discontinue your participation in the study at any time without prejudice or effect on your medical care."

Dr. Ressling and Mr. Wise spent the next 30 minutes explaining all of the details of the study protocol and possible harms and benefits to Mr. Almquist. As he returned to his cell, Mr. Almquist wrestled with his basic mistrust of health care in general and his desire to get out of the crowded cell block in which he was housed. On the one hand, Mr. Almquist reasoned, it would look good on his parole record if he participated in the study. Also, he might actually be doing something that could help other people, maybe someone in his family. Yet, he didn't like the idea of taking medication, especially if he didn't need it and wasn't really sick. On the other hand, the chance to go outside two times a day was very tempting. Mr. Almquist weighed all of these factors as he decided whether to sign the consent forms.

Commentary

Pharmacist Stuart Wise has become part of a research project, a clinical trial of a new blood pressure medication. The general questions of the ethics of clinical trials will be discussed in Chapter 14 and those of informed consent in Chapter 15. Here, the issue of debate is whether Jared Almquist is a substantially autonomous person for the purposes of deciding whether to participate in the proposed research.

Research involving prisoners raises special questions about their capacity to give an adequately informed and free consent. New federal guidelines governing research with prisoners were issued May 23, 2003.[7] These regulations cover all federally funded research involving prisoners. The research being proposed to Mr. Almquist is funded by a pharmaceutical manufacturer and so may not technically be governed by these requirements, but many researchers associated with manufacturers and universities routinely strive to meet federal requirements even if they are not technically required to do so.

These guidelines require that for purposes of review of prison research the institutional review board (IRB) include a "prisoner, or a prisoner representative with appropriate background and experience to serve in that capacity," and that a "majority of the IRB (exclusive of prisoner members) shall have no association with the prison(s) involved, apart from their membership on the IRB." Regarding incentives for prisoners to participate in research, "any possible advantages accruing to the prisoner through his or her participation in the research, when compared to the general living conditions, medical care, quality of food, amenities and opportunity for earnings in the prison, are not of such a magnitude that his or her ability to weigh the risks of the research against the value of such advantages in the limited choice environment of the prison is impaired."

There is no reason to believe that he lacks the innate capacity to understand the information presented or to process it. He lacks none of the factors inherently necessary to be an autonomous person. He is not mentally ill, retarded, or ill to the point that he cannot think clearly. The real question is whether the external constraints within his environment keep his decisions in this setting from being substantially autonomous ones.

There is evidence in the case that Mr. Almquist probably would not consent to be part of this study if he were not incarcerated. He does not like the idea of taking medication, especially if, in his words, he really is not sick, which presumably is the case if he does not have symptoms that bother him. It seems clear that the only reason Mr. Almquist would agree to participate is because he is incarcerated.

But does the incarceration present external constraints on his behavior that make his choice nonvoluntary? Mr. Almquist is presented with two options, returning to his present life in the crowded cell block or moving to the new, more comfortable surroundings and taking a chance he will get the medication he does not really want. Is that an unacceptable offer? If so, is it simply because it is irresistibly attractive?

Consider someone who is dying from cancer who is told that the only chance she has of a cure is to agree to a nauseatingly unpleasant chemotherapeutic agent. Presumably that agent is at least as troublesome to the cancer patient as the blood pressure medication is to Mr. Almquist. Yet the offer must appear to be irresistibly attractive considering the alternative (death). Yet we do not normally argue that the cancer patient cannot consent to the chemotherapy because the offer is so attractive. If someone tried to ban the offer because it is so attractive we would probably protest—precisely because the offer is so attractive. People should have access to very attractive options even when their choices are very limited.

What is the difference between the prisoner's case and the cancer patient's? The prisoner's choices are "artificially constrained" by the incarceration. Yet let us assume that Mr. Almquist is justifiably imprisoned. Should he not be allowed to make limited choices, say between two different work details, even though his environment is artificially confining? If so, should he not be allowed to choose a "work" option of being a research subject, even if the offer is terribly attractive? Is he less autonomous if he is given the additional option that is very attractive? Would it be more ethical to conduct the research if the living conditions were made much worse, say, as bad as those in which he would otherwise be living?

Overriding the Choices of Autonomous Persons

Up to this point this chapter has dealt with persons whose autonomy is debated, either because of inherent lack of the internal capacity to make substantially autonomous choices or because of external constraints that could make specific choices nonautonomous. Some persons, however, are substantially autonomous. They both possess the internal capacity to make choices according to their life plan and live in an environment that offers them reasonable freedom to choose without external constraints. Still, the choice they make may seem to be very foolish. It may seem to offer risks of harms far exceeding any benefits to be gained. Assuming a person is substantially autonomous, is there ever a time when it is ethically justified to constrain his or her actions for the individual's own good? Or does the principle of autonomy always win out? Must an autonomous individual's own choices be respected as long as it is only that individual's interests being jeopardized?

CASE 6-4 Compulsory Education About STDs

Because of his work with the County Board of Health, Marc Billet, Pharm.D., was keenly aware of the incidence of sexually transmitted diseases (STD), especially in the adolescent and young adult population. Thus, Dr. Billet decided to do something positive in his community practice setting, Sunrise Pharmacy, to decrease the number of STDs. He moved all of the condoms to behind the counter and put up a sign that asked, "Need condoms? Just ask your pharmacist." Dr. Billet instructed all of his professional staff to offer advice and counseling on the proper use of condoms and the dangers of STDs whenever a patient asked for condoms.

Cody Abbott was surprised when he saw the sign where the condoms had been previously shelved in Sunrise Pharmacy. He wanted to purchase condoms, but he didn't want to ask for them. He also didn't want to take the extra time to go to another pharmacy. Mr. Abbott asked Dr. Billet for a box of condoms then stated, "I'm 21 years old. I don't think I should have to ask someone if I can buy condoms."

"I'm just concerned about your health and the health and well-being of others," Dr. Billet replied and then quickly proceeded to deliver his "lecture" on the potential harms of STDs.

Commentary

Dr. Billet seems to have grasped the idea all too well that the pharmacist should take seriously the education of the patient about health risks. He has developed a plan whereby the education is, in effect, compulsory. The implication seems to be that Mr. Abbott and other potential purchasers of condoms are not adequately informed about the risks of their sexual practices and therefore are not really making adequately autonomous choices.

It is normally held that, for a choice to be autonomous, the one making it must have enough information to compare alternative courses and know about the risks and benefits. Presumably, that applies to sexual choices such as those related to condoms. Yet, Mr. Abbott is 21 years old. He is presumed to be capable of making such choices and may believe he possesses enough information about sexually transmitted diseases. The notion that autonomous choice requires adequate information does not imply that the decision-maker must have "full" or "total" information. It is possible that Mr. Abbott feels adequately informed for the purposes of the purchase he is contemplating.

Dr. Billet's plan of making Mr. Abbott ask for the condoms and making their purchase contingent on hearing the lecture on STDs is a mild form of paternalism. It forces Mr. Abbott to receive the information—perhaps more information than he believes necessary—for what Dr. Billet believes is Mr. Abbott's own good. Undoubtedly, this action is not a dramatic example of paternalism, but it is paternalism nonetheless. Two questions are raised. First, how likely is Dr. Billet to be correct in his assumption that his customers are better off getting this information whether they want it or not? Second, assuming it is reasonable to believe many of them would really be better off, does that justify forcing them to receive it in order to make their purchase? Should substantially autonomous adults have the authority to decline such "benefits" that the pharmacist has to offer?

CASE 6-5 Overriding Patient Autonomy: Hiding the Side Effects of Chemotherapy

Aretha Pals had been diagnosed with Hodgkins lymphoma stage IIA 2 weeks ago. Ms. Pals is a 30-year-old, single advertising executive. Ms. Pals began radiotherapy and single-agent chemotherapy in the hospital and was scheduled to continue these treatments on an outpatient basis after discharge. Yasmin Raku, Pharm.D., is the clinical pharmacist in the outpatient oncology program where Ms. Pals was scheduled to receive her chemotherapy.

On her first visit, Dr. Raku noted that despite her current illness Ms. Pals was an alert, amiable woman. Upon settling in the chair for administration of her chemotherapy, Ms. Pals told Dr. Raku, "Just look at this; my hair is falling out at the lower part of my scalp. That's from the 'mantle' radiation treatment I'm getting, but it is only temporary, thank God. I told the doctors that I wouldn't undergo any treatment that would cause me to lose all of my hair. I plan to continue in my work, and my looks are extremely important to me. I have to look upbeat, healthy, and attractive if I want to successfully sell ideas to customers. I can cover this little problem with the rest of my hair. It isn't that noticeable, is it?" Dr. Raku reassured Ms. Pals that her hair loss was not that noticeable and went to get her chemotherapy.

After hearing Ms. Pals's speech about her feelings about hair loss, Dr. Raku was surprised to see the orders for "ABVD" combination chemotherapy to be administered to Ms. Pals on 4-week cycles. When used alone, each drug employed in the combination (doxorubicin, bleomycin, vinblastine, and dacarbazine) was active against limited-stage Hodgkin's disease. Dr. Raku understood that the selection of these independently effective agents in combination achieved a "synergistic antitumor effect" that was not attainable with a single agent. ABVD chemotherapy was standard first-line therapy. However, the general side effects of the four drugs included temporary nausea and vomiting, peripheral nervous system toxicity, bone marrow suppression, and most importantly as far as Ms. Pals was concerned, alopecia.

Dr. Raku asked Ms. Pals, "Did your physician talk to you about the new chemotherapy that he ordered for you?" Ms. Pals replied, "He mentioned that this combination of drugs would work better than the one I was on in the hospital. That's about all he told me except that I might get nauseated and that I might have a tendency to bruise more easily."

Dr. Raku called Ms. Pals's physician, Dr. Vernon Pritchford, and asked if he had explained the risks of the ABVD chemotherapy, especially the great likelihood of alopecia.

CASE 6-5   *Continued.*

Dr. Pritchford responded, "I really don't think its necessary to explain all of the risks of the drugs, particularly those that are not life-threatening. I am more concerned that she knows the problems associated with bone marrow suppression than hair loss. This combination of drugs provides cure in most cases. We cannot hope to attain as good results if we avoid agents that cause alopecia. She'll get over the hair loss when she appreciates the fact that we can cure her disease."

Dr. Raku was not convinced that Ms. Pals would see things in this light based on her comments about her appearance. If Ms. Pals knowingly consented to the ABVD chemotherapy, Dr. Raku thought she could dispense it, but in this case, Ms. Pals had not consented to the specific risk of hair loss, which was al most guaranteed within 3 weeks of therapy. Dr. Raku was not certain she could prepare the chemotherapy under these conditions.

Commentary

There is no reason to believe that Ms. Pals lacks any innate capacity to understand the decision to add extra drugs to her regimen. She is clearly constrained by external forces but not by any environmental constraints, such as a prison in the previous case. One might argue that legally there is no consent to treatment because the patient does not have an adequate awareness of the treatment options and their likely effects.

But prior to the legal questions of informed consent, there arises an ethical question. Given that Ms. Pals has the intellectual ability to make an autonomous choice and is not under any necessary external constraints, should Dr. Raku become a collaborator in the paternalistic decision made by Dr. Pritchford? The physician seems to believe that he can figure out what is best for his patient. He believes that it would be morally wrong to worry her needlessly with an explanation of the risks of the combination chemotherapy. He is convinced that the added agents might help her and that the side effects are worth it.

In the cases of Chapter 4 we examined how difficult it is for someone else, a pharmacist or a physician, to know what is really in the best interest of a patient. It may not be correct that her interests are served by the course that provides the best possibility of prolonging her life. She seems to have given signals that she does not favor the burdens for the extra chance of benefit the added agents will provide.

We can imagine, however, that Dr. Pritchford is really right. Ms. Pals might be the sort who would worry endlessly and needlessly over the risks even though, by some imagined objective standard, they were worth taking. If Dr. Pritchford is not as reliable at estimating Ms. Pals interests as she is, then even on grounds of the principle of beneficence, she needs to be consulted. Suppose, however, that Dr. Pritchford is really right about Ms. Pals's interest. She really will be better off getting the extra agents without being told the side effects, than she would be if she were told about them and permitted to choose. (She might even acknowledge later that she had been mistaken in her worries about the hair loss.) Assuming that is the case, is that sufficient to justify Dr. Pritchford's action? To one who supports the dominance of the principle of beneficence it would be. To advocates of the principle of autonomy, however, the fact that Dr. Pritchford could really know what is in his patient's interest would not settle the matter. Ms. Pals would still have a moral right to be self-determining (and therefore have a right to the information needed to be self-determining) even though she would be worse off for it. Should autonomy or beneficence prevail in such situations?

CASE 6-6   Overriding Patient Autonomy (to Save a Life)

The consultation team of the hospital ethics committee was convened only when there were urgent and complex cases. Sara Mueller, Pharm.D., was a member of the consultation team and worked in the critical care areas of the hospital. Dr. Mueller received a message to meet as soon as possible in the hospital emergency room for an ethics consultation. The emergency room physician told the consultation team that the patient in question was a 25-year-old woman who had sustained massive injuries in a motor vehicle accident and lost a large amount of blood. The patient was a Jehovah's Witness and clearly expressed her wishes *not* to receive any sort of blood product. Although the ethics committee had read numerous articles about just this type of case, this was the first time it had faced an actual patient with these religious beliefs. Dr. Mueller knew that Jehovah's Witnesses believe that consuming blood can lead to losing eternal salvation. (They see it as violating the biblical injunction against "eating" blood.) Based on these tenets, they refuse all blood products. Alternatives other than blood products can be used but are not always as effective. The emergency room physician wants to override the patient's decision because he firmly believes that she would not survive surgery without a blood transfusion.

It was the habit of the consultation team to meet with as many of the individuals immediately involved in an ethical problem as soon as possible, including the patient. The patient's husband supported his wife's decision even though he was distraught at the thought of losing her. The couple had no children, so that was not a consideration. The patient was coherent enough to talk to the consultation team and said, "I understand that I might die. I don't want to leave my husband and friends, but my relationship to God is more important to me than my life."

Dr. Mueller was impressed by the patient's courage and clarity. However, she was also moved by the emergency room physician's argument that a transfusion would dramatically improve the patient's chance for survival. If the patient died she would leave her husband and friends behind as well. This also troubled Dr. Mueller, and she wondered if this was a strong enough concern to override the patient's decision.

Commentary

This case in many ways resembles the previous one. They both involve what appear to be competent patients who clearly want to refuse treatments that their physicians consider reasonable. There are important differences, however. For one, the stakes may be higher in this case. In the Hodgkins lymphoma case, changing from a single chemotherapeutic agent to the ABVD chemotherapy combination improves the patient's chance of survival, but not as much as the transfusion does in the present case. Also, the "side effect" of the treatment is quite different. In the cancer case, the side effect of the combination regimen is hair loss, which the patient considers serious but that the physician seems to think is trivial. He believes the patient will come to adjust to the effects. In this case, if the patient's religious beliefs turned out to be correct, she loses something anyone would consider terribly important—eternal salvation. However, if the physician's understanding is correct, the transfusion will have no impact at all on salvation. We are not told his religious belief but presumably he is either a secular-minded person who holds no positive beliefs in this area or a religious person who believes one's salvation is unaffected by transfusion.

This poses an unexpectedly complicated problem. On the one hand, we generally accept the right of adults not only to hold any religious belief they choose, but also to act on those beliefs provided their actions do not have an unacceptable impact on others. Since the patient's beliefs are of a religious nature, this might lead us to honor her position. On the other hand, the patient's belief is about a purported factual matter: the conditions under which one receives eternal salvation. The physician, as a medical scientist, may feel there simply is no empirical basis for these beliefs. If the patient expressed some other beliefs about the nature of reality that did not have the trappings of religion as the basis for her position, the physician might be inclined to try to have a judge declare her mentally incompetent. If she, for example, claimed she heard voices telling her to refuse blood, or if she believed without further evidence that the blood contained poison, he would say she grossly misunderstands reality. Should he reach the same conclusion about someone who believes transfusions change one's future throughout all eternity?

The law in such cases is quite clear. Competent adults who are refusing life-saving blood transfusions for themselves have the right not to be transfused.[6] In the case of parental refusal for a minor, the courts have intervened to order blood if it is likely to be lifesaving. In some cases in which parents are attempting to refuse blood for themselves but their death will leave a minor without a caregiver, the courts have ordered intervention in order to protect the physical welfare of the minor. They have not intervened, however, in the case of adults without dependents.

The physician and Dr. Mueller must first, however, face the ethical question. They must decide whether ethically they would be justified in doing what they believe will save a patient's life. They might decide to do so, even though it would be illegal. If they believed strongly that they had a duty to benefit the patient and also that they knew what would benefit, then they would be morally compelled to act. However, if they gave priority to the principle of autonomy, this would be a case in which they would have to stand by even though they believed a great and unnecessary harm would result.

Notes

1. For good discussions of the principle of autonomy and related concepts see Feinberg, Joel. "Legal Paternalism." In his *Rights, Justice, and the Bounds of Liberty: Essays in Social Philosophy*. Princeton, NJ: Princeton University Press, 1980, pp. 110–129; Dworkin,

Gerald. "Moral Autonomy." In *Morals, Science, and Society*. H. Tristram Engelhardt and Daniel Callahan, Editors. Hastings-on-Hudson, NY: The Hastings Center, 1978, pp. 156–171; Faden, Ruth, and Tom L. Beauchamp, in collaboration with Nancy N. P. King. *A History and Theory of Informed Consent*. New York: Oxford University Press, 1986; and Beauchamp, Tom L., and James F. Childress, Editors. *Principles of Biomedical Ethics*. Fifth Edition. New York: Oxford University Press, 2001, pp. 57–103.

  2. See the extended discussion of this approach in The Hastings Center. *Guidelines on the Termination of Life-Sustaining Treatment and the Care of the Dying*. Briarcliff Manor, NY: The Hastings Center, 1987, pp. 20–29.

  3. Mill, John Stuart. *On Liberty*. New York: Liberal Arts Press, 1956.

  4. Areen, Judith. "The Legal Status of Consent Obtained from Families of Adult Patients to Withhold or Withdraw Treatment." *Journal of the American Medical Association* 258 July 10, 1987): 229–235; Veatch, Robert M. "Limits of Guardian Treatment Refusal: A Reasonableness Standard." *American Journal of Law and Medicine* 9, no. 4 (1984): 427–468.

  5. Appelbaum, Paul S., Charles W. Lidz, and Alan Meisel. *Informed Consent: Legal Theory and Clinical Practice*. New York: Oxford University Press, 1987, pp. 66–69.

  6. Moore, Maureen L. "Their Life Is in the Blood: Jehovah's Witnesses, Blood Transfusions, and the Courts." *Northern Kentucky Law Review* 10, no. 2 (1983): 281–304; Byrn, Robert M. "Compulsory Lifesaving Treatment for the Competent Adult." *Fordham Law Review* 44 (1975): 1–36; Meisel, Alan. "The Legal Consensus about Forgoing Life-Sustaining Treatment: Its Status and Its Prospects." *Kennedy Institute of Ethics Journal* 2 (1992): 309–345.

  7. http://www.hhs.gov/ohrp/humansubjects/guidance/prisoner.htm, accessed July 19, 2006. For the actual regulations see *Code of Federal Regulations*, Title 45, Public Welfare Department of Health and Human Services, Part 46, Protection of Human Subjects, revised June 23, 2005; effective June 23, 2005, http://www.hhs.gov/ohrp/humansubjects/guidance/45cfr46.htm.

7

Veracity

Dealing Honestly with Patients

In the previous chapter pharmacists were in positions in which they had to choose between doing what they thought was best for a patient and respecting the patient's autonomy. The moral principle of autonomy was in conflict with the principle of beneficence. We saw that some people held that respect for autonomy can take precedence over doing good for the patient.

Respect for autonomy is an element of the more general moral concept of respect for persons. Respect for persons, according to this view, sometimes requires moral choices that do not maximize the patient's well-being.

Another element of respect for persons deals with honest disclosure. Traditional ethics holds that it is simply wrong morally to lie to people, even if it is expedient to do so, even if a better outcome will come from the lie. According to this view, lying to people is morally wrong in that it shows a lack of respect for them. Holders of this view claim that veracity or honesty or truth telling is per se a moral principle, that dishonesty in actions or practices is an element that makes those actions or practices inherently wrong. As with justice and autonomy, there may also be other dimensions that tend toward making actions right. For example, the fact that a lie produces good results would tend to make it right. However, holders of this view maintain that, nevertheless, the lie itself is an element that makes the action wrong. It is, according to this approach, prima facie wrong, that is, wrong insofar as the lying dimension is considered.

It is striking that even though many common moral systems treat lying as wrong in and of itself traditional professional health care ethics has not. Thus the Hippocratic Oath does not require that physicians deal honestly with patients. Many professional medical ethicists have, in fact, maintained that it is right for a physician to lie to a patient when doing so will spare the patient agony. In this sense professional medical ethics has focused on the consequences of actions, not on any inherent moral element, whether it be respecting autonomy or telling the truth.

By contrast, the code of the American Pharmacists Association has for many years considered truthfulness part of the essential character of the pharmacist. The 1969 version of the APhA Code of Ethics states that a pharmacist "should strive to provide information to patients regarding professional services truthfully, accurately, and fully and should avoid misleading patients regarding the nature, cost, or value of these professional services."[1] The 1995 revised code states that a pharmacist "acts with honesty and integrity in professional relationships." This provision is followed with an interpretation that reads, "A pharmacist has a duty to tell the truth and to act with conviction of conscience."[2]

Ethics that focus on consequences, such as the Hippocratic Oath, accept lies when they produce more good than harm. Classical utilitarian ethics assesses the acceptability of a lie based on the total consequences. It considers the benefits and harms for all parties.[3] By contrast, traditional health professional ethics looks only to the consequences for the patient.[4] For example, in past eras when pharmacists were expected to be paternalistic, if asked by a patient the purpose of a medication they might refuse to answer, saying that the patient should ask the physician; but if the patient asked, "Isn't it true that I am taking this because I have advanced cancer?" the pharmacist likely would have considered telling a benevolent "white lie." Likewise, if a pharmacist were asked the ingredient in a placebo, he probably would have dishonestly told the patient the name of the medication that the placebo was mimicking. The cases in this chapter present situations in which pharmacists or other health professionals believe that they can benefit their patients by lying or at least withholding the truth.

While ethics that focus on consequences evaluate whether to lie by trying to determine whether a lie will produce positive benefits, ethics that emphasize features other than consequences, such as respect for persons, hold that there is something simply wrong about lying. Immanuel Kant, the eighteenth-century philosopher, is most closely identified with this view.[5] Twentieth-century thinkers agreed.[6] While physicians traditionally accepted the legitimacy of lying to patients in order to protect them,[7] more recent developments suggest that physicians are changing, perhaps placing greater emphasis on the patient's right to be told the truth.[8] We have seen that, in contrast, the American Pharmacists Association has been committed to truthfulness for many years.

The cases in this chapter begin with the special problem of what patients should be told when the pharmacist is not yet sure what the facts are. This is followed by a series of cases that explore the problem of lying to patients in order to benefit them and, then, by cases in which the pharmacist considers lying to the patient in order to benefit others. We will then take up two special situations involving veracity: cases in which first the patient and then the patient's family ask not to be told. The final case explores disclosure to patients who ask to see their medical records.

The Condition of Doubt

Before discussing the ethics of disclosure, it is important to get some sense of exactly what it is that might be disclosed. In health care a problem arises frequently that can be referred to as the "condition of doubt," that is, when the health care provider is in real doubt about what the facts are.

The confusion may be in regard to a diagnosis about which the health care professional has only a preliminary suspicion. It may arise when innovative therapies are contemplated and the pharmacist is not clear about what the effects of the treatment will be. He or she may not even know whether the doubt is from personal ignorance of the current literature or because even the leading authorities are unclear.

In pharmacy the condition of doubt may stem from the pharmacist having only a limited understanding of a patient's condition as well as the knowledge that someone else on the health care team is better informed. In such cases, even someone who is in principle militantly committed to dealing honestly with the patient may not know exactly what should be said. The first case in this chapter raises this problem.

CASE 7-1   The Duty to Disclose Doubtful Information

The orthopedic/rehabilitation ambulatory clinic where Jean Thrailkill, Pharm.D., works handles its fair share of fractures and other types of sports injuries. Also, because they are very beneficial to physical therapy patients, enhancing the outcome of rehabilitation treatment, Dr. Thrailkill fills many prescriptions for nonsteroidal anti-inflammatory agents (NSAIDs). So she was not surprised when Julie Schulte handed her a prescription for Ibuprofen 800 mg tablets for the management of postoperative pain. Ms. Schulte, a 22-year-old volleyball player for the local college, had recently sustained a long bone fracture that had been surgically repaired.

As Dr. Thrailkill began to fill the prescription, she suddenly recalled a recent survey article that addressed the controversy surrounding the issue of the effect of NSAIDs on bone healing. She remembered that preclinical evidence had shown that NSAIDs delay fracture union during early stages of healing, though it was not determined whether these preclinical results applied to humans. She understood that NSAIDs also increase the negative effects of smoking on bone healing. The possibility that NSAIDs may delay bone healing had not been confirmed by any high-quality clinical study. Dr. Thrailkill had to decide whether she should disclose this possible remote risk to Ms. Schulte when she was doubtful about data to support this conclusion.

Commentary

If a study had been completed and had shown at a high level of statistical significance that NSAIDs caused delayed bone healing in patients, then Dr. Thrailkill would have no difficulty in deciding what Ms. Schulte should be told. In fact, she might face the new problem of whether to modify the protocol for pain management in patients with fractures to prohibit the prescribing of NSAIDs in the clinic.

But Dr. Thrailkill's situation is quite different. Consider the truthful statements that she might have said about NSAIDs and bone healing.[9] She could have said, "There has been a recent publication showing a discrepancy in findings regarding the effect of NSAIDs on bone healing following surgery." Or she might have said, "There are some data that show an association between your NSAID prescription and bone healing." Either way she would have been stating the truth.

The real problem here seems to be that Dr. Thrailkill is confronted with a situation in which she really does not know if NSAIDs delay bone healing. She has some reason to believe there might be some risk but no firm evidence. Moreover, she is not even sure she remembers exactly what the survey article indicated. Dr. Thrailkill is in a condition of doubt.

Many people who generally believe there is a moral duty to tell the truth also recognize that there are situations in which it is too early to tell what the truth is. If a pharmacist sees a patient who is a smoker and who has a persistent cough, laryngitis, and fever, the diagnosis of lung cancer may enter her mind, but that does not mean she should blurt out to the patient that he or she could have lung cancer. Not only is there real doubt about the diagnosis at this point, but there also is doubt that the pharmacist should be the one to raise the issue.

Dr. Thrailkill must decide what counts as truthful, meaningful communication about a preliminary suggestion of a link between NSAIDs and bone healing. It should be clear that no one wants what could be called the full truth. An infinite number of things could be said. No reasonable patient wants to know everything: the hypothesized mechanism of the link between NSAIDs and the various cells involved in bone healing, various trials that might be conducted to establish or refute the suggested link, the theories of statistical testing, all of the educational credentials of all the participants involved in suggested linkage, the capabilities of the manufacturer of ibuprofen, or the predictive nature of animal studies on human reaction to specific drugs.

What is usually expected is that information be "reasonably meaningful." The problem in this case is that it is not clear exactly what is reasonably meaningful. Surely some suggestions in the literature are so tenuous and the effects so trivial that patients would not consider them meaningful. In fact, supplying too much trivial, unneeded information will actually make the consent process more confusing and therefore inadequate.

Dr. Thrailkill's problem is compounded because she faces two different kinds of uncertainty. First, there is the uncertainty in the published information itself. The data are preliminary. Second, there is her doubt about whether she knows adequately what is in the literature. She probably does not remember the exact details of the article she read. Even if she did, she would never know for sure whether newer, more definitive studies had appeared in the literature that she simply had not seen. If she did an exhaustive search of the literature—something she cannot realistically do for the special conditions of each patient presenting in the clinic—she still would not know whether she had covered all the data. She will have to learn to live with the uncertainty.[10] Is she being dishonest if she omits marginal information of this sort? These questions as they arise in the consent context will be discussed in more detail in Chapter 15.

Lying in Order to Benefit

Resolving doubt about what is the truth is not all that is at stake in the ethics of truth telling. In some cases the health care provider may know the truth but fear that disclosing it to the patient will do the patient or someone else significant harm. Often it turns out that telling the truth is also beneficial, but the interesting moral cases are those in which honesty involves risk of hurting someone. In such cases, is there still a moral duty to tell the truth, or is it right to be honest only in those cases in which telling the truth is expected to be beneficial? The following cases are ones in which someone is worried about hurting another person by being honest.

Protecting the Patient by Lying

Often it is the patient who could be injured—psychologically or physically—if the health care provider is completely honest. Among the issues presented in the following case are (1) is avoiding the truth any different morally than telling an outright lie? (2) how can the pharmacist know what the consequences will be? (3) can the

---

CASE 7-2   Placebos for Addiction Withdrawal

Harvey Silversmith, Pharm.D., a recent graduate from pharmacy school, was newly employed at Main Pharmacy, an independent store in a small Midwestern town that struggled to fill 20 prescriptions a day. He received a telephone call from a woman who identified herself as Mrs. Abraham's nurse. She asked for a refill of Mrs. Abraham's sleeping pills and gave Dr. Silversmith the number.

When he checked the file, he discovered it was for Seconal placebo, No. 30. The record indicated that it had been refilled almost monthly for at least the past 2 years. There was then a reference to an earlier number indicating that the prescription was even older.

He asked Mr. Tolson, the proprietor of the store, about it when he came in that afternoon. Mr. Tolson said Mrs. Abraham had been getting the prescription filled for years. It turns out she had had a malignancy of the colon 4 years previously. Surgery had corrected the problem, but in the emotional and physical distress that followed, Mrs. Abraham had a terrible time sleeping. She had received a prescription for the Seconal from her oncologist to help her sleep and continued taking them to the point at which she could not sleep without them. Her physician after several months realized that he had caused her to become addicted and felt that it was his duty to break her of her habit. He had arranged with Mr. Tolson to take Seconal capsules and gradually replace more and more of the active ingredient until some months later she was on pure lactose packaged in the distinctive Seconal capsules. She now claimed she could not sleep without her sleeping pills.

Dr. Silversmith understood the purpose but felt uncomfortable about the compounding he was being asked to undertake. He was concerned about potential legal implications of mislabeling by placing the drug name on the prescription label. He was concerned about the fact that Mrs. Abraham was paying monthly, even though he saw that the charge was modest, barely covering the cost of the capsule ingredients that were being discarded. But most of all he was concerned about whether he was being asked to participate in something that was dishonest. Do placebo prescriptions, such as Mrs. Abraham's, involve lying, and, if so, are they morally wrong?

problem be avoided by referring the patient to the physician for disclosure? and (4) what is the nature of the duty to be honest?

Commentary

Dr. Silversmith is facing the classical ethical dilemma of the conflict between medical paternalism and the principle of veracity. According to the traditional ethical health care ethics based on the duty to be beneficent to the patient, placebos were considered an important therapy in the armamentarium of the health care provider. Patients in situations such as Mrs. Abraham's occasionally become addicted. If the physician is convinced that the drugs are now doing more harm than good and has tried other more direct methods of withdrawing his patient without success, then the graded reduction in dosage, often done without the patient's knowledge, was judged by the provider to be the best course for the patient.

If it is a physician who reaches that conclusion and his action is to write a placebo prescription, then the pharmacist, if he fills the prescription, is willy-nilly brought into the act. A first level of problem might arise if the pharmacist does not agree that the placebo is the best course. He might, for example, believe that referral to a psychiatrist or a plan for decreasing dosage involving the full knowledge of the patient would be a better course for her. If he subscribes to a similar Hippocratic, beneficence-driven ethic, then his duty is diametrically opposed to that of the physician. The question then becomes, what should two paternalistically oriented health professionals do if they are jointly involved in the care of a patient but perceive they have conflicting duties? Is there any reason to assume that the physician's judgment about the placebo being the best course should prevail?

Dr. Silversmith's conflict seems somewhat different, however. He may agree that the placebo is in Mrs. Abraham's best interest but feel that he is still doing her wrong by continuing the practice of filling the prescription with an inert substance. This clearly generates costs for Mrs. Abraham, but that may not be the main concern. He may feel it is simply dishonest to imply to his patient that she is getting something that she really is not. Some, including those who reason like Immanuel Kant, believe that there is simply something unethical about telling such lies—even when everyone is better off for the lie being told. People who hold such a view believe there is a moral principle that it is wrong to lie regardless of the consequences. This principle, sometimes called the principle of veracity, identifies all knowing wrongful statements as unethical, at least in regard to the lie.

Dr. Silversmith may see the dispensing as an implicit lie. He may consider the labeling an outright lie as well as a legally suspect practice. First, consider the distinction often drawn between lying and failing to tell the truth. Can Dr. Silversmith reason that dispensing without false labeling was not lying but merely withholding the truth about the placebo?

Even if all outright dishonest statements are morally wrong, no one has a moral duty to say everything he knows to other people. Could Dr. Silversmith solve his ethical dilemma by omitting the directly false information?

Outright lying is different morally from simply failing to tell the whole truth. In normal human interactions, out of courtesy we sometimes fail to tell the whole truth—for instance about the appearance of someone who is not terribly attractive. Lying always involves failing to respect persons in a way that merely withholding part of the truth does not.

At the same time, health professionals have a duty to make sure that patients are adequately informed so they can make autonomous choices about treatment options. Informed consent requires that patients be given truthful, relevant information. This suggests that health professionals have an obligation to disclose relevant information even though ordinary citizens do not have such an obligation. Here the duty of veracity is interconnected with the principle of fidelity. Those who are committed to the respect-for-persons perspective would probably claim in this case that the pharmacist owes it to the patient with whom there is a bond of fidelity or loyalty not only to refrain from making false statements, but also to provide all potentially relevant information honestly. Holders of this view might reach that conclusion even when it conflicts with the duty to do what the provider believes is best for the patient.

Protecting the Welfare of Others

In the previous case a health care provider contemplated lying or withholding the truth because he thought it would be better for the patient not to know. Sometimes it is not the patient, but someone else—a colleague or friend—whose welfare could be protected if the truth were withheld. In the following cases, pharmacists are asked to lie to protect others.

CASE 7-3   Reporting a Colleague's Innocent Mistake

James Naughton, Pharm.D., was tired after a 12-hour shift in the critical care pharmacy that was responsible for dispensing and delivering first-dose medication to the medical and surgical intensive care units. Dr. Naughton saw that he would have to make one more trip to the medical intensive care unit before he left for the day. The medication orders were for Cecily Traverda, a 45-year-old woman with an acute inferior wall myocardial infarction. Her physician, Dr. Franz Neuhaus, had ordered a stat 35 mg bolus IV push dose of esmolol over 1 minute, followed by a double-strength esmolol drip at 3.5 mg/min. The double-strength infusion comes prepared as a 20 mg/ml ready-to-use bag.

Dr. Naughton prepared and delivered the esmolol bolus and drip to the patient's room. Melaine Walters, RN, gave the esmolol bolus and hung the drip at 21 cc/hr, as directed by Dr. Naughton's instructions on the bag. Dr. Naughton spoke briefly to Michelle Tonn, Pharm.D., the next clinical pharmacist on duty. Dr. Naughton ran through the few orders he had not completed and left.

About an hour later, Dr. Tonn reread the instructions that Dr. Naughton had prepared for the double-strength esmolol drip and was surprised to find an error. Although the esmolol double-strength bag was provided correctly, Dr. Naughton had made an error in the instructions he wrote for the administration of the esmolol drip. Dr. Naughton had failed to decrease the drip rate by half. The 3.5 mg/min infusion should be at 10.5 cc an hour, but Ms. Traverda was incorrectly receiving a 7 mg/min infusion.

Dr. Tonn raced to the unit to check on Ms. Traverda's status and the actual drip rate. The IV was running at 21 cc/hr, but fortunately, according to the nurse, Ms. Traverda had not demonstrated any signs of cardiac disturbance. The nurse slowed the drip rate to 10.5 cc an hour and corrected the instructions on the label.

CASE 7-3   *Continued.*

> While Dr. Tonn is in Ms. Traverda's room, Dr. Neuhaus enters the room and notices Dr. Tonn examining the esmolol drip. Dr. Neuhaus asks, "Is anything wrong?" Dr. Tonn knows that Dr. Naughton is normally highly competent and believes that no good would come from reporting this error to Dr. Neuhaus. In fact, Dr. Neuhaus could cause a great deal of harm to Dr. Naughton by discrediting his contributions to the critical care team in the future. Furthermore, Ms. Traverda had not experienced any apparent harm. Dr. Tonn contemplates how she should respond to Dr. Neuhaus.

CASE 7-4   Revealing Alcoholism on a Job Application

> As far as Marcus Heywood, Pharm.D., could tell, the whole interview process had gone very well. Dr. Heywood was one of the final candidates for the position of regional manager for a national pharmacy chain. Jonathan Gurran, the chief operating officer stated, "We think you are the right person for the job, and we want to make you an offer."
>
> Dr. Heywood was thrilled, "I accept. I know you've made the right choice."
>
> "Good," Mr. Gurran responded. "Now I have just a few more questions. Have you ever participated in a drug-rehabilitation program? We verified all of your start and end dates from previous employers and notice a gap for about a year. So, Marcus, why the year gap in your employment?"
>
> Dr. Heywood stopped and thought. Over 10 years ago, when the twins were just infants and he had been working two jobs to pay off loans and take care of his new family, he had started to drink to relax. It was not long after that he knew the drinking was getting out of hand. Dr. Heywood had watched his father die an early death from alcoholism. The awful memories of his childhood frightened him enough that he had voluntarily checked himself into a 10-month rehabilitation program. He had been sober ever since and continued to participate in Alcoholics Anonymous.
>
> Dr. Heywood had worked steadily since that time to reach this point in his career. Now his chance to really make something of his life and secure a future for his five children seemed to be in jeopardy if he told the truth. Who would want to hire a regional manager with a history of alcoholism? Should he tell Mr. Gurran the truth about the gap in his employment history or not?

Commentary

These two cases each involve pharmacists in situations in which they believe that serious harm could be done to someone if the truth were told while no real purpose is served by speaking honestly. In Case 7-3 James Naughton made a potentially serious mistake but one that apparently caused no harm. His colleague, Dr. Tonn, caught the mistake and knows that Dr. Naughton is generally a competent, careful practitioner. She believes he could be hurt if she answers the physician's question in a straightforward, honest way. In contrast to Case 7-2, where the pharmacist contemplated being dishonest in order to benefit the patient, Dr. Tonn has to decide whether lying to benefit a colleague is justifiable.

It is part of the nature of being in a profession that bonds of loyalty to one's colleagues are important. This includes not only providing aid and assistance, but also taking steps to deal with a colleague's deficiencies, whether they are a misunderstanding, a lack of knowledge, or even a substance abuse problem. Here, however, Dr. Tonn believes that her colleague's error was an innocent one, one unlikely to be repeated. She also fears what will happen to Dr. Naughton if she reports his error to the physician. Her calculation of the benefits and harms to all parties seems to lead to the conclusion that more good overall will be done if she hides her colleague's mistake.

Two kinds of counterargument must be considered. First, are we sure Dr. Tonn has calculated correctly? It may be important that the error occurred at the end of a 12-hour shift. There may be a structural or system reason for Dr. Naughton's mistake that should be fixed. It may turn out that the only way to fix that system problem is to report the error so that some adjustment can be made to address the effects of long shifts. If Dr. Tonn is to base her choice on benefits and harms, should she rely on her own judgment about those benefits and harms, or should she ask for more formal reviews that might be stimulated by telling the physician, Dr. Neuhaus, what happened?

Assuming that this is a problem to be addressed by calculating benefits and harms, Dr. Tonn must decide whether is it acceptable to include benefits to Dr. Naughton in the calculation or follow the more traditional route of considering only potential benefits and harms to the patient. A case could be made that in this situation it is only the patient's welfare that should count and that more good for patients is likely to result if Dr. Tonn reveals the events so that in the future similar mistakes can be avoided. A classical social utilitarian would take into account the effects on all parties—including Dr. Naughton—while a Hippocratic ethic would include only the welfare of the patient or patients.

In Case 7-4, the one involving Dr. Heywood's history of treatment for alcoholism, the problem of whose benefits to include is even more dramatic. The classical social utilitarian, taking into account benefits and harms to all parties, would include the benefits to Dr. Heywood himself if he tells a lie to the chief operating officer, Mr. Gurran. If benefits to the one who responds dishonestly cannot be included in the calculation of benefits and harms, it will be much harder for Dr. Heywood to argue that his lie is justified on grounds of consequences.

He might claim that the lie is justified to benefit his children, but, then, other applicants might also take the welfare of their children into account in deciding how to answer questions during an interview. It will be hard for Dr. Heywood to show that more good is done this way. However, if he should focus in Hippocratic fashion only on the welfare of patients, it is hard to see how the lie would be justified. He would apparently have to argue that his getting the job is so beneficial to the patients of the pharmacy chain that the lie is justified—hardly an easy case to make.

Even if the consequences in this case would justify the dishonest response during the interview, a second line of argument must be confronted. As we have seen in the previous cases in this chapter, some people interpret the principle of veracity to require honesty even when it can be shown that greater good will come from lying.

Some reach that conclusion by considering what would happen if everyone acted on the rule that they could lie, for instance on applications, whenever they thought more good would come from the lie. These people, sometimes called rule utilitarians, believe that the chance of a mistake being made by permitting lies whenever it appeared to do more good would be so great that it is better in the long run to have a flat rule prohibiting lying.

Others reach the same conclusion but on different grounds. They believe that lying violates the integrity of personal relations, even if the consequences are no worse and even if, as in this case, the consequences might actually be better. They see dishonest communication as threatening the respect for persons that is essential to maintaining good human relations. They would insist in all the previous cases that the morally right thing to do is to tell the truth, even if the pharmacist believed that better consequences would come from avoiding it.

Special Cases of Truth Telling

Although the usual cases of truth telling involve situations in which the pharmacist contemplates lying or withholding the truth in order to benefit the patient or benefit someone else, some special cases occur in which lies, deceptions, or the withholding of information are motivated by other concerns, such as respect for someone who is believed to have authority to decide that the truth should be withheld. These include cases in which the patient or some member of the family requests that the truth be withheld.

Patients Who Don't Want to Be Told

Sometimes a patient is said to fear bad news or, for other reasons, desires not to know some aspects of his or her condition. When being seen for a diagnosis of a potentially fatal disease, the patient may explicitly ask the provider to avoid disclosing the bad news. A pharmacist may, as in the following case, contemplate a plan of pharmaceutical care that includes educating the patient about the side effects of a medication only to discover that the patient does not want the information.

CASE 7-5   Refusing to Learn the Risks of Chemotherapy

Terra Ramsey, an unmarried, 25-year-old patient with advanced squamous cell carcinoma of the cervix, was supposed to start therapy with cisplatin and mitomycin-c. Patricia Griem, Pharm.D., a clinical pharmacist on the oncology service was assigned to explain the proposed treatment and answer any questions Ms. Ramsey might have about cisplatin and mitomycin-C. As Dr. Griem began explaining the reason for her visit, she was surprised when Ms. Ramsey cut her off by saying, "Look, I am an educated person. I know enough about all of these chemotherapy drugs from what I've seen on television or read in magazines to know that I can expect some problems. But you need to know that I do much better without knowing exactly what to worry about. If you tell me, 'You could get

CASE 7-5 *Continued.*

dizzy.' I will. So just don't tell me. I don't want to hear about the risks involved. I've already made that clear to my physician and the nurses."

Dr. Griem responded, "I respect your right to refuse information, but are you sure that you don't want to know about some of the unique risks of this particular drug?" Dr. Griem was specifically thinking about the fact that cisplatin and mitomycin-C may be hazardous to the fetus. Although these drugs could be used in pregnant patients in life-threatening situations, that was presently not the case with Ms. Ramsey. Dr. Griem wanted to make sure Ms. Ramsey did not become pregnant while on the drug. Furthermore, Ms. Ramsey would have to use effective contraception during treatment and for a few months past treatment. Dr. Griem knew of several cases in which cancer patients under treatment had become pregnant. At this point, Dr. Griem did not know if Ms. Ramsey was sexually active or not.

Ms. Ramsey replied, "I'm sure. I do not want to be bothered with the details." Dr. Griem left Ms. Ramsey's room troubled by her sense of obligation not only to Ms. Ramsey, but in this case to her potential children. Didn't they have a right to be protected from the risk involved with the drug? Did Ms. Ramsey have a right to waive information under these circumstances?

Commentary

While earlier cases in this chapter involve health care providers who are inclined to withhold potentially traumatic information from patients, Dr. Griem faces the opposite problem. She is not only willing to disclose the details of the chemotherapy, she appears to feel morally obliged to do so.

Ms. Ramsey, the 25-year-old woman with cervical cancer, appears less interested. She has a right to the truth, but does she have a duty to get it? The rights associated with autonomy and veracity, with consent and informing patients, are what can be called alienable rights. The one who has the right to information also may, at least in some circumstances, waive the right. Sometimes we might waive the right to information to which we are entitled because it seems too trivial. People leading busy lives cannot possibly stop to process all the details of the information to which they are entitled. But is it ethically acceptable to decline information about momentous, life-and-death events like treatment for cancer?

Assuming that Ms. Ramsey continues to insist that she does not want to know the details, that is, that she waives her right to know, Dr. Griem has to decide whether to cooperate in the treatment of the uninformed patient. Some would claim that pharmacists have the legal right to refuse any patient, but when they refuse, they do so within a health care system that may create psychological and social pressures. The real issue here, however, is whether there is any moral reason why Dr. Griem should refuse to cooperate.

One reason why Dr. Griem might object to continuing with Ms. Ramsey's treatment is that the welfare of other parties could be at sake, thus changing the moral situation. Not only might Ms. Ramsey put her own life in jeopardy, she might also jeopardize the life of any child she conceived while on cisplatin and mitomycin-C. Keeping in mind that traditionally the clinician's moral duty has been to the patient and the patient alone, are these third-party interests relevant in deciding whether

Ms. Ramsey has a duty to know the truth about the risks of her treatments? If so, is it because pharmacists today must consider all benefits and harms, not just those involving the patient? Or is it the special nature of the relationships these patients have with third parties that generates an obligation on their part to learn the truth about their treatments?

In some cases the family plays a different role, that of demanding that the patient not be told certain information. It is to that kind of case that we now turn.

Family Members Who Insist That the Patient Not Be Told

A second kind of special case involves a patient whose family insists that the patient not be told. Now it is the family member who is claiming the authority to waive the right to know. In some cases, such as the one that follows, it can be argued that the patient would be hurt, psychologically or physically, if he or she knew the threatening information. Nevertheless, the question persists whether there is anyone who has the authority to overturn the patient's claim on information.

CASE 7-6   When the Family Asks Not to Tell

Allen Younger, Pharm.D., works at an ambulatory geriatric clinic. For the past 6 months he has been refilling prescriptions for donepezil for Cory Banyon, a 72-year-old man with moderate Alzheimer's disease who resides with his daughter. Dr. Younger participated in the initial interdisciplinary workup of Mr. Banyon to determine his diagnosis. His recollection is that Mr. Banyon had all the usual signs of what was probably Alzheimer's disease, such as forgetfulness, sleep disturbances, moderate word finding difficulties, trouble getting dressed, and at least 2 episodes of getting lost. Mr. Banyon was started on donepezil and appears to be tolerating the drug well. However, whenever the prescription is refilled the daughter, Victoria Banyon, picks it up. Mr. Younger asked Ms. Banyon how her father was doing and if Mr. Banyon needed any counseling. The daughter responded, "He is doing fine. I'd rather you didn't talk to him about his drugs or mention that he has Alzheimer's disease. The diagnosis would scare him to death, and there is so little that can be done that it seems kinder not to tell him. We've asked the doctor not to say anything either, and he agrees."

Dr. Younger has just been informed by the clinic receptionist that Mr. Banyon's daughter has dropped him off at the clinic entrance and that Mr. Banyon is asking for that "nice pharmacist." It seems he has a question about his "medication." Mr. Banyon is waiting to speak to Dr. Younger while his daughter parks the car and then joins him for his appointment with the physician.[11]

Commentary

In some ways this case is like Case 7-5. Someone believes that the patient is better off not knowing. Yet in this case it is not the patient who is waiving the right to be informed. Recently in health care ethics, patients have been given the right to appoint a surrogate (sometimes called a durable power of attorney) to make decisions when the patient is no longer capable. The issues of surrogate appointment and decision-making will be explored in more detail in the cases of Chapter 16. In some ways, Mr. Banyon's daughter is acting as if she were her father's legal surrogate with the authority to make decisions, such as consenting to the medication treatment now being undertaken. Has her father given her that authority? Is there any reason to believe that the daughter can assume it without her father's approval?

The exact policies for surrogate decision-making are still evolving. In some cases we all accept the role of certain family members acting as surrogates without any formal procedures. Parents act as surrogates for their children, but the law clearly presumes they have that authority. If a patient is without any doubt incompetent—is unconscious or delirious—health providers normally assume that the next of kin is capable of making decisions. But it is in just those cases that it is not possible to tell the patient relevant information.

In this case, Mr. Banyon appears competent enough to want to ask questions about his medication and has asked to speak to the pharmacist even though he has a diagnosis of Alzheimer's disease. Merely having a diagnosis of Alzheimer's disease is hardly a clear indication that he is mentally incompetent and that his daughter can be presumed to be his surrogate. In such cases, are there circum-stances in which the daughter can act as her father's surrogate? For instance, what if Mr. Banyon had said during an earlier visit that he wanted his daughter to make all decisions for him? Would that count as an acceptable transfer of authority? Are there any conditions in this case under which the daughter could assume that role without her father designating her for it? When we are dealing with infor-mation transfer, do parents, a spouse, adult children, or others concerned about the patient ever have the right to protect the patient from potentially traumatic information in cases that, unlike the previous cases, do not involve the patient's waiver of the right to know?

A related issue worth discussing is how the daughter came to find out about the diagnosis and treatment in the first place without Mr. Banyon knowing. The traditional ethics of confidentiality requires that information about a patient not be disclosed without the patient's permission. The daughter apparently learned of her father's diagnosis from the physicians caring for her father. There is no evidence that Mr. Banyon gave permission to disclose his diagnosis to his daughter before he found out about it. Does that constitute a violation of the ethics of confidentiality? Confidentiality will be discussed further in the cases of the next chapter.

The Right of Access to Medical Records

Closely related to the ethics of truth telling is the question of the right of access of a patient to his or her medical records. This is a problem for medical records adminis-trators but also for all other health care providers, including pharmacists, especially those in a hospital setting. If the patient has the right to be told all that is potentially meaningful about his or her medical condition and treatment, does that also imply a right to see his or her medical records or at least to know what they contain?

CASE 7-7   The Right to Health Records

Eric Mendelsohn, a 27-year-old patient recently diagnosed with HIV+/AIDS, was recovering from lymphocytic interstitial pneumonia. Lauren Quist, Pharm.D., a clinical pharmacist on the infectious diseases service was in the process of winding up a discussion with Mr. Mendelsohn about his medication regimen when he asked, "You've really answered all of the questions I had about my medications, but I still have a few other questions about my lab values and prognosis."

Dr. Quist responded, "It probably would be better to discuss those types of questions with your physician, but I would be happy to try and find the information for you if I can." So saying, Dr. Quist went to the computer station just outside Mr. Mendelsohn's door and pulled up the most recent lab results.

Mr. Mendelsohn stated, "I probably know as much about this disease as anyone taking care of me. I think I can understand and interpret any information in my chart as well as you can. Please print me a copy of my lab results, and I'll let you know if I have any questions."

No one had ever asked Dr. Quist to see what was in the medical record before. Dr. Quist was not certain if Mr. Mendelsohn, or any patient for that matter, had the right to see his medical record.

Commentary

Mr. Mendelsohn's request poses a doubly complicated problem for Dr. Quist. First, even if the request had been made of Mr. Mendelsohn's physician it would raise issues that many physicians have not faced. Second, in this case it raises the question of whether a pharmacist or any other member of the health care team other than the physician should be allowed to share information in the record with the patient.

A traditional consequentialist would ask whether the information would, on balance, be beneficial to the patient. The answer in this case is not obvious. There is information at stake that is potentially important to his current health care and peace of mind. Moreover, many AIDS patients, including apparently Mr. Mendelsohn, learn a great deal about their disease and can understand even complex medical accounts. However, traditionally health providers have believed that patients are likely to be confused and potentially distressed at seeing the actual medical record. The same arguments confronted earlier in this chapter pertaining to disclosing diagnoses orally are likely to arise when the actual data from the clinical record are shared with the patient. The physician or other members of the health care team may have entered notes about the patient's mental state or other potentially embarrassing information they did not expect the patient to see. Basing an assessment just on the consequences, it may not be clear whether the patient will, on balance, be helped or hurt by seeing his record.

Now look at the case from the point of view of the rights of the patient. Assuming that Mr. Mendelsohn has the right to information potentially meaningful in making medical decisions, it would seem that he would have a right to the information even if it is, on balance, likely to harm him. Increasingly, courts are granting the right of patients to see medical records,[12] and many state legislatures have passed laws granting patients the right to see their records.[13] Patient advocacy groups are pressing for a right of access.[14] Physicians and others examining the psychological and medical effects of granting a right of access are increasingly more positive about such access.[15]

Even if, in general, Dr. Quist accepts the idea of giving patients access to their records, she faces a second problem: is the pharmacist the person best situated to share the information with the patient? Certainly the easiest solution would be to indicate to Mr. Mendelsohn that this request will have to be taken up with his physician. However, there is also reason to consider whether that is the only course or the best one. Dr. Quist may know that the physician retains more traditional paternalistic attitudes about such matters. Deferring to the physician may, de facto, be blocking the patient's right of access. Moreover, Dr. Quist may be in a better position than the physician to discuss the contents of parts of the record. Does Dr. Quist defer or make the decision on her own to share the information? If she does share the record with Mr. Mendelsohn, what obligations does she have to make sure the patient understands its content?

This completes our exploration of cases dealing with the ethical principle of veracity. Autonomy and veracity, the focus of the previous chapter and this one, respectively, were the first two principles related to respect for persons. We now turn to the third such principle: fidelity.

Notes

1. American Pharmaceutical Association. "Code of Ethics." Washington, DC: American Pharmaceutical Association, 1969. This provision was not changed in the amendments of 1975 or the revision of 1981.

2. It continues, however, with a possible opening to the more traditional Hippocratic paternalism when it adds that a pharmacist "avoids . . . actions that compromise dedication to the best interests of patients." See American Pharmaceutical Association. "Code of Ethics for Pharmacists." Washington, DC: American Pharmaceutical Association, 1995.

3. Sidgwick, Henry. *The Methods of Ethics.* New York: Dover Publications, Inc., 1966 [1874].

4. Meyer, Bernard. "Truth and the Physician." *Ethical Issues in Medicine.* E. Fuller Torrey, Editor. Boston: Little Brown, 1968, pp. 159–177.

5. Kant, Immanuel. "On the Supposed Right to Tell Lies from Benevolent Motives." Translated by Thomas Kingsmill Abbott. Reprinted in Kant's *Critique of Practical Reason and Other Works on the Theory of Ethics.* London: Longmans, 1909 [1797], pp. 361–365.

6. Ross, W. D. *The Right and the Good.* Oxford: Oxford University Press, 1939.

7. Oken, Donald. "What to Tell Cancer Patients: A Study of Medical Attitudes." *Journal of the American Medical Association* 175 (April 1, 1961): 1120–1128.

8. Novack, Dennis H., Robin Plumer, Raymond L. Smith, Herbert Ochitill, Gary R. Morrow, and John M. Bennett. "Changes in Physicians' Attitudes toward Telling the Cancer Patient." *Journal of the American Medical Association* 241 (March 2, 1979): 897–900.

9. Biederman, R. E. Pharmacology in Rehabilitation: Nonsteroidal Anti-inflammatory Agents. *Journal of Orthopedics Sports and Physical Therapy* 35, no. 6 (June 2005): 356–367.

10. Good discussions of the problems of uncertainty faced by health professionals are Fox, Renée C. "Training for Uncertainty." In *The Student-Physician.* Robert K. Merton,

George Reader, and Patricia L. Kendall, Editors. Cambridge, MA: Harvard University Press, 1957, pp. 207–241; Fox, Renée C. "Medical Uncertainty." *Second-Opinion* (Nov 1987): 91–105; and Bosk, Charles. *Forgive and Remember: Managing Medical Failure.* Chicago: University of Chicago Press, 1979.

11. Haddad, Amy. "Leading Students to Care: The Use of Clinical Simulations in Ethics." *Journal of Pharmacy Teaching* 12, no. 1 (2005): 61–79.

12. McLaren, Paul. "The Right to Know: Patients' Records Should Be Understandable by Patients, Too." *British-Medical-Journal* 303, no. 6808 (Oct 19, 1991): 937–938; Bruce, Jo Anne Czecowski. "Access of Patient to Health Records." In her *Privacy and Confidentiality of Health Care Information.* Second Edition. Chicago: American Hospital Publishing, 1988 pp. 161–182; Kirby, Brian J. "Patient Access to Medical Records." *Journal of the Royal College of Physicians of London* 25 (July 1991): 240–242; Gilhooly, Mary L. M., and Sarah M. McGhee. "Medical Records: Practicalities and Principles of Patient Possession." *Journal of Medical Ethics* 17 (Sept 1991): 138–143; de-Klerk, Anton. "Should a Patient Have Access to His Medical Records?" *Medicine and Law* 8 (1989): 475–483; Klugman, Ellen. "Toward a Uniform Right to Medical Records: A Proposal for a Model Patient Access and Information Practices Statute." *UCLA Law Review* 30 (Aug 1983): 1349–1385; Fox, Lloyd A. "Medical and Prescription Records—Patient Access and Confidentiality." *U.S. Pharmacist* 4, no. 2 (1979): 15–16+.

13. "Summary of Selected Statutes concerning Confidentiality of and Patient Access to Medical Records." *State Health Legislation Report* 9, no. 1 (May 1981): 13–23; Annas, George J., Daryl B. Matthews, and Leonard H. Glantz. "Patient Access to Medical Records." *Medicolegal News* 8, no. 2 (April 1980): 17–18.

14. Public Citizen Health Research Group. *Medical Records: Getting Yours.* Washington, DC: Public Citizen Research Health Research Group, 1986.

15. Schade, Hugh I. "My Patients Take Their Medical Records with Them." *Medical Economics,* March 8, 1976, pp. 75–81; Giglio, R., B. Spears, David Rumpf, and Nancy Eddy. "Encouraging Behavior Changes by Use of Client-Held Health Records." *Medical Care* 16 (1978): 757–764; Shenkin, Budd N., and David C. Warner. "Giving the Patient His Medical Record: A Proposal to Improve the System." *New England Journal of Medicine* 289 (1973): 688–692.

8

Fidelity

Promise-Keeping and Confidentiality

The cases in the previous chapter included a number of situations in which pharmacists did not propose to overtly lie to patients but nevertheless contemplated withholding the truth. We noted that the principle of veracity treated the intentional telling of false information as a moral infringement but that it was less clear how to treat the withholding of information. It seems clear that no one has a duty to tell all the truth to anyone who happens along. At the same time, certain people seem to have a duty not only to avoid lying, but also to tell certain things to others. In general, pharmacists who are in an ongoing relation with a patient or patients have a duty to disclose what they would reasonably want to know or find meaningful in making a decision related to care.

We might attribute such a duty to the principle of veracity (truthfulness, honesty, correctness, and accuracy), but it can also be associated with what we will call the *principle of fidelity*. When people exist in special relationships with others, they take on special duties. Parents have duties to their children, spouses to each other, that they do not have with other people. Likewise, when a pharmacist enters a special relation with a patient or patients, certain special obligations are created. This relationship is more than a legal contract. It is not just a matter of a business interaction. A moral contract is established generating mutual obligations. This contract in the pharmaceutical care literature is often referred to as a "covenant."[1] As part of the contract or "covenant" that establishes the relationship, commitments are made that generate new and special obligations. The duty to disclose potentially meaningful information is one such duty, but there are many others.

In general, when one party promises something to another party, such a special relationship is established. That promise can be as routine as promising to return something one has borrowed or as distinctive as establishing a relationship between provider and patient. Usually, promise-making is reciprocal: each party both offers something and agrees to be bound by mutual agreement. In health care, promises are made in scheduling appointments, agreeing to fee schedules, and in keeping records. More fundamentally, promises are made when a patient-provider relationship is established that includes a pharmacist's pledge of loyalty to the patient—to abide by a code of ethics and to stay with the patient in time of need. Among the promises made is the promise to keep information confidential.

All promises are made with implicit or explicit limits. The commitment to establish a provider-patient relation normally carries with it an implied limit that either party can break the relationship under certain conditions: adequate notice, justifiable reason, and—in the case of the pharmacist—arrangement for a colleague to assume responsibility.

The contract, covenant, commitment, or promise that establishes the relationship between provider and patient rests, in part, on the ethics of keeping promises. The principle underlying the idea that one has a duty—other things being equal—to keep a commitment once it is made is sometimes called the principle of fidelity. The cases in this chapter look at situations in which pharmacists are faced with problems of what the moral limits are on keeping commitments once they are made. In particular, we will face cases in which the pharmacist has made some sort of commitment and later discovers that, in the pharmacist's estimate, the patient or someone else would be better off if the commitment were not kept. The general problem is, thus, one of the conflict between the principle of beneficence and the principle of fidelity.

The first cases involve general notions of fidelity to explicit and implicit promises. The second section of the chapter deals with the more specific area of the promise of confidentiality and its limits. Finally, we look at fidelity in terms of professional obligations and loyalty when dealing with incompetent, impaired, or dishonest colleagues.

The Ethics of Promises: Explicit and Implicit

We all learn very young that it is immoral to break a promise. Unfortunately, soon thereafter we also learn that there are cases when one can give strong reasons why promises should not always be kept. There are promises that it is in one's self-interest to break. Normally, however, we do not confuse self-interest with ethics. The interesting case is the one in which a promise has been made but one comes to believe that it will serve the welfare of others to break it. These other-regarding reasons for breaking promises may pose a legitimate moral dilemma.

Sometimes, as in the first case in this section, the promise is explicit, and yet the one to whom the promise is made will be hurt only modestly if the promise is not kept while someone else will benefit enormously if it is violated. The question raised in the following case is whether that counts as an acceptable reason to break the promise.

CASE 8-1   Keeping a Promise to a Medical Colleague

Callista Upwood, Pharm.D., dreaded calling Lyndon Dorfer, M.D., to clarify yet another one of his prescriptions for a frail, elderly woman, Emily Wilkens. Dr. Upwood often had to call Dr. Dorfer. She suspected that his undecipherable handwriting was just a cover-up for a lack of knowledge of contemporary pharmacotherapy. Dr. Upwood thought that Dr. Dorfer should have retired years ago. Although he was kind to his patients, he was terribly out of touch with modern medical practice. More than once, she had found an error and suggested the correct dose or drug. What made the phone calls so unpleasant was that Dr. Dorfer initially blamed the problem on the pharmacist who called. When the drug or dosage was corrected, Dr. Dorfer became conciliatory and often ended the conversation by stating, "We'll just keep this little mix-up to ourselves, okay?" None of the errors were harmful just not appropriate or helpful, so Dr. Upwood kept his "mistakes" to herself.

This time, it looked like Dr. Dorfer had written a prescription for chloral hydrate, ii tsp q 4hr/po. This didn't sound at all right to Dr. Upwood based on Ms. Wilkens's history, so she asked Ms. Wilkens, "What did Dr. Dorfer tell you this prescription was for?" Ms. Wilkens replied, "Oh, I have a little cough that bothers me at night, and he said this would help."

Dr. Upwood steeled herself and dialed Dr. Dorfer's office. When Dr. Dorfer came to the phone, he once again complained that he didn't have time to do his job and the pharmacist's too. Dr. Upwood stated, "I just have to be certain what you have written on this prescription. Did you mean to order chloral hydrate for Ms. Wilkens?" "Heavens, no," Dr. Dorfer huffed. "Can't you read?" he stated. "What could I have meant, do you think?" Dr. Upwood knew that this was his way of allowing her to correct the prescription, so she hazarded an educated guess, "Well, Ms. Wilkens says she has a cough. Could you have written the prescription for 'terpin' hydrate?"

"That sounds good," Dr. Dorfer responded. Dr. Upwood could think of many cough remedies that were more effective than terpin hydrate and suggested them to Dr. Dorfer. He stated, "No, no. Let's stick with the old favorites." After the prescription was changed, Dr. Dorfer once again ended the conversation by asking Dr. Upwood to keep the matter to herself. Dr. Upwood casually acknowledged that she would.

When Dr. Upwood returned to the counseling counter with the terpin hydrate, Ms. Wilkens asked, "Is something the matter with the prescription? I heard you speaking to Dr. Dorfer." Dr. Upwood was sorely tempted to break her promise to Dr. Dorfer and tell Ms. Wilkens about his incompetence. Ms. Wilkens would clearly benefit from a competent, up-to-date internist because she had numerous medical problems. It is possible that Dr. Dorfer's reputation would suffer if Dr. Upwood expressed her misgivings about him to Ms. Wilkens. However, if Ms. Wilkens knew, she could then seek out a better qualified physician.

Commentary

In this case two relationships exist on which we need to focus, one between pharmacist and patient and another between pharmacist and physician. Both involve fiduciary relations, that is, a relationship in which trust is expected. For many generations pharmacists and physicians have maintained working relations in which mutual trust is assumed. Sometimes that has led to one party protecting the other when embarrassing or innocent mistakes are made. At an earlier time, some professional codes of ethics even included provisions not to speak critically of colleagues to outsiders, such as patients.

Here the pharmacist, Dr. Upwood, has maintained a trusting relationship with the physician, Dr. Dorfer, by helping him clarify prescriptions that were written unclearly (sometimes even incorrectly). The problem is that Dr. Upwood also has a fiduciary relationship with the patient, Ms. Wilkens. The APhA Code of Ethics refers to this as a "covenant relationship."[2] The pharmacist is historically committed to working on behalf of the benefit of the patient. In this case, working for Ms. Wilkens's benefit seems to require not only getting the prescription corrected, but also dealing with the fact that it is increasingly clear that her physician is deficient and out-of-date. It seems clear that conveying to her that another physician might serve her better would be in Ms. Wilkins's interest.

Thus, Dr. Upwood seems to have made two promises that cannot both be kept at the same time. She has promised Dr. Dorfer to keep his incompetence between them and has promised Ms. Wilkens that she will work for her benefit. By the time two conflicting promises are made, there is probably no completely clean way out. The problem is made more complex because Dr. Upwood made an explicit promise to Dr. Dorfer to keep the matter between the two of them. Dr. Upwood no doubt made this commitment out of a respect for the relationship with the physician (as well as perhaps having a financial interest in staying on Dr. Dorfer's good side). Even if there is no general duty to refrain from criticizing a professional colleague to outsiders, an explicit duty of promise-keeping is created when Dr. Upwood agrees not to tell.

One strategy might be to claim that no real promise was made to Ms. Wilkens; at best the promise was implicit. Dr. Upwood never said in so many words that she would do whatever would help the patient. Whether such a promise was made is a complicated issue. Dr. Upwood undoubtedly never made an explicit promise to her patient. She might, however, have posted the APhA code, including its provision that a pharmacist "promotes the good of every patient." Even if she had not done so one could argue that, by accepting a license to practice pharmacy, there is an implied commitment to work for the good of the patient.

One might at this point try to claim that implicit promises must be subordinated to explicit ones. It is possible that such a claim might work in some legalistic framework, but this is unlikely to resolve Dr. Upwood's problem satisfactorily. In the end, Dr. Upwood has no easy solution once she has made the commitment that contradicts her fundamental obligation to work for the welfare and rights of the patient. Some would attempt to resolve the issue by examining the relative harms of breaking each promise. Breaking the promise to Dr. Dorfer will, no doubt, damage the relationship between the pharmacist and the physician, but failing to keep the promise to the patient could have terrible consequences not only for Ms. Wilkens, but possibly for other patients as well. One might also attempt to resolve the conflict by asking which promise was made first, claiming that the later promise was invalid insofar as it conflicted with the earlier one. There may be times when the principle of promise-keeping has to be violated. Times when two conflicting promises are made is just one of those situations.

Promise-keeping is not the only moral implication of the principle of fidelity. Dr. Upwood has fiduciary relations with others as well. These might include present and future patients and the profession of pharmacy as a whole. Do any of these relationships generate obligations on Dr. Upwood's part to take action to address what appears to be a colleague's impairment? If so, does this justify breaking the promise made to her?

The Limits on the Promise of Confidentiality

One of the most traditional elements of an ethic for health professionals is confidentiality. Almost all people, health professionals and laypeople, have heard of the notion of confidentiality and believe there is a general duty to keep from disclosing information about the patient to others. There are cases in health care, however, in which we have second thoughts about following the notion of confidentiality. The codes of ethics are actually remarkably different on the question of when, if ever, confidences may be broken. Some, such as the Declaration of Geneva of the World Medical Association, usually believed to be a modern version of the Hippocratic Oath, contains an exceptionless rule regarding confidentiality. It states simply, "I will respect the secrets which are confided in me, even after the patient has died."[3]

Others would permit exceptions under certain circumstances. While the Declaration of Geneva would permit no exceptions, the original Hippocratic Oath seems to envision them on occasion. It says, "What I may see or hear in the course of the treatment or even outside of the treatment in regard to the life of men, which on no account one must spread abroad, I will keep to myself holding such things shameful to be spoken about."[4] While this commits the Hippocratic health professional to certain confidences, it also implies that some things should be "spoken abroad." Typical modern interpretations determine what should be disclosed by applying the core Hippocratic principle that the clinician should always work for the patient according to his or her ability and judgment, thus permitting breaking of confidences whenever the clinician believes the patient would benefit. This can be called the paternalistic exception because it provides an exception for the good of the patient. That, for example, was the position of the code of the American Pharmaceutical Association (APhA, now called the American Pharmacists Association) prior to 1995. That code states that a pharmacist "should respect the confidential and personal nature of professional records; except where the best interest of the patient requires or the law demands, a pharmacist should not disclose such information to anyone without proper patient authorization."[5] Other codes in related health professions used to contain similar paternalistic exceptions, but many of them have now been changed.

When the APhA approved its revised code in June 1995, it appears to have dropped the patient-benefit exception clause. Now its view is that a pharmacist "promotes the good of every patient in a caring, compassionate, and confidential manner."[6] There may be, however, some doubt about whether this is really an abandonment of the traditional paternalism because this sentence is in a paragraph that begins with a commitment to promote "the good of every patient."

Other codes contain another kind of exception (or add to the paternalistic one). They would permit confidences to be broken when doing so would benefit third parties. (We could call this the other-benefiting exception.) That is a possible interpretation of the earlier APhA Code when it authorized breaking confidences when the law demands. The courts in some jurisdictions have required a health professional to break confidence when a patient offers what is believed to be a credible threat to seriously harm another person.[7] The current version of the APhA Code as revised in 1995 differs from the codes of its affiliated professions in not explicitly recognizing an exception to the duty of confidentiality when there is a serious threat to the interests of others. It does, however, state in more general terms that "the obligations of a pharmacist may at times extend beyond the individual to the community and society."[8]

This later exception is not paternalistic; it focuses on benefits to others, not to the patient. The exception when the law requires disclosure is perhaps indirectly based on utilitarian reasoning, that is, on the idea that the law will specify exceptions only when it seems clear that great good to other parties would be done, as, for instance, when there is a serious threat of grave bodily harm. The compulsory reporting of sexually transmitted diseases, gunshot wounds, and perhaps HIV+ diagnoses might be considered to fall under this exception. The two following sections present cases calling for possible exceptions to the confidentiality rule, first, for paternalistic reasons and, second, on grounds of benefit to others.

Breaking Confidence to Benefit the Patient

Sometimes a pharmacist comes to believe that the patient very much needs to have someone else know some important but perhaps embarrassing or controversial fact. If the patient agrees to the disclosure there is no problem, but what happens if that patient refuses to agree?

CASE 8-2   The Adolescent on the Pill: Maintaining Confidentiality When the Patient May Be Harmed

---

Merilee Domolakes, Pharm.D., was certain she had not met the young woman standing nervously at the prescription counter before her, yet she recognized the last name when the technician repeated it. The girl was in the process of paying the pharmacy technician for the prescription when Dr. Domolakes asked the girl, "Are you related to George and Anita Fellowes?" The girl was startled by the question but was able to reply, "Yes. They're my mom and dad." At this the girl quickly left the pharmacy, prescription in hand. Dr. Domolakes began to wonder why the girl was presenting her own prescription. Dr. Domolakes knew the Fellowes, especially George Fellowes, but not their children. However, she seemed to remember that they had three sons who were in college and a daughter still in high school. Dr. Domolakes guessed the girl to be 16 or 17 years old.

Since a colleague had filled the prescription, Dr. Domolakes looked at the package insert to see what the prescription was. She was surprised to discover that it was for birth control pills. Dr. Domolakes became concerned. Not only was she concerned that the Fellowes might be unaware that their daughter was taking birth control pills, she also was worried about the pharmacological side effects of the pills. A mother of adolescent daughters herself, Dr. Domolakes was worried about Ms. Fellowes's "moral health."

CASE 8-2   *Continued.*

Two days later, Dr. Domolakes saw George Fellowes in the pharmacy. She asked him about his family in general and then specifically if his daughter had plans for marriage. "Marriage?" Mr. Fellowes snorted, "We'd like her to finish high school first. Why, she's only 16. Why would you ask a question like that?" Dr. Domolakes replied, "I asked because your daughter had a prescription filled for birth control pills this week. I thought you should know." Later in the day, Shashi Banakar, R.N., a family nurse practitioner, called Dr. Domolakes and chastised her on the phone. Ms. Banakar, who had prescribed the oral contraceptives for Ms. Fellowes, exploded, "Whatever happened to confidentiality?" Dr. Domolakes defended herself by stating that she knew confidentiality was important to a point. "I was convinced," Dr. Domolakes stated, "that her physical and moral health required me to disclose the information to her father. The health and welfare of my patients is my only consideration."

Commentary

The pharmacist in this case, Dr. Domolakes, had confronted the ethics and legality of confidentiality in a most dramatic form. She understood the general idea that information about a patient, particularly about a practice as intimate as using oral contraceptives, should not be disclosed to third parties, even the patient's parents. But in this case she had real worries about the welfare of her patient. She believed that the patient's welfare was in jeopardy and that only by disclosing to her father could the risk be confronted and perhaps avoided.

One might be tempted to resolve this conflict by asking what the law requires. That is difficult question to answer. Federal HIPAA (Health Insurance Portability and Accountability Act)[9] law provides some protection of confidentiality, including confidentiality of medical information pertaining to adolescents.[10] However, not all medical care is governed by HIPAA. (In fact, this case occurred outside of HIPAA jurisdiction.) More critically, the focus of our concern here is what the ethical action is; not only what is legal. If it turned out that Dr. Domolakes's behavior was ethically required but illegal in the jurisdiction in which she practiced, the implication would seem to be that the law should be changed. Hence, the basic issue is whether it was ethical for her to disclose in order to protect her patient.

We might doubt that Dr. Domolakes figured the consequences correctly. She seems to have given considerable attention to what she called the patient's "moral health." Social, psychological, and moral well-being are broad, complex issues. Dr. Domolakes hardly knew Ms. Fellowes. She may have misjudged the social consequences of Ms. Fellowes's use of birth control pills. Failure to use it could lead to an unintended pregnancy, disruption of her education, and so forth. Others who decided that overall the consequences were, on balance, better for her than if she did not use the pills would not face the conflict between patient welfare and confidentiality.

Others might criticize Dr. Domolakes on the grounds that she should stick to worrying about the patient's medical interests. Even considering the pharmacological effects of the pill, the medical risks to Ms. Fellowes seem minimal, and if one balances them against the medical risks of pregnancy, others may not share Dr. Domolakes's judgment.

Should a pharmacist trying to promote the welfare of the patient consider only the medical welfare, or should total patient welfare be the goal? Some codes, such as the Declaration of Geneva, call for the health professional to promote the *health* of the patient. Does that mean *medical* well-being in the narrow sense, or should the focus of the pharmacist be broader? While some would press for excluding moral and psychological considerations, others insist that enlightened health care takes into account broader considerations. The World Health Organization, for example, defines health as total physical, psychological, and social well-being.

As we saw in the introduction, The Code of the American Pharmaceutical Association in existence in 1979 said that a pharmacist "should respect the confidential and personal nature of professional records; *except where the best interest of the patient requires or the law demands,* a pharmacist should not disclose such information to anyone without proper patient authorization" (emphasis added).[11] If that is Dr. Domolakes's duty, then she should consider the patient's interest.

It is a further question whether she would be obligated to do what *she thought* was in her patient's interest or what was *actually* in her interest. In the traditional ethics of American pharmacy, the clinician's own judgment about what will promote the patient's welfare should be the controlling factor. That is essentially the same moral stance taken by the author of the Hippocratic Oath, which says that the health professional should benefit the patient, according to his or her "ability and judgment." Taken literally, this would require Dr. Domolakes to disclose the information to Ms. Fellowes's father provided she really believed, according to her ability and judgment, that doing so would be best for her patient.

While some might disagree by arguing for a different assessment of the consequences or by insisting that only certain consequences, the "medical" ones, count, there are other reasons why Dr. Domolakes might be expected to maintain confidentiality. Some hold that confidentiality is a duty in the patient-professional relationship even if, hypothetically, the patient's interests could be promoted by disclosing. Thus, even though the Declaration of Geneva states that the health of the patient is the first consideration, it also says that there is a duty to keep confidences. In contrast to the Hippocratic Oath, no exception is made in the Declaration of Geneva for cases when the patient's interests would be promoted by breaking confidence. The duty is apparently exceptionless. This, as we saw in the introduction to this chapter, is apparently also the stance of the APhA in its revision of its code of 1995. Just as in some ethical systems it is simply one's duty to tell the truth, so it may be that it is simply the duty of the pharmacist to keep information about the patient confidential.

One reason sometimes given for this duty is that there is an implied promise by a health professional that information learned about the patient will not be disclosed. If one believes that a principle of fidelity is part of ethics and that that principle makes it one's duty to keep promises regardless of the consequences, then to the extent that such a promise has been made, either explicitly or implicitly, there is a moral reason to keep it. Dr. Domolakes is faced with the question of whether the decision to disclose should be based on her judgment about benefits and harms to the patient or on the basis of a promise of confidentiality.

While many confidentiality cases involve conflicts between judgments of patient welfare and promises of nondisclosure, in other cases, such as the ones to which we now turn, the welfare of others is what leads pharmacists to consider breaking confidence.

Breaking Confidence to Benefit Others

While breaking confidence paternalistically in order to benefit the patient is one of the traditional justifications for disclosure, serving the welfare of other parties is also put forward as a reason why a pharmacist might reveal information about a patient. According to a rigid application of the traditional Hippocratic ethic, all actions of the pharmacist should be solely for the welfare of the patient. Of course, this means that any action for the purpose of serving other individuals or the society as a whole would be unethical. This would not only make public health interventions, research medicine, and cost containment unethical, it would also make it unethical to disclose confidential information for the benefit of another. In the array of codes of ethics in the health professions we have quite a variation of statements concerning the matter of breaking confidence in order to benefit others.

The following case poses the question of whether the promise made by the pharmacist should be to keep medical information confidential no matter what or whether an exception should be made when there are risks to others that can be prevented only by breaking a confidence.

CASE 8-3   The Policeman with Bipolar Disorder: When Others May Be
            Harmed

When Monica Landeo, Pharm.D., greeted the next patient waiting at the counseling desk in the community pharmacy where she worked, the first thing she noticed was that he was a police officer. The patient, Sam Giantello, quietly introduced himself and asked for his prescriptions. Dr. Landeo recalled that the prescriptions were for lithium and valproate. As Ms. Landeo counseled Mr. Giantello about the need to take the medications with meals to avoid gastrointestinal upset, she noted that he seemed disinterested and in a hurry to leave. As soon as she finished, he murmured "thanks" and left.

Dr. Landeo was disturbed that Mr. Giantello was a police officer and taking maintenance drugs for what was obviously a bipolar disorder. She went back to the computer and called up Mr. Giantello's full medication history. She could ascertain that Mr. Giantello had a long history of mental illness by the various types of antidepressants that had been tried over the past 5 years and the lithium and valproate for the past year. Dr. Landeo also noticed that Mr. Giantello paid for his medications out of pocket rather than through the city's drug card program. Dr. Landeo believed she had an obligation to tell the appropriate person in the police department hierarchy about her findings, since she thought there was a strong possibility of treatment resistance. It made Dr. Landeo extremely uneasy to think of Mr. Giantello in high-stress situations armed with a weapon. At a minimum, she felt someone in authority at the police department should be monitoring Mr. Giantello's mental status. She wondered if the interests of others in the society justified disclosing Mr. Giantello's medical history.

Commentary

Dr. Landeo has reason to be concerned. In contrast to the previous case, however, it is not the welfare of the patient that motivates her concern; it is the welfare of other parties that may be at risk if Mr. Giantello's bipolar disorder is not adequately controlled. If pharmacists have made an absolute promise of confidentiality, such as is implied in the Declaration of Geneva and perhaps in the most recent APhA Code as well, then they are prohibited from disclosing not only in cases in which they are motivated by the welfare of the patient, but also in cases in which the concern is the welfare of third parties. Is that promising more than pharmacists can deliver? Can they anticipate that they may someday find themselves in a position in which there are such dramatic and immediate threats to others in the society that confidences must be disclosed?

A straight utilitarian would assess the problem by asking about the total benefits and harms of alternative courses of action. In this case, Dr. Landeo's options seem to come down to disclosing to an employer and keeping silent. A third possibility—asking Mr. Giantello for permission to disclose or to make the disclosure himself—could potentially eliminate any moral conflict for Dr. Landeo, but it seems likely that Mr. Giantello would not authorize the disclosure if he were asked. In that case, Dr. Landeo would be back to the two options of keeping an implied commitment of confidentiality or breaking it in the name of producing the greatest possible good.

One problem with the utilitarian approach is that it seems to make disclosure too easy. It would support disclosure as soon as the total anticipated good exceeded the harm to Mr. Giantello or others. Granted that Mr. Giantello's interests could be severely compromised with the disclosure (and perhaps some of his family's as well), many people would resist the conclusion called for by utilitarianism that Dr. Landeo is not only permitted to disclose, but also morally required to do so as soon as the anticipated benefit of the disclosure to others exceeded the harm.

Another, less directly utilitarian, approach treats this as a problem of conflicting duties. On the one hand, according to this view, there is a duty to benefit others; on the other hand, there is a duty to keep confidences, at least in the normal case. This latter duty to keep confidences might rest on an implied promise made, such as by posting the APhA Code or by the general notion in the health care professions that there is a duty of confidentiality.

Some would claim that when these two duties conflict, the competing claims must be balanced. In this case, only very substantial harms to others could defeat the presumption that there was a duty of confidentiality. This may be the reasoning that has led the American Medical Association to adopt its provision that confidences may be broken only when "a patient threatens to inflict serious bodily harm to another person and there is a reasonable probability that the patient may carry out the threat."[12] Pharmacist codes of ethics do not contain such a provision, but, presumably, they are governed by the same law.

In one famous California court case, a psychologist who had been told by a patient that he planned to murder a former girlfriend was found to have a duty to warn not withstanding the traditional professional ethical duty of confidentiality.[13] It was important in that decision that the psychologist was himself convinced that his patient was going to carry out the threat and that the risk was a substantial one.

It is a matter of judgment whether the risks to society posed by Mr. Giantello are sufficient that disclosure would be required either by law or by various ethical stances. It may be that the main pharmacy codes do not authorize disclosure in cases such as Mr. Giantello's but that the law, nevertheless, would require the disclosure. In such cases, Dr. Landeo would have to decide whether her ethical judgment would follow the APhA, perhaps requiring her as a matter of conscience to break the law, or whether she could ethically conform to what the law requires.

Incompetent, Impaired, and Dishonest Colleagues

The principle of fidelity has thus far been applied to the areas of the making and breaking of promises and, in particular, the keeping of confidences. Those who recognize an independent principle of fidelity believe there is something intrinsically immoral about breaking a promise, including the promise to keep medical information confidential.

There are other implications of the principle of fidelity. One of the most significant regards loyalty to colleagues, especially when it conflicts with loyalty to the profession as a whole or loyalty to the patient. Many of the professional codes require reporting of incompetent or dishonest practices. This seems consistent with serving the welfare of patients as well as showing loyalty to the profession of which one is a member. However, in life we are also expected to be loyal to our friends and colleagues. If a colleague appears to be incompetent, impaired, or dishonest, as in the following cases, the health care worker is often put in a situation of conflict.

CASE 8-4   Careless Parenteral Preparation: Marginally Competent Colleagues

As George Kimiko, Pharm.D., watched his coworker Emelda Hall, Pharm.D., put the finishing touches on a minibag of an antibiotic, the words of his parenteral products instructor in pharmacy school echoed in his head, "Don't make it if you won't take it." Dr. Kimiko was a staff pharmacist in a home-care agency that specialized in parenteral products, including total parenteral nutrition (TPN), antibiotics, and pain medications. Dr. Kimiko took his instructor's words to heart in his work preparing solutions in the sterile environment of the laminar flow unit. Dr. Kimiko was so concerned about contaminating a solution or making a mistake in the numerous calculations required in the preparation of many of the prescriptions, that if he was called away from his work while in the middle of preparing a solution, he would discard what he had been working on and begin anew.

Dr. Hall was not as concerned as Dr. Kimiko about technique. In fact, Dr. Kimiko had seen her make numerous small errors or breaks in aseptic technique that he would not have tolerated. For example, he had seen her replace strands of her hair under the paper "bonnet" staff were required to wear in the sterile preparation room and then return to her work without washing her hands. One day, he was shocked to see her bring a can of soda into the clean room and place it under the hood where she was working! He noticed that she frequently worked on more than one prescription at a time, moving back and forth between them. One time this resulted in the mislabeling of a solution intended for a

CASE 8-4 *Continued.*

home-care patient, Mr. Johnson. Fortunately, the home-care nurse caught the error before leaving for the patient's home. Because Dr. Hall was on her lunch break, the nurse brought the mislabeled bag to Dr. Kimiko. Dr. Kimiko has tried to talk to Dr. Hall about improving her technique, but each time the changes are only short-lived and she returns to marginally competent work. Dr. Kimiko has even talked to the supervisor about his concerns. Not knowing that Dr. Kimiko was the one who went to the supervisor, Dr. Hall confided in him that the supervisor warned her, "One more mess up and you're out of here."

Dr. Kimiko feels a sense of responsibility to all the patients of the home-care agency, thus he simply cannot ignore Dr. Hall's incompetence.

* This phrase is displayed above each laminar flow hood in the parenterals laboratory of Kenneth Keefner, Ph.D., associate professor in the School of Pharmacy and Health Professions at Creighton University, Omaha, Nebraska, and is used here with his permission. The original source is uncertain, but Dr. Keefner recalls one of his instructors in pharmacy school using a similar warning phrase when he was a student.

Commentary

Dr. Kimiko is confronted with a colleague who does not perform up to his standards. Although his standards may be particularly high, the lapses manifested by Dr. Hall are hard to defend. He feels an obligation to serve his patient's best interest as well as a loyalty to a colleague whose interests would be jeopardized if Dr. Kimiko acted aggressively and reported Dr. Hall to a supervisor or took other action to get her to clean up her act.

Were the problems with Dr. Hall's behavior gross and dramatic, Dr. Kimiko might face less difficulty in deciding what to do. While Dr. Hall's practice is decidedly substandard, it is not as overwhelmingly incompetent as it could be. Nevertheless, the duty to serve the patient's *best* interest would seem to call for some action.

One issue here is whether Dr. Hall should be viewed as culpably negligent for her behavior—whether she should understand that her behaviors are inadequate. Is she in a position where she should clearly realize that she is failing to meet the standard of professional conduct? This may well determine whether Dr. Kimiko and others hold Dr. Hall responsible, whether they hold her accountable for her conduct.

Whether she is blameworthy or not, some intervention may be required. Before Dr. Kimiko can decide what that intervention would be, however, he will first need to determine whether he has any duty to Dr. Hall to serve her interests, whether as a colleague he has a duty to protect her reputation and career, or whether his sole duty is to future patients who could be injured by her conduct. What options are available for Dr. Kimiko?

In the case we have just discussed the pharmacist raised problems of competence. Similar problems arise when the pharmacist is impaired by mental problems or substance abuse as in the following case.

CASE 8-5   The Impaired Colleague: The Colleague in an Emotional Crisis

Claudia Renaldo, Pharm.D., has worked with Melinda Jenkins, Pharm.D., for 3 years in the busy critical care area of a large medical center hospital. Dr. Renaldo has noticed that since Dr. Jenkins went through a stormy divorce 3 months ago that she has been behaving very erratically. Dr. Jenkins doesn't work as quickly and efficiently as the rest of the clinical pharmacists. Dr. Renaldo knows for certain that Dr. Jenkins has made several mistakes in dispensing and documentation in the last week alone.

Dr. Renaldo decides to confront Dr. Jenkins with her concerns about her performance. Dr. Jenkins states, "Everyone has a bad week—even you. I'm just so depressed. I'm taking some medication so maybe I'm not functioning one hundred percent. Please give me another chance. Promise me you won't tell anyone, and I promise it won't happen again." Dr. Renaldo agrees to be quiet for the time being.

However, 2 weeks later, Dr. Renaldo notices that Dr. Jenkins is even more forgetful and sometimes sits down on a stool in the corner and falls asleep. Other coworkers have noticed her lack of attention to detail and her strange behavior. Dr. Renaldo's supervisor, Farley Powell, Pharm.D., approaches her and states, "Dr. Jenkins comes to work in a terrible mood. Then she goes to the restroom and comes out all smiles and acting oddly. You're close to her. Do you know what's wrong with her?"

Commentary

Dr. Jenkins is a colleague and friend of Dr. Renaldo. In some sense she is a patient (or potential patient), but the relationship between the two pharmacists is not one of pharmacist and patient, it is that of two professional colleagues. It might be argued that whatever Dr. Renaldo has learned about Dr. Jenkins's medical and psychological status, she has not learned it in a pharmacist-patient relationship.

That clearly does not settle the confidentiality issue, however. One approach would be to ask what obligation normal colleagues in employment would have in such a situation. Is there a duty of confidentiality among employee colleagues, and if so, does it apply in this case?

The problem is made more complex because Dr. Renaldo made an explicit promise not to tell anyone. Even if there is no general promise of confidentiality among colleagues in a work environment, an explicit duty of promise-keeping is created when Dr. Renaldo agrees not to tell.

That promise, however, seems to have been part of a deal struck. Dr. Jenkins says, "Promise me you won't tell anyone, and I promise it won't happen again." This resembled a mutual promising. Is the implication in such a situation that each party is bound only so long as the other keeps her promise? Or is each promise binding, independent of the other?

Promise-keeping is not the only moral implication of the principle of fidelity. Dr. Renaldo has fiduciary relations with others as well. These might include present and future patients and the profession of pharmacy as a whole. Do any of these relations generate obligations on Dr. Renaldo's part to take action to address what appears to be a colleague's impairment?

Many health professional organizations as well as groups from outside the professions believe that members of a profession have an obligation to protect the integrity of the profession as well as the welfare of patients by reporting or otherwise taking actions to deal with colleagues who are dishonest, impaired, or incompetent. The APhA states in its interpretation of its code that the pharmacist must "maintain knowledge and abilities as new medication, devices, and technologies become available and as health information advances,"[14] but it does not address matters of impaired, incompetent, or dishonest colleagues. How does fidelity to a colleague relate to fidelity to the profession and to patients in a case like this one?

In this case, should "impairment" be understood as a mental problem? Whether such impairments should be referred to as a mental illness is a matter of dispute. One of the classical characteristics of illness is that society ought not to view the ill person as responsible for his or her condition. In some illnesses, especially mental illnesses, the impairment is such that the individual cannot even recognize the abnormal behavior involved. Dr. Jenkins seems to have some degree of awareness but perhaps not sufficient that she should be considered responsible for taking actions to remove herself from practicing in an impaired state. This lack of responsibility and lack of awareness may be relevant to Dr. Renaldo's decision about how to handle the case.

The ambiguity about personal responsibility of pharmacists for their impaired or incompetent conduct is removed in the case of some pharmacists who are unambiguously dishonest in their practices. That is the issue in the final case in this chapter.

CASE 8-6   Dishonest Colleagues: Intentionally Shorting Tablet Counts

After Lorine Lance, Pharm.D., counseled Ferris Janowski, an elderly patient, about his 3 cardiac maintenance medications, she was surprised by Mr. Janowski's final question, "Would you please open these prescriptions and count them for me so that I know I'm getting what I paid for? There was a letter in my favorite advice column last night that told about how you can get shorted on your prescriptions, so I just want to make sure all the pills are there. No offense meant, you understand. I just can't afford to pay for pills and not get them."

Mr. Janowski's prescriptions had been filled by the owner of the pharmacy, Glen Battin, R.Ph., who would not be in for several hours. Dr. Lance decided to humor Mr. Janowski and opened the first bottle. To her dismay, the prescription was four tablets short. She made up the difference. The remaining two prescriptions were also short by the same amount—four pills each. Dr. Lance remedied the shortage in these two and returned all three prescriptions to Mr. Janowski. "I guarantee you that these are filled accurately and fully," Dr. Lance told Mr. Janowski as she handed him his medications.

Mr. Janowski was not the only patient with concerns about shortages that day. Evidently, several patients were prompted by the newspaper article to count their pills and found less than there should have been. Dr. Lance took numerous calls from angry patients and tried to determine if the caller might have miscounted, lost a pill, or took more than they should have, all reasons that the prescriptions could appear short. She noted that all of the prescriptions that patients claimed were shorted were for maintenance drugs and that Mr. Battin had filled them.

CASE 8-6 *Continued.*

When Mr. Battin arrived at the pharmacy, an exhausted Dr. Lance told him about what she had discovered and the number of dissatisfied patients that called to complain about shortages. She was certain Mr. Battin would have a reasonable explanation. He stated, "It's really a shame that advice column printed that letter. We'll have to stop short-ing maintenance prescriptions for a while until people get over the excitement and the need to count every prescription."

Dr. Lance could not believe what she was hearing. "You mean that you *have* been shorting prescriptions?" Mr. Battin shrugged, "Just the maintenance prescriptions and only on the higher-end products. People don't miss three or four pills a month and the phar-macy recoups a steady amount. Besides, they always come in for a refill before they run out, so the patients aren't harmed." Dr. Lance had always admired Mr. Battin, but his nonchalant admission of guilt instantly changed her appraisal of her employer. She had never knowingly shorted a prescription. How could she work for someone who did it as a matter of course? Furthermore, what should she do about this dishonest behavior?

Commentary

Glen Battin, the owner of the pharmacy who is routinely shorting patients on their medi-cation, spares us the problem we encountered in the two previous cases of determining whether the practitioner understands and is responsible for what he is doing. He non-chalantly acknowledges to Lorine Lance what he is doing. He seems to think that as long as he limits his practice to maintenance prescriptions and his patients get them refilled before they run out, he is not causing any harm and that his behavior is tolerable.

Of course, patients can be injured financially as well as medically. They are here being cheated out of four tablets for which they are paying. Even if it is an insurer that is bearing the extra costs, someone is paying for something the patient is not getting. Mr. Battin also needs to take into account the fact that his dispensing practice consti-tutes a deception to the patient if not an outright lie. If ethics is a matter of keeping faith with patients as well as making sure that their interests are served, at minimum this practice presents a challenge to fidelity in the pharmacist-patient relationship.

The more subtle ethical issue raised by this case is what the implications of the principle of fidelity are for his employee, Dr. Lance. If she is operating strictly on the Hippocratic principle of protecting the patient's interests (especially if it is an insurer who is paying the bills), she might conclude that her employer's practice is not hurt-ing the patient. No harm, no foul. However, she may understand her responsibilities to be more complex. Even if Mr. Janowski is not paying directly for the medication, he may pay indirectly in the form of extra premiums required to support Mr. Battin's practice (and other similar practices to which the insurer is exposed). Moreover, even if Mr. Janowski is insured through a public Medicare or Medicaid program for which he bears essentially no financial burden, somebody is paying the costs of this practice. If Dr. Lance is a utilitarian concerned about burdens to others as well as to her patient, she will have cause for concern.

Most critically, Dr. Lance may feel that she has an obligation to maintain trust with her patient. The trust of the community in the profession of pharmacy is jeopardized by Mr. Battin's practice. If there are duties of fidelity incumbent upon a pharmacist, Dr. Lance owes it to her profession and to patients in general to challenge the dishonest practice of one member of the profession.

Pharmacists also have some kind of duty of fidelity to colleagues. A collegial relationship commands loyalty that is grounded in the principle of fidelity. Is there any sense in which a colleague's duties of loyalty require remaining silent about dishonest practices, especially those that seem not to jeopardize a patient's welfare in any dramatic and direct way? Is there any case to be made for remaining silent in the face of incompetent, impaired, and dishonest practices, such as those in these last three cases? If not, what action can Dr. Lance take?

Notes

1. Hepler, Charles D., and Linda M. Strand. "Opportunities and Responsibilities in Pharmaceutical Care." *American Journal of Pharmaceutical Education* 53, no. 5 (1989): 7s–15s.

2. American Pharmaceutical Association. "Code of Ethics for Pharmacists." Washington, DC: American Pharmaceutical Association, 1995.

3. World Medical Association. "Declaration of Geneva." *World Medical Journal* 3, supp. (1956): 10–12. Reprinted with revisions in *Encyclopedia of Bioethics*. Revised Edition. Vol. 5. Warren T. Reich, Editor. New York: Simon and Schuster, 1995, pp. 2646–2647.

4. Edelstein, Ludwig. "The Hippocratic Oath: Text, Translation, and Interpretation." *Ancient Medicine: Selected Papers of Ludwig Edelstein*. Owsei Temkin and C. Lilian Temkin, Editors. Baltimore, MD: Johns Hopkins Press, 1967, p. 6.

5. American Pharmaceutical Association. "Code of Ethics." Washington, DC: American Pharmaceutical Association, 1981.

6. American Pharmaceutical Association. "Code of Ethics for Pharmacists." Washington, DC: American Pharmaceutical Association, 1995.

7. *Tarasoff v. Regents of University of California.* 17 C.3d 425, 131 Cal. Rptr. 14, 551 P.2d 334, 1976. In Shannon, Thomas A., and Jo Ann Manfra, Editors. *Law and Bioethics: Texts with Commentary on Major U.S. Court Decisions.* New York: Paulist Press, 1982, pp. 293–319.

8. American Pharmaceutical Association, "Code of Ethics for Pharmacists,"1995.

9. Health Insurance Portability and Accountability Act of 1996. Public Law 104–191. 104th Congress. August 21, 1996.

10. Maradiegue, A. H. "Applying HIPAA to Minors." *Nurse Practitioner* 27, no. 5 (2002): 24.

11. American Pharmaceutical Association, "Code of Ethics," 1981.

12. American Medical Association. Council on Ethical and Judicial Affairs. *Code of Medical Ethics: Current Opinions with Annotations.* Chicago: American Medical Association, 1994, p. 72 (opinion originally issued 1983; revised 1994).

13. *Tarasoff v. Regents of the University of California.* 17 C.3d 425, 131 Cal. Rptr. 14, 551 P.2d 334, 1976. In *Law and Bioethics: Texts with Commentary on Major U.S. Court Decisions.* Thomas A. Shannon and Jo Ann Manfra, Editors. New York: Paulist Press, 1982, pp. 293–319.

14. American Pharmaceutical Association. "Code of Ethics for Pharmacists." Washington, DC: American Pharmaceutical Association, 1995.

9

Avoidance of Killing

The principles examined in the preceding chapters—beneficence, nonmaleficence, justice, autonomy, veracity, and fidelity—cover most of the moral considerations that arise in one-on-one personal moral decisions involving pharmacists. But before turning to some special topical areas in Part III, we should look at one additional moral consideration. Many moral controversies in health care hinge on claims that are variously based on the notion that human life is sacred or that killing a human is morally wrong. In this chapter, we look at cases involving pharmacists who are put in positions in which they need to know exactly what is implied by these notions. With the emergence of the legalization of physician-assisted suicide (often by prescription medication), pharmacists will increasingly be put in a position in which they will be parties to patient suicides. At least in the state of Oregon, patients who meet certain criteria, including mental competence, can now legally get prescriptions filled for the express purpose of killing themselves. In this chapter we explore the ethical implications of pharmacist participation in this emerging practice.

For all of us, killing of another is usually wrong if for no other reason than that normally people want to live. Killing does people harm in the most dramatic way. The principle of nonmaleficence (not harming) counts strongly against killing in most cases. But there are special cases when it is not as obvious that killing would be perceived as a harm by the individual. Some patients are suicidal. While many suicidal persons are so seriously depressed that they are not mentally competent, others may have an accurate grasp of their life-prospects and have decided that their future will, on balance, offer more burdens than benefits. Others are so racked with the pain of a chronic, perhaps terminal, illness that they would plead to be killed or to be aided in dying.

Killing is a complex and ambiguous term. Some people imply that the word always conveys a negative moral judgment—that to say something is a killing is to say it is morally wrong. However, we sometimes speak of *justified killings,* such as in cases of justified war, police actions, self-defense, and perhaps merciful euthanasia. There are many ways in which society, both secular and religious, has condoned the taking of another person's life, some of these against that person's will. The wide prevalence of the death penalty, ethnic cleansing, jihads, and even assassinations makes clear that throughout history humans have believed that killing can be justified.

It seems that not all behavior that is causally related to the shortening of life is classified as killing. For example, as we show in this chapter, most people do not consider refusing life support to be a suicide and, in some cases, withdrawal of another person's life support is not considered a killing, even though such refusals and withdrawals will lead to death. Moreover, even if an action is deemed to be a *killing,* the use of that term does not automatically imply that the action is morally wrong. For example, accidental killings, such as from a lethal idiosyncratic reaction to a prescription, are not always morally wrong.

Even among actions that are directly intended to terminate the life of another, we can distinguish killing for merciful motive from other kinds of killing. We can also distinguish self-killing (suicide) from the killing of another (homicide). We can distinguish killing with the consent of the one killed from those that are involuntary (against the victim's wishes) and those that are nonvoluntary (without the approval or disapproval of the one who is killed). Finally, we can distinguish homicide on request (in which the health provider or other acquaintance of the patient will kill on the patient's request) from assisted suicide (in which the health provider supplies information or materials (such as medication) but patients themselves take the last decisive step in ending their own lives).

Our traditional religious and secular values have dictated that even in cases in which the motive is merciful and the patient requests the action, it is wrong to kill. But why? If the killing relieves severe suffering, especially if it is requested by a competent patient, can it not count as a good and noble thing to help those who are suffering end it?

We have seen that some people hold that in ethics the consequences are the only morally relevant factor. Utilitarians, for example, hold this view. So do those who subscribe to the Hippocratic principle, which requires the health professional to always act only so as to benefit the patient. Although many health providers do not realize it, the Hippocratic principle by itself could permit or even require the health provider to cooperate in killing a patient when it would, on balance, do more good than harm.

However, the Hippocratic Oath also contains a specific provision that is usually interpreted as prohibiting active killing. Technically it proscribes "giving a deadly drug, even if asked." But usually in modern readings that is taken to prohibit generally any physician participation in killing. Insofar as the oath can be extended to all health professionals, it would prohibit pharmacists from participating as well. Since most pharmacists are not normally in positions where they would seriously contemplate mercifully killing patients on their own, the codes of pharmacists generally do not mention a prohibition on killing, but one can assume that such actions would be opposed by the traditional pharmacist organizations. In fact, as we see in the cases in this chapter, pharmacists do actually encounter situations where they are asked to participate in forgoing treatment and some are now actually placed in positions where they could consider whether to cooperate in an assisted suicide.

The interesting problem is why such a prohibition on killing exists if the goal of the provider is always to benefit the patient. One possibility, of course, would be that the authors of the oath considered it always a net harm to the patient to end the patient's life. Many people, however, are willing to concede that, at least in rare cases, the patient may be worse off if he or she continues to live. Normally, that would involve cases of intractable, severe suffering. If some patients occasionally would actually be "better off dead," then there are two other possible justifications for proscribing merciful killings.

First, as we have seen in previous chapters, some people who base moral judgments on consequences do not believe it is right to directly calculate the consequences in each individual case. Instead they consider possible alternative moral rules or policies. They assess the net consequences of the alternative rules or policies and choose the rule or policy that they believe will do more good than any alternative. These people are called *rule-utilitarians*.[1]

They may do this for a number of reasons. First, some are worried about the risk of error if individuals were permitted to make the calculations on the spot for each case. Especially in highly emotionally charged situations where rapid decisions have to be made and especially when those doing the calculating may not know the individuals affected very well, the danger of miscalculation may be great. These critics of merciful killing believe that in the long run more good may be done (and more harm prevented) if we simply apply the rule against killing because on balance it will produce more good than any alternative.

Second, some people, not necessarily persuaded that the risk of error is this great, may still hold that it is just the nature of morality that practices are established by evaluating alternative rules or policies and choosing the set that produces the greatest net good.[2] They may favor a rule against merciful killing because they consider it the utility-maximizing rule, that is, they may believe that the rule prohibiting such killing produces more good outcomes than any other rule they can imagine. For either of these reasons, some consequentialists, those who are rule-consequentialists, may favor a rule that prohibits health professionals from participating in killing.

There is a second reason why the Hippocratic Oath may prohibit active killings for mercy. As we have seen in previous chapters, there may be moral principles other than beneficence and nonmaleficence that determine whether an act is right or wrong. We have already seen that some people hold that autonomy, veracity, and fidelity to promises help determine the rightness of actions regardless of the consequences. Is it possible that killing is just inherently wrong—even if the one who is killed is better off than if he or she had lived? If so, avoidance of killing could be an independent principle that helps shape the rightness and wrongness of human conduct. We might refer to it simply as the *principle of avoidance of killing*. It is not clear whether the writer of the Hippocratic Oath believed this. If so, he was not a pure consequentialist.

Whether the Hippocratic author believed that killing people was inherently wrong, clearly other moral traditions are committed to this view. Judaism considers life to be sacred, a gift from God. Killing a human, at least an innocent human, is always wrong. In fact, Judaism has even gone beyond the view that killing, at least killing of the innocent, is wrong to the view that all human life is sacred. According to this perspective, it is always wrong for humans to make decisions, such as deciding to withdraw life support, which will predictably shorten a patient's life.

Catholicism considers killing an intrinsic wrong, but, as we shall see, this tradition does not extend its condemnation to all actions that will shorten life. It accepts certain forgoing of life support. Other moral traditions, both religious and secular, condemn killing as well.[3] They at least view it as prima facie wrong, that is, wrong insofar as the action involves killing (although that wrongness might, on occasion, be offset by other moral considerations). If killing is always a wrong-making characteristic of an action, then avoidance of killing can be thought of as another moral principle that must hold beneficence and nonmaleficence in check.[4] The cases in this chapter help clarify how pharmacists should evaluate possible attempts to relieve patients of their misery by putting them to death. In later sections of the chapter, participation in active merciful killing will be compared and contrasted with decisions to forgo treatment (to withhold or withdraw treatment).

Active Killing Versus Letting One Die

Both religious and secular traditions in the West have held that it is always morally wrong to actively kill a human being, even if the killing is done for a merciful motive. For example, some terminally ill patients appear to be in pain. They may be inevitably dying rapidly and could be spared the misery of the dying if someone actively intervened with an injection of a drug to hasten death. Some argue that such intervention would be the humane and moral thing to do, but others claim that there is something intrinsically wrong with killing—that life is sacred and to be preserved or that at least it should not be ended directly by human hand. The following case, fictionalized, but based on real events in several states, raises the question of whether there is any significant moral difference between actively killing someone who is dying and simply stepping aside and letting nature take its course.

CASE 9-1 Prescriptions for Suicide: Forming a Policy for Pharmacy

Eun Peet, Pharm.D., had breathed a sigh of relief when the state's newly passed ballot measure allowing citizens the option of assisted suicide (in the form of a prescription for a lethal dose of a drug) was not allowed to go into effect because of legal challenges. Dr. Peet was the current chair of a liaison committee representing all pharmacy organizations in the state. She had the unenviable task of sitting through endless debates on the bill trying to reach consensus. The APhA Code of Ethics for Pharmacists wasn't a great deal of help in this area. There was no statement in the code prohibiting active killing or assisted suicide. There was also no statement or position paper in pharmacy publicly stating the

CASE 9-1   *Continued.*

profession's position as there was in the American Nurses Association and the American Medical Association. The American Society of Health-System Pharmacists Statement on pharmacist's decision-making and assisted suicide allowed each pharmacist to make his or her own decision about whether or not to participate in assisted suicide.[5]

Now that the ballot measure was in legal limbo, Dr. Peet hoped that the liaison group could explore just what the pharmacist's role in assisted suicide might be should the law go into effect. There were certainly practical and procedural concerns regarding the law even by those who supported it. The means of assisting in the suicide outlined in the law was a prescription for a lethal dose of medication or combination of medications. Although pharmacists are capable of recommending proper therapeutic doses of medications, would they be able to determine what dosage would be lethal for a particular patient? Would they be expected to counsel patients on how to properly take their medications so that death, not permanent injury, was the outcome? These practical questions were almost eclipsed by the comments of opponents of the law concerning the inherent wrongness of being involved in any way with active killing or assisting in suicide. Members of the liaison committee who opposed active killing and assisted suicide were not appeased by the conscience clause in the law that allowed pharmacists the right to refuse to participate. The opponents of the law wanted the liaison committee to issue a clear statement that the collective voice of pharmacy, at least in this state, opposed the law.

The reprieve that Dr. Peet thought she would have to wrestle with these divergent views turned out to be short-lived when she opened the morning paper and read that the state supreme court would not block the law. The legal barriers that delayed the implementation of the law appeared to be gone. Dr. Peet knew that her phone would start to ring any moment with questions about the pharmacy profession's position either for or against the law.

CASE 9-2   Deciding Whether to Fill a Lethal Prescription

Although the so-called death with dignity law legalizing assisted suicide had been in place for a year, this was the first time that Moe Jamison, Pharm.D., had actually received a lethal prescription from a terminally ill patient. Dr. Jamison actually knew the prescription was coming since the patient's physician had called earlier in the day to talk with Dr. Jamison about his recommendations for the most effective combination of drugs to result in certain death. Dr. Jamison believed that a person had the right to choose his or her own manner of death and that there should be laws to legalize medication for assisted suicide. He also believed that pharmacists should have a role in advising the prescriber on the choice and dose of drugs used. Furthermore, he thought it was essential that pharmacists be informed about the intended purpose of prescriptions for assisted suicide so that they could decide whether to participate in dispensing or not.

Now that he was holding the prescription in his hand and could see the slender, frail patient waiting on the other side of the counter, Dr. Jamison wasn't certain he could take this last step and dispense the medication for assisted suicide and counsel the patient on its appropriate use.

Commentary

Dr. Peet is facing a problem that many pharmacists may have to face as soon as assisted suicide becomes legalized either by court order or by statute. The writers of these proposals seem to worry about granting physicians the right to conscientiously refuse to participate, but there is real doubt whether pharmacists and other health care team members also have that right. Traditionally, it is a moral, and perhaps a legal, duty for a pharmacist to fill a valid prescription. It is an open question whether a pharmacist may refuse on grounds of conscience. Dr. Peet is being asked to formulate a position on behalf of the pharmacy organizations in her state regarding pharmacist participation in assisted suicide through the act of filling a valid and legal prescription.

The first issue raised is whether this is a matter about which pharmacists can and should speak with one voice. Is there a single view on such controversial matters that should be held by all pharmacists? Is there a practice of pharmacy to which all pharmacists should subscribe that must either include or exclude filling such prescriptions? One possibility here is that pharmacists of Dr. Peet's state will simply agree that there is more than one possible answer to such controversial questions, that either participation or refusal would be acceptable, as in the case in the ASHP statement on assisted suicide. This is another way of saying that there may be more than one acceptable conception of the practice of pharmacy and that the state pharmacy coalition should not enter into taking a position on exactly which conception of the practice is best.

Even so, Dr. Peet and the other pharmacists of the state will have to decide what they can do ethically when presented with such prescriptions. One issue pharmacists must face is both conceptual and moral. Is there a significant difference between active killing for mercy when the killing is done by another on the request of a patient (homicide on request) and assisted suicide, in which the patient kills himself or herself with the help of another?

Some are claiming that a line can be drawn between the two. They may be pointing to the concern that homicide on request sometimes raises the issue of whether the homicide was really requested by the patient and, if so, whether the patient was competent when the request was made. There is concern that such actions would be open to serious abuse, as it would be hard to verify that the request was truly voluntary since the patient will be dead by the time the question arises.

Others, however, say that even in the case of assisted suicide the patient could be forced, pressured, or manipulated into taking the lethal medication. In any case, they claim, even if there are pragmatic differences having to do with degree of certainty that the request from the patient was actually made, there is no difference in principle between homicide on request and assisted suicide. In both, the patient would not die but for an action of someone else. That action is a decisive event in the causal chain leading to the patient's death. They say that if one is wrong, then the other is as well.

One approach to these issues focuses on the consequences. Some would approach the question in traditional Hippocratic fashion by insisting that the pharmacist's moral duty is to benefit the patient. Then the question becomes one of whether it is ever possible to benefit someone by killing them or by helping them kill themselves.

Defenders of active killing, including physician-assisted suicide, claim that killing does no harm in such cases and may actually prevent future harm (that is, patient suffering). They argue that, if the active intervention shortens the period of suffering, it may actually be morally preferred over simply stepping back and letting the patient die.

Critics of such practices also raise arguments based on consequences. They claim that the consequences of a policy authorizing active killing may be different from those of a policy that accepts the forgoing of life-sustaining treatment. Some of these critics are what in the introduction we called *rule-utilitarians*. They believe that morality is based on certain practices or rules, and they assess the consequences of general rules rather than those related to specific choices in individual cases. They believe that even if Dr. Peet or a colleague can correctly determine the consequences in a particular case, the risk of abuse of a policy endorsing active killing is too great. They worry that eventually those who are unwanted, unloved, or unattached to others will be done away with through misguided or uncaring decisions to kill in a purportedly merciful way or, in the case of assisted suicide, that these patients will be unduly pressured into requesting assistance. This concern about the consequences of accepting assistance in suicide leads them to prefer a rule against it, claiming it will have better consequences even if in some individual cases the results are not as good.

In contrast to rule-utilitarians, *deontologists* believe there is more to morality than simply calculating consequences. They believe that certain characteristics of actions, such as lying or breaking promises, make actions wrong even if they would produce better consequences than alternative actions. Some people approach the question of mercy killing and assisted suicide from this perspective. They believe that calculating the consequences of killing for mercy or assisting in a suicide will not necessarily settle the matter. There are those who believe that killing another human is simply wrong, regardless of whether it relieves suffering. This principle is sometimes expressed, especially by the religious, as the *principle of the sacredness of life*.

Holders of this view, however, must confront the issue of whether it is equally wrong to assist in a suicide and even to forgo life-sustaining treatment. Some people, for instance some Jews, hold that life is sacred in its every moment so that forgoing life-sustaining treatment is just as wrong as actively killing. They would see active killing of another, assisting in suicide, and forgoing life-support all as moral violations.

Others, including many Roman Catholics, affirm that forgoing life-sustaining treatment is morally acceptable if the intention is not to kill the patient, but only to put an end to treatment that is no longer fits the patient's condition. Holders of this view sometimes say that the withdrawal of treatment does not kill the patient, that the underlying disease does (if they are honest, though, they admit that the patient would have died differently and not as quickly had the life-sustaining intervention been continued). They usually find both assisting one to commit suicide and actually killing someone else for the sake of mercy as unacceptable. Both acts are intentional killings in a way that merely forgoing life-support need not be.

The list of right-making characteristics of those who see active killing as intrinsically wrong could thus be said to contain an additional principle, along with veracity, autonomy, and fidelity: the *avoidance of killing*. This principle could comprise a prohibition on both active killing and forgoing treatment or, as is common in U.S. law and much ethical thinking, extend only to prohibiting active killing. It could include suicide and assisting in suicide as well. If Dr. Peet held such a view, she would conclude that it is unacceptable for pharmacists to participate in such actions and would oppose the filling of prescriptions designed to be used for killing, even self-killing.

Even if Dr. Peet's committee concluded that pharmacist participation in assisted suicide was acceptable, individual pharmacists, such as Dr. Jamison, will have to decide for themselves whether they can participate or should exercise a right of conscientious objection based on personally held beliefs and values. It is hard to conceive how pharmacists could be forced to participate against their conscientiously held views, especially if physicians are given a right to refuse to participate.

Recent discussions of these issues have introduced an additional complication. Some have pointed out that if there is a significant difference, legally or ethically, between actively intervening to kill and simply letting someone die, there is a strategy that would guarantee a quick and painless death while still not technically involving active killing. This approach is sometimes referred to as *terminal sedation*.[6] It is defined as administering drugs to keep patients in deep sedation or coma until death. Recently it has been suggested that terminal sedation, combined with the withdrawal of nutrition and hydration, a ventilator, or a life-prolonging antibiotic, would accomplish everything desired by those advocating active killing for mercy or assisted suicide while still not crossing the line to active killing.[7] This controversial proposal raises serious questions about whether withdrawal of nutrition and hydration or these other life-prolonging interventions really should be considered active killing. The following case deals with the complicated issues surrounding terminal sedation.

CASE 9-3   The ALS Patient: Does Voluntary Choice Justify Terminal Sedation?

The first symptoms of the disease had been so innocuous. Kirk Cornelius could remember the day he noticed difficulty swallowing and a certain awkwardness in using his fingers. The diagnosis of amyotrophic lateral sclerosis (ALS) had been devastating. He was 35 years old at the time, and the disease had steadily progressed until now, 4 years later, he was not only ventilator dependent, but also had to use a computer-assistance device to communicate with his caregivers. He had a gastrostomy tube for nutrition and hydration since he was no longer able to swallow safely. Lately Mr. Cornelius has become increasingly frustrated, depressed, and angry about his failing health. He is less willing to cooperate with caregivers and talks more and more of his impending death. His wife continues to be a strong source of support and is often present during the morning rounds of the attending physician and the rest of the health care team.

On this particular day, Winifred Roskens, Pharm.D., was participating in the rounds of the critical care team. Dr. Roskens knew Mr. and Mrs. Cornelius well, as she served as the clinical pharmacist for the medical critical care unit. Mrs. Cornelius greeted the team by asking them to listen to what her husband had to say to them. "Kirk has come to a difficult decision, and I want you all to know that I support him," Mrs. Cornelius said.

Mr. Cornelius painstakingly produced the following message on his computer, "I have lived with this disease long enough. I would like you to withdraw the ventilator, but I am

CASE 9-3 *Continued.*

terrified of not being able to breathe. I would like you to give me something to put me to sleep permanently before you disconnect the ventilator."

Mrs. Cornelius added, "I don't want him to suffer, and he would certainly suffer if you turned off the ventilator and he felt like he couldn't get any air."

Dr. Roskens had heard of the use of barbiturates and opioids to ease the withdrawal of ventilators from dependent patients, but she felt that the use of a lethal dose would be different. Dr. Roskens said as much to Mr. Cornelius and the rest of the treatment team. "I think that the use of sedatives, such as the benzodiazepines and such analgesics as morphine sulfate, can decrease air hunger and anxiety so that you will be comfortable. I can recommend the proper dosage and titration so that we make you comfortable but avoid hastening death."

Mr. Cornelius returned his attention to the computer and responded, "Why wait? I know that I can ask to have the ventilator removed. If I can request that, why can't I request a single, massive dose to end things? The outcome is the same."

Commentary

The use of terminal sedation has become more common in recent years. It relies on the distinction between active killing and forgoing life-support that is central to current legal and moral traditions. Dr. Roskens accepts the position that it would be wrong to give Mr. Cornelius a lethal dose of barbiturates but recognizes that withdrawal of the ventilator is acceptable legally and that many people believe it is also morally acceptable. As we shall see in later cases in this chapter, many people also believe that it is acceptable to give patients medications that will keep them comfortable during the withdrawal of life support. This could involve the administration of analgesics or the use of sedatives. When sedatives are given at the end of life when life-support is being withheld, the term *terminal sedation* is sometimes used.

The moral issue for Dr. Roskens is whether the combination of withholding life-support and terminal sedation to render the patient unconscious doesn't amount to the same thing as active killing. The consequences are surely about the same. Terminal sedation begins to appear like an ambiguous case on the border between active killing and forgoing life-support. Is terminal sedation simply active killing dressed in clothing to make it appear legal and ethical?

Withholding Versus Withdrawing Treatment

While the distinction between killing and simply omitting life-sustaining treatment in order to let the patient die has a long history and is well understood by most clinicians, there is an intermediate case that generates confusion. If a therapy has begun, withdrawing it could seem to be morally similar to not having provided it in the first place, and yet to many health care providers, it may feel, psychologically, much closer to actively doing something to cause the patient's death. The following case asks how we should assess the withdrawal of a treatment that was begun in an effort to be beneficial but is now being removed because it is believed not to offer benefits exceeding the burdens.

CASE 9-4   Withdrawing an Antibiotic: Is It Active Killing?

As Rosaria Obowa, Pharm.D., stood beside Shawna Blash's bed, she noticed the label on the intravenous antibiotic "cefepime hydrochloride" that was being steadily administered by an infusion pump. Dr. Obowa noted the date on the IV label and counted backwards, calculating that this was the third day the antibiotic had been given. Ms. Blash was resting, though resting was not exactly the appropriate term, as she had to use all of her accessory muscles to breathe. Ms. Blash was 18 years old and thus in this jurisdiction a legal adult. She had been diagnosed with cystic fibrosis as a child and because of aggressive therapy, excellent care, and a determination to live, had survived well beyond initial expectations. As is common for children with chronic diseases, Ms. Blash was an expert on her symptomatology and treatments. Until she was old enough to legally decide for herself, Ms. Blash's parents had been the decision-makers regarding her medical care, although since she was old enough to express herself they had always sought her input.

Dr. Obowa only wanted to check on Ms. Blash's status without disturbing her sleep, but Ms. Blash woke up just as Dr. Obowa turned to leave the room. "I'm glad you're here," Ms. Blash said softly. "Drugs are your area, so I wanted you to be the first to know about my decision. I realize that I said I'd try another course of antibiotics, but I've changed my mind. I want it stopped."

Dr. Obowa questioned Ms. Blash's understanding of the course of antibiotic therapy and cautioned her that perhaps she needed to wait a while longer in order for the therapy to reach maximal effectiveness. Ms. Blash responded, "I'm not stopping the antibiotic because it hasn't worked yet; I just have had enough. I know more about my disease than anyone. I understand the consequences of my decision." With that, Ms. Blash shut her eyes, exhausted from the effort to speak.

Dr. Obowa took the news of Ms. Blash's decision to discontinue the antibiotic to the treatment team conference at their meeting later that day. The nurse on the treatment team responded, "I think we have an obligation to continue with this course of therapy since we started it in the first place. It seems to me that by taking away a treatment that might prove to be life-saving that we are somehow shortening her life. I don't want to be a part of that." The rest of the treatment team was divided on the decision, but the attending physician was willing to support Ms. Blash's choice. Dr. Obowa agreed with the nurse. Dr. Obowa had been the one on the team to suggest this particular course of treatment, and now she was being asked to agree to stop it before it had had a chance to work. If they hadn't started the antibiotic in the first place, Dr. Obowa reasoned, that would be an entirely different story. Stopping potentially beneficial treatment seemed more like active killing to Dr. Obowa, and she was certain she did not want to participate in such an action.

Commentary

The agony of realizing that removing the antibiotic will be the immediate cause of the death of her patient might well be traumatic for Dr. Obowa. The psychological impact is in some way linked to the moral issues, but in some sense it must be kept separate.

The first issue is whether removing an antibiotic at the request of the competent adult patient is morally any different from not starting it in the first place. The question is whether it is an instance of active killing or an instance of forgoing treatment, which is legal and widely considered to be ethical. At least until state laws are changed, active killing is illegal in the United States and most other jurisdictions. The only exceptions are the Netherlands and Belgium. It is also widely considered to be unethical,

The law makes a clear distinction between withdrawing life-sustaining treatment and active killing, treating killing as illegal while treating the withdrawal of treatment at the competent patient's request as not only legal, but required. One approach to the problem is to view the decisions from the perspective of what is required by the doctrine of informed consent. Patients cannot be treated without consent, as we saw in the cases of Chapter 6. The autonomous patient has a right to agree to or refuse any medical intervention. Presumably Ms. Blash did this when the antibiotic was initiated. When she did, it presumably made sense, because she believed it would offer a significant chance of benefit. Otherwise, it is hard to see why she would have agreed to it.

But no rational consent would be open-ended; no rational person would agree to the use of a drug forever and ever until death just because it seemed to make sense for a time. In fact, many clinicians are recognizing that time-limited trials of possibly beneficial therapies often are more reasonable than some open-ended commitment that might lead caregivers to mistakenly believe that the patient's permission goes on indefinitely. In the use of an antibiotic, therefore, it is often wise to specify for how long the treatment will be tried. If no time limit is specified, the only reasonable conclusion is that if the patient has the authority to give permission to try a treatment, she also has the right to withdraw the permission and stop the treatment. Once the consent is withdrawn what else can the provider do but take the treatment away?

In addition to the moral basis for removing such treatments, a pragmatic argument has been given for this approach. If the rule were that once an authorization for treatment was given it could not be withdrawn, a strong incentive would exist to not try an intervention unless one was very sure it would work. It seems irrational to avoid trying possibly effective life-prolonging interventions unless they were sure to succeed. The alternative is to permit patients or their surrogates to withdraw permission once the trial treatment is found wanting.

While the consent doctrine can force a provider to stop a treatment in just the same way it can force the provider not to begin, it can never force the provider to actively intervene to kill the patient. From the point of view of the consent doctrine, withdrawing treatment is much more like withholding it than it is like active killing.

Direct Versus Indirect Killing

The distinction between active killing and forgoing treatment is sometimes confused with another distinction that has become important in deciding whether it is morally wrong to kill another human being. Roman Catholic moral theology has long distinguished between directly intended evil and evil that is not intended. Theologians within this tradition (and many people in the secular world as well) have held that there are certain evils that are intrinsically wrong (such as killing an innocent person) and that it is always wrong directly to intend such evils. They have long recognized, however, that sometimes what they consider to be evil may occur even though it is not intended. Sometimes the one causing the evil may have no reasonable way of knowing that the evil would result, as when a health professional produces a fatal anaphylactic reaction by giving penicillin to a patient who is not suspected to be allergic. Surely, there is a sense in which the one who gave the unexpectedly dangerous drug killed the patient, and yet, just as certainly, the death was not intended. The health provider would have done anything to avoid the death, if only he had known. These "killings" are active killings, yet they are unintended; they are sometimes called *indirect killings*.

A more complicated case involves situations in which the evil is anticipated but not desired. Some drugs are known to have undesirable side effects so that the health provider knows she is taking a risk by administering the drug. In some cases she may even know for sure that the side effect will occur but consider the effect worth it. It may be known that giving an antihistamine will make the patient drowsy but that, on balance, the antihistamine will benefit the patient. If it is given, we would not say that the provider intended to make the patient drowsy; rather, it was foreseen and unavoidable, though not intended.

Likewise, Catholic theologians have held that something as evil as a death may be morally tolerable if it is unintended, even if it is foreseen. If the patient dies from respiratory depression resulting from a heavy narcotic dose given to control pain, the death can be called an indirect killing, that is, one that, though foreseen, was not intended.

Those who accept this distinction between directly intended and indirect killing hold that, even though direct (that is, intended) killings are never acceptable, under certain circumstances indirect killings are morally acceptable. To be acceptable, the evil must not be intended. Also, the good that is done, such as the relieving of pain, must be at least as great as the evil. Finally, the evil cannot be the means to the good end.[8] This notion that unintended bad consequences are morally tolerable when these conditions are met is referred to as the *doctrine of indirect or double effect*.

Thus according to Catholics, who believe that abortion is evil, it is unacceptable to abort a fetus to produce the "good" of relieving a pregnant woman's anxiety about becoming pregnant because the evil (the abortion) would be the means to the good. However, it might be acceptable to remove a cancerous uterus even if the woman with the cancer happened to be pregnant at the time. In the case of the cancer, the death of the fetus would not be a means to removing the cancer; it would be a foreseen but unintended side effect. Catholics and others who recognize these distinctions conclude that the removal of the uterus to save the pregnant woman's life is morally tolerable even though it will result in the death of the fetus because the death was merely foreseen and not intended. While some people do not accept this distinction, it has been the prevailing view in American law and professional codes of ethics.

In the care of terminally ill patients, sometimes a medication dispensed by a pharmacist may actively kill a patient in a way that is foreseen but unintended. In the following case, the issue is whether the fact that the death was not intended makes a moral difference.

CASE 9-5   Unintended but Foreseen Killing with Morphine

"I didn't say that I wanted to end her life! Although, if there was ever a solid case for active euthanasia, I think this is the one. All I wanted to do is relieve her pain," Dr. Sebastian Lombardo firmly stated. The conference room was silent for a moment as the treatment team waited for the counter argument from Cory Eden, Pharm.D. The physician and the clinical pharmacist were deeply embroiled in a disagreement about the pain management of Sadie Alsharif. Mrs. Alsharif, a 54-year-old woman, was in the terminal stages of breast cancer with metastases to the bone. Dr. Lombardo, an oncologist and director of the hospital's hospice program, began Mrs. Alsharif's pain-management therapy with a nonopioid analgesic and a COX-2 inhibitor. When neuropathic pain developed, Dr. Lombardo added a tricyclic antidepressant and oral morphine around the clock. He also ordered a form of immediate-release morphine to manage breakthrough pain. Mrs. Alsharif made it clear from the outset that she did not want to suffer unnecessarily.

As the disease progressed, Mrs. Alsharif became weaker and in more pain. She required higher and higher doses of morphine to relieve her pain. The dose was titrated until she was comfortable. The present situation that provoked the team conference is that if the team continues to increase the dose of morphine, it will cause respiratory depression and, quite possibly, subsequent death. Dr. Eden is the clinical pharmacist on the treatment team and is as adamant as Dr. Lombardo about his own position.

"I know you want to relieve her pain. So do I. But you want to relieve her pain permanently, by killing her. It is immoral to kill a patient, I don't care how compassionate your reasons," Dr. Eden retorted, breaking the silence.

"I know that respiratory depression is a side effect of opiates. That's unfortunate, but one of the harms I am willing to accept in order to fulfill my promise to keep her as pain-free as possible," Dr. Lombardo countered.

"Besides," Dr. Lombardo continued, "I'm not entirely convinced that opiates are the cause of respiratory depression in terminally ill patients who have developed a tolerance. When death is imminent, perhaps the respiratory rate naturally decreases. In that case, there would be no reason to withhold analgesia because of fear of respiratory depression. However, the research is not definitive in this area, so I return to my previous position that pain relief is of utmost importance, even if the outcome is death."

Commentary

Dr. Lombardo and Dr. Eden are locked in a dispute that is in part technical—what the link is, if any, between the opiate use and the respiratory depression. However, they also appear to have a moral disagreement. The respiratory distress is not unexpected. They can agree on that. They also can agree that the respiratory depression may be so severe that it will cause death. Primarily in dispute is whether the fact that the intention or desire of the clinicians is to relieve pain rather than cause death makes the risk morally tolerable.

The first question to address is what the intention of the physician was and whether the intention matters morally in deciding whether he would be doing wrong if he administered the narcotic. One possibility is that he simply intended to kill the patient in order to relieve her suffering. Had that been his intention, he certainly would be guilty of an illegal act, and most people seem to have concluded that such intentional, active killing of the patient is morally wrong as well.

But it might also be that his real intention was only to relieve the pain by whatever means were available and effective. If that was his intention, he would try to titrate the dose of the narcotic to avoid killing the patient. But suppose he realizes that he is approaching dangerously close to the point at which respiration would be fully suppressed. If he believes that approaching that point is necessary in order to achieve the intended goal of controlling pain, is the physician doing a moral wrong that is comparable to intended killing? Is a foreseen but unintended evil morally equivalent to an intended one?

Catholic theology insists that such risk of unintended, but foreseen, evil is tolerable. The *Ethical and Religious Directives for Catholic Health Care Services* (ERDs) states the position of the U.S. Council of Catholic Bishops as follows: "Medicine capable of alleviating or suppressing pain may be given to a dying person, even if this therapy may indirectly shorten the person's life so long as the intent is not to hasten death."

Other groups, however, dispute this conclusion. They might take the more liberal stance that holds that even active, intended killing for mercy (what the ERDs call "euthanasia") is acceptable provided that, all things considered, it is the only way to relieve the suffering and does more good than harm. Other, more conservative, groups take a position that may be similar to Dr. Eden's. They hold that active, intended mercy killing is morally wrong but that it is just as wrong to give the drug if death is foreseen, even if unintended. A death is a death, according to this view.

Some who take this position emphasize that we must distinguish between the assessment of the moral blameworthiness of the actor and the moral rightness of the act. They might acknowledge that intention is important in assessing the character of the actor and conclude that it is a person of worse moral character who intends the death compared to one who merely foresees that the death is a possibility while relief of pain is his sincere intention. Those who reject the distinction between direct and indirect (intended and foreseen) killing, however, say that when we are assessing the act itself, the same effect occurs, regardless of the intention. If it is wrong to intend death; it is just as wrong to act in such a way that one foresees that death will result even though it is not the direct intention of the act. The pharmacist seems to take a position like this while the physician is either directly intending the death or, more likely, indirectly causing the death that he foresees but does not intend.

This is relevant to the related problem of what the physician should say on the death certificate. If administering this dose of narcotic analgesia is the moral equivalent of intending the death of the patient, then it makes sense to view the narcotic as the immediate cause of the death and to mention it on the death certificate, perhaps listing the breast cancer as an underlying or secondary cause. If, however, lack of intention justifies treating such deaths as morally different (even if they are foreseen), then perhaps we should view the cancer as the cause of death rather than the narcotic. Many defenders of the distinction between intended and foreseen effects claim that interventions in which death is not intended should not be viewed as "causing" the death.

Since these rather esoteric distinctions can lead to confusion and perhaps hide controversial behaviors (for example, if the physician fails to disclose that the narcotic contributed to the death), some people are now advocating that these contributing factors to a death should be reported even if they are not considered the cause of the death. If the physician is convinced that administering the narcotic was justifiable, he should be willing to defend his position publicly. This has led policy-makers in the Netherlands to insist that the administration of lethal agents at the request of dying patients, a practice accepted in the Netherlands, be listed on the death certificate. In the Netherlands, however, death is the intention of the physician when lethal agents are administered. Does the fact that Dr. Lombardo does not intend Mrs. Alsharif's death, make his decision morally more acceptable?

Justifiable Omissions

The previous case suggests that for one reason or another many people believe that active killings are morally unacceptable, at least if they are directly intended. The distinction between active killing and omitting treatment (sometimes referred to as the commission-omission distinction or the active-passive distinction) has grown to great importance in the debate over the care of the terminally ill. That is why it has been so important to figure out whether withdrawing treatment is more like withholding it or more like active killing. Even if some treatments are justifiably omitted, clearly not all of them can be. The next case raises the issue of what is necessary to justify omission of treatment. In particular, are there certain kinds of treatments that can be forgone even though others never can be, or is the criterion for justifying an omission based on assessment of benefit and harms?

CASE 9-6   Can an Antibiotic Be an Extraordinary Means of Saving Life?

Mr. Wyatt looked much older than his age of 67 years, Matt Postki, Pharm.D., had to silently admit to himself. Dr. Postki was consulting with Mr. Wyatt about his decision to refuse medications to treat his pneumonia. Mr. Wyatt fit the stereotype of nursing home transfers to the acute-care setting, i.e., frail, dehydrated, malnourished, yet he differed in that he generally retained not only clarity of thought but also a sense of humor. Dr. Postki could not believe that Mr. Wyatt would refuse something as simple and effective as a first-line cephalosporin. Although Mr. Wyatt gave up smoking several years ago, he had all of the classic signs and symptoms of chronic obstructive pulmonary disease (COPD). He was dependent on oxygen, "barrel chested," and chronically short of breath. However, Dr. Postki was convinced that Mr. Wyatt's pneumonia was treatable even though his COPD was not. Without the antibiotic, Mr. Wyatt would surely succumb to the respiratory failure that would be the outcome of untreated pneumonia in such a fragile, chronically ill patient.

Dr. Postki felt it was his obligation to convince Mr. Wyatt that his refusal of the antibiotic was wrong, that it would result in his death. No matter that Mr. Wyatt's physician, Dr. Maria Conklin, agreed with Mr. Wyatt's decision and had entered orders for do-not-resuscitate status and supportive care, Dr. Postki believed that withholding an easily administered, relatively painless treatment like an intravenous antibiotic was

CASE 9-6 *Continued.*

tantamount to murder. He could understand if Mr. Wyatt was refusing to be placed on a ventilator if he should go into respiratory failure. After all, ventilators are complicated, expensive, and, from what patients had told him, uncomfortable.

Dr. Postki asked Mr. Wyatt if he understood that not receiving the antibiotic would probably result in his death. Mr. Wyatt had to recover from a fit of coughing before getting enough breath to reply, "I've had my share of medications, and I know how they are supposed to work. I believe you when you say the drug would make me better, but that doesn't change my mind. The drug will only prevent the inevitable. I am exhausted from fighting for each breath. If this pneumonia is what will be the cause, so be it."

Upset, Dr. Postki left the room. He wondered if he had a moral obligation to take the case to the hospital ethics committee or even to seek judicial review.

Commentary

Both secular and religious sources acknowledge that some treatments are so "extraordinary" that they are expendable.[10] We often think of high technology treatments, such as ventilators, dialysis machines, chemotherapy, or major surgery, as treatments that might be expendable because they are viewed as being extraordinary, that is, statistically unusual or technologically complex.

Those who traditionally used the term *extraordinary* did not really have in mind the unusualness or complexity of the treatment. After all, it does not make much sense to consider a treatment expendable simply because it is unusual or complex. Something may be very unusual but just right for a patient with an unusual condition. It may be high tech but still very beneficial. The authorities that used to speak of extraordinary means of treatment now have tended to abandon that language because of this confusion. Instead, they make clear that treatments are expendable or required morally based on consideration of the benefits and burdens.

If the benefits exceed the burdens, then the treatment is acceptable; if they do not, then it makes no sense to require it. This notion of the relative amount of benefits and burdens is now generally referred to as the *criterion of proportionality*. If the burdens equal or exceed the benefits, then there is no moral necessity to provide the treatment. This is true for even simple treatments, such as antibiotics, cardiopulmonary resuscitation (CPR), and routine nursing protocols, such as those specifying when patients should be turned.

One remaining area of controversy is how the benefits and burdens are assessed. While some have traditionally believed that the benefits and the burdens can best be known by the physician, more recent commentaries have emphasized the subjective nature of these assessments. Hence, they have stressed that the physician has no special expertise in deciding whether an effect is a benefit and, if so, how beneficial it is. Likewise, the physician cannot have any special knowledge in deciding whether an effect is a harm and, if so, how harmful. Similar positions are being taken in pharmacology. While most pharmacology texts used to freely describe the benefits and burdens of treatments, sometimes even labeling certain drugs as "drugs of choice," increasingly these are seen as value judgments based on how various people perceive the effects of treatment rather than as labels that can be derived directly from the science. According to this view, pharmacological research can tell us about the various effects of a chemotherapeutic agent but not whether those effects are good or bad or how good or bad they are. These latter judgments require somebody's value system. There is no reason to believe that pharmacologists are uniquely skilled in making such value judgments.

If we apply this reasoning to our present case, the critical question becomes, "Is the cephalosporin for Mr. Wyatt a treatment that will likely produce more benefits than burdens?" From pharmacist Matt Postki's point of view it certainly is. Recent movements insist, however, that it is not the pharmacist's or the physician's assessment of benefits and burdens that is definitive. It is the patient's. Clearly, Mr. Wyatt has reached the conclusion that this treatment is not worth it to him. Mr. Wyatt gives quite realistic reasons for his judgment: he is tired of fighting for air and realizes that curing the pneumonia would only delay the inevitable. Do they count as reasons that could be compatible with a patient who is mentally competent?

Voluntary and Involuntary Killing

In the previous cases we have seen that there is room for disagreement over whether some patients would be better off if they were dead. Those who focus exclusively on consequences would, logically, favor killing if they believed that the patient would be better off. However, those who accept that there is something inherently wrong with killing might continue to oppose active, direct killing even if they accepted the legitimacy of withholding or withdrawing treatment. There is one additional ethical principle that needs to be factored in. Especially if the decisions about what counts as a benefit or a harm are subjective, there may be good reasons to give moral weight to the autonomous choices of patients when it comes to deciding about whether to forgo life-sustaining treatment. In the following case, we shall explore the role of the autonomous choice of the patient in such decisions.

CASE 9-7   Assisted Suicide and Chronic Depression

Gloria DeSilva was a 63-year-old woman who lived by herself in a small town in Oregon. She had never married and had no close friends or relatives. She came to Mr. Rubinoff at the pharmacy for a refill of her prescription for citalopram hydrobromide (Celexa), the antidepressant she had been taking for over a year.

Her mood was somber. She looked, as she had for some time, withdrawn and without affect. When she approached Mr. Rubinoff she said she had a question she needed answered. She asked him if he knew which physicians in the area were prescribing barbiturates for people who were tired of living.

Mr. Rubinoff knew the internist Ms. DeSilva had been seeing, the one who had prescribed the Celexa. Mr. Rubinoff had never seen a prescription for this purpose from

CASE 9-7   *Continued.*

that internist and believed he probably would not cooperate if Ms. DeSilva asked him for a prescription to end her life. It was very likely that Ms. DeSilva would not qualify for a prescription for a lethal agent in any case because she had no diagnosed terminal illness unless, chronic depression could be construed as qualifying. Mr. Rubinoff, in fact, knew one physician who would likely be willing to prescribe for her and get a colleague to confirm his actions. He knew he was legally required to assure that Ms. DeSilva had given an adequately informed consent for her medication and that the consent process included providing information about the alternatives that were available. It occurred to Mr. Rubinoff that referral to the physician who might prescribe was an alternative. Should Mr. Rubinoff give Ms. DeSilva the physician's name?

Commentary

There is increasing controversy over the role of the health professional in assisting a patient in bringing about his or her death. Physician killing based on persistent requests from a competent patient is widely practiced in the Netherlands and is tolerated by the law. Legislative and judicial efforts are underway in several states that would legalize physician efforts to end a dying patient's life actively and intentionally. One feature of these efforts, both in the Netherlands and in the United States, is that, if a physician is authorized to kill patients for a merciful motive or assist in a suicide, the plans carefully restrict such killing to patients who have made a voluntary request while they are mentally competent and, hence, able to make substantially autonomous choices.

The issue here is whether Ms. DeSilva's request is voluntary and, if so, whether that is a sufficient reason for Mr. Rubinoff, to cooperate. First, is Ms. DeSilva capable of making a voluntary choice? If so, she would have to have the mental capacity to understand the nature of her choice and be substantially free from internal and external forces that would make her choice involuntary. Is she a substantially autonomous agent? What do you make of the fact that she has been on an antidepressant for a year? Is that enough to make her incompetent to make a voluntary choice?

Assuming that she is substantially autonomous in her choice, does the principle of autonomy provide a moral basis for overcoming our general reluctance to cooperate in active killing of another human being, or does the moral prohibition on killing, insofar as there is one, carry over to cases in which the patient has made a conscious, voluntary choice to end her life? There are two separate issues here: whether autonomy provides a defense of suicide by autonomous persons and whether it provides a defense of the involvement of other people, such as the pharmacist, Mr. Rubinoff. The principle of autonomy holds that it is wrong to interfere with the actions of others who have made substantially autonomous choices based on their own life plans. Some would argue that this principle supports the choice of suicide by substantially autonomous people. Even that conclusion is controversial. Some people have made commitments to others (such as their children) that they would be breaking if they ended their lives. That Ms. DeSilva lives alone and has no family minimizes that concern. In addition, if there is something inherently wrong with killing humans, even self-killing might be seen as violating that notion. Religious people believe that their own lives are really not theirs to dispose of and that we are merely stewards of our lives. Some secularists also believe self-killing is wrong.

Regardless, the principle of autonomy cannot settle the question of whether someone else should cooperate in the killing. Ms. DeSilva would be able to kill herself by taking prescribed medications, but even in a state like Oregon, where assisted suicide was legal, she would need a physician's assistance. She would also need to have others involved, in this case a pharmacist.

Even if we conclude that Ms. DeSilva has the right to kill herself, it does not necessarily follow that Mr. Rubinoff, as the pharmacist who would be involved in referring her to a willing physician and possibly in preparing the medication, has the moral right or duty to cooperate. Some would argue that even if, in theory, active mercy killing and suicide are legitimate, still health professionals ought not be involved. They maintain that there is something about the role of being a health professional that is incompatible with killing, even at the request of the patient and even if the killing is done for mercy. All parties recognize that Ms. DeSilva, assuming she is competent, would have the right to insist that life-supporting interventions, such as a ventilator, be withdrawn. They seem to agree that it is acceptable to give medication to make patients comfortable while they die, even if the medication hastens the death as a side effect. Is there any reason why, assuming she has voluntarily chosen the course, that the prescription should not be modified to end her life more directly? For most terminally ill patients suicide is an option, although perhaps an unpleasant and unethical one. For Ms. DeSllva, however, this would be difficult and probably require some burden. If she is deemed mentally lucid and competent, is there any reason why she cannot have the assistance she appears to contemplate?

The principles of avoidance of killing and autonomy seem to pull us in different directions in this case. In order to resolve the matter we may have to appeal to our general theory of how to resolve conflict among principles. Does one of the two deserve priority such that it is ranked above the other, permitting a ready formula for resolving the conflict? Or do both deserve consideration so that they are "balanced against each other" or in some other way combined to reach a final answer to the question of what Mr. Rubinoff's duty is?

This problem of conflict among the major principles of bioethics arises in many areas of health care ethics. In Part III of this volume we will look at some of those areas to see how the principles can be integrated to resolve potential conflicts.

Killing as Punishment

Standard discussions of the ethics of killing usually include consideration of certain killing that is not done for merciful motive. They take up killing in war and police activity. They also include capital punishment. While most of these discussions are outside the realm of health professional ethics, capital punishment has emerged as a problem that health professionals must face. In the past decade many states have become troubled by the inhumaneness of traditional execution of criminals by electrocution, hanging, and other techniques increasingly seen as barbaric. They have moved to what they call *medical execution,* the use of lethal injection of barbi-turates or other chemical agents intended to kill quickly and painlessly. Pharmacists potentially can play a key role in the preparation of these agents and in determining the most effective dose regimens. Deciding whether ethically one can participate will be an issue facing every pharmacist, either as a direct participant or as a citizen debating state policy.

CASE 9-8   Participation in Capital Punishment

Although Roland Kenefick, Pharm.D., worked with the inmates on death row for the past 6 years, no one had been scheduled for execution. The inmates and their attorneys were constantly caught up in endless appeals so that it seemed the death penalty could be delayed forever. This was not going to be the case for one inmate, Charles Autry, who was scheduled for execution at the end of the month. Mr. Autry's execution was the first one in the state since the adoption of lethal injection as the sole means of execution.

Dr. Kenefick believed in his work as the prison pharmacist, but involvement in the execution of an inmate seemed to him to be distinct from his general duties as a phar-macist. He did not have any qualms about recommending appropriate pharmacotherapy for sedatives and tranquilizers for inmates who were anxious about the possibility of an upcoming execution. However, when he was approached by the warden to consult with a physician and nurse anesthetist to design the protocol for lethal injection for Mr. Autry's execution, Dr. Kenefick felt that his involvement had moved to a different level. On the one hand, if the execution was inevitable, and it appeared to be, then his involvement in planning the protocol could ensure that the right combination of drugs was used to make the execution as benign as possible. At a minimum, he believed he knew enough about toxicology to ensure that the result would be a quick and painless death. Dr. Kenefick had read about executions that took as long as 10 minutes for the inmate to die, during which time the inmate was conscious, moving about and in pain. No one should have to die that way, Dr. Kenefick thought. On the other hand, Dr. Kenefick believed that killing was wrong. Furthermore, participation in an execution seemed to him to lie far outside standard pharmacy practice. Yet, Dr. Kenefick worked directly for the state penitentiary and, therefore, for the state criminal justice system. The execution was serving the pur-poses of the state, but what was its place in regard to the profession of pharmacy and, more specifically, to Dr. Kenefick's practice?

Commentary

Dr. Kenefick will have to reach some moral decisions if he is to continue in his pres-ent employment as a prison pharmacist. Probably the first issue he should confront is his overall moral views about capital punishment. Many are increasingly critical, raising issues of whether it is too cruel and inhumane, even if done using a physically painless and certain medical method. Others argue that there seems to be something incon-gruous if a society punishes terrible crimes, such as murder, by taking another human life. They are concerned that institutionalizing such a practice will corrupt the society, making it the kind of community that is not as noble as it could be. Still others point

to the irreversibility of capital punishment and express fear that the inevitable erroneous convictions will eventually leave some innocent person dead. They point out that
juries and courts cannot be infallible and that we can never be completely certain that
those executed were really mentally capable of being responsible for their actions.
They believe that the necessary doubt about the certainty of the criminal's responsibility should leave society with a way of reversing its judgment.

However, those defending capital punishment can point to the terrible crimes
that have been committed. They argue either in terms of the general or specific
deterrence of capital punishment or appeal to notions of retribution, claiming that
the most vicious criminals, such as those who have consciously taken innocent life,
should pay with their own lives.

The position one takes on capital punishment will depend in part on one's
interpretation of the principle of avoiding killing. If it is understood to mean that
it is morally wrong to kill in all circumstances—that life is sacred to use the more
religious language—then, of course, capital punishment will be unacceptable. The
most radical interpretation views killing even of those who have committed serious
offenses in war or civil life as unacceptable. If holders of such views are consistent,
they are pacifists. Others interpret the principle of avoidance of killing to be only
a prima facie duty that can be offset by other principles. Certain interpretations of
the principle of justice provide a basis for killing as retribution for the most serious
wrongs. Some interpretations of beneficence might provide a basis for killing as a
general or specific deterrence.

If Dr. Kenefick concludes that capital punishment is morally unacceptable under
any circumstances, he may have to take the position that as a matter of conscience,
he cannot participate. However, it is conceivable he might claim that, even though
he considers capital punishment unacceptable, he owes it to the criminal to see
that the inevitable is done humanely and competently, leading him to participate.
Of course, if he ends up concluding that, on balance, the deterrent or retributive
arguments in favor of the practice win out, then that also could make him decide in
favor of participation.

He also raises the question of whether participation is compatible with his professional identity as a pharmacist. It is possible that Dr. Kenefick could conclude that a
society has a right to execute its most evil criminals but that pharmacists, as members
of the healing professions, cannot participate. That could lead him to the conclusion
that, although capital punishment is acceptable, someone else will have to be the
source of the knowledge needed to carry it out. Some physicians have argued that
their profession must separate itself from capital punishment because the practice
is incompatible with the role of the healer. Professional pharmacy associations have
once again left this decision to individual conscience, adding that pharmacists should
not be put at risk for disciplinary action if they refuse to participate in capital punishment.[17] However, if execution is to be accepted as appropriate public policy, someone will be needed who has the skills of a pharmacist, such as Dr. Kenefick.

If Dr. Kenefick decides he can participate, should he limit himself to consulting?
Would it be any less acceptable to play a direct role in the preparation of the agents
to be used? If he decides he cannot participate, who should the state rely on for this

role? Must he leave his position of employment to separate himself entirely from a practice he finds morally unacceptable?

These are very practical questions that will require considerations not only of the principle of avoidance of killing, but also all the other principles discussed in this part of the book. Many other practices in which pharmacists may be asked to participate also raise questions that involve the careful balancing of two or more principles. Some of these areas are addressed in the chapters in Part III.

Notes

1. Rawls, John. "Two Concepts of Rules." *Philosophical Review* 44 (1955): 3–32; Lyons, David. *Forms and Limits of Utilitarianism* (Oxford: Oxford University Press, 1965); Ramsey, Paul. *Deeds and Rules in Christian Ethics,* New York: Charles Scribner's Sons, 1967; Brandt, Richard B. "Toward a Credible Form of Utilitarianism." *Contemporary Utilitarianism.* Michael D. Bayles, Editor. Garden City, NY: Doubleday & Co., 1968, pp. 143–186.

2. Ramsey. *Deeds and Rules in Christian Ethics.*

3. For example, see Kant, Immanuel. *Groundwork of the Metaphysic of Morals.* H. J. Paton, Translator. New York: Harper and Row, 1964.

4. For a development of this view see Veatch, Robert M. *A Theory of Medical Ethics.* New York: Basic Books, 1981, pp. 227ff.

5. American Society of Health-System Pharmacists. "ASHP Statement on Pharmacist's Decision-making on Assisted Suicide." *American Journal of Health-System Pharmacy* 56 (1999): 1661–1664.

6. Craig, Gillian. "Is Sedation without Hydration or Nourishment in Terminal Care Lawful?" *Medico-Legal Journal* 62, pt. 4 (1994): 198–201; Kenny, Nuala P.; and Gerri Frager. "Refractory Symptoms and Terminal Sedation of Children: Ethical Issues and Practical Management." *Journal of Palliative Care* 12, no. 3 (1996): 40–45; Mount, Balfour. "Morphine Drips, Terminal Sedation, and Slow Euthanasia: Definitions and Facts, Not Anecdotes." *Journal of Palliative Care* 12, no. 4 (1996): 31–37; Wilson, William C., Nicholas G. Smedira, Carol Fink, James A. McDowell, and John M. Luce. "Ordering and Administration of Sedatives and Analgesics during the Withholding and Withdrawal of Life Support from Critically Ill patients." *Journal of the American Medical Association* 267, no. 7 (1992): 949–953; Truog, Robert D., John H. Arnold, and Mark A. Rockoff. "Sedation before Ventilator Withdrawal: Medical and Ethical Considerations." *Journal of Clinical Ethics* 2, no. 2 (1991): 127–129; Rietjens, J. A., J. J. van Delden, A. van der Heide, A. M. Vrakking, B. D. Onwuteake-Phillipsen, P. J. van der Maas, and G. van der Wal. "Terminal Sedation and Euthanasia: A Comparison of Clinical Practices," *Archives of Internal Medicine* 166, no. 7 (2006): 749–753.

7. Bernat, James L., Bernard Gert, and R. Peter Mogielnicki. "Patient Refusal of Hydration and Nutrition." *Archives of Internal Medicine* 153 (December 1993): 2723–2728; Miller, Franklin G., and Diane E. Meier. "Voluntary Death: A Comparison of Terminal Dehydration and Physician-Assisted Suicide." *Annals of Internal Medicine* 128 (1998): 559–562.

8. McCormick, Richard A., and Paul Ramsey, Editors. *Doing Evil to Achieve Good: Moral Choice in Conflict Situations.* Chicago: Loyola University Press, 1978; Curran, Charles E. "Roman Catholicism." *Encyclopedia of Bioethics.* Second Edition. Vol. 4. Warren T. Reich, Editor. New York: Free Press, 1995, pp. 2321–2330; for secular treatments of the

indirect or double-effect doctrine see Foot, Philippa. "The Problem of Abortion and the Doctrine of the Double Effect." *Oxford Review* 5 (1967): 5–15; Graber, Glenn C. "Some Questions about Double Effect." *Ethics in Science and Medicine* 6, no. 1 (1979): 65–84.

9. U.S. Conference of Catholic Bishops. *Ethical and Religious Directives for Catholic Health Care Services.* Fourth Edition. Washington, DC: U.S. Conference of Catholic Bishops, 2001.

10. Pope Pius XII. "The Prolongation of Life: An Address of Pope Pius XII to an International Congress of Anesthesiologists." *The Pope Speaks* 4 (Spring 1958): 393–398; President's Commission for the Study of Ethical Problems in Medicine and Biomedical and Behavioral Research. *Deciding to Forego Life-Sustaining Treatment: Ethical, Medical, and Legal Issues in Treatment Decisions.* Washington, DC: U.S. Government Printing Office, 1983.

11. Congregation for the Doctrine of the Faith. "Declaration on Euthanasia." Rome: Sacred Congregation for the Doctrine of the Faith. Issued May 5, 1980; cf. President's Commission, *Deciding to Forego Life-Sustaining Treatment,* p. 88.

12. Van Der Mass, Paul J., J. M. Johannes, Loes Pijnenborg Van Delden, and Casper W. N. Looman. "Euthanasia and Other Medical Decisions concerning the End of Life." *The Lancet* 338 (Sept. 14, 1991): 669–674.

13. Jonsen, Albert R. "Initiative 119: What Is at Stake?" *Commonweal* 118, no. 14, supp. (August 9, 1991): 466–469; *Compassion in Dying v. Washington.* Docket No. 94-35534, D.C. No. CV-94-119-BJR. U.S. Court of Appeals for the Ninth Circuit, 1994; *Quill et al. v. Vacco et al.* Docket No. 95-7028, U.S. Court of Appeals for the Second Circuit, 1995.

14. For a more thorough discussion of the ethics of capital punishment general analyses can be found in Stanley E. Grupp, Editor. *Theories of Punishment.* Bloomington: Indiana University Press, 1971; Walter Berns. *For Capital Punishment: Crime and the Morality of the Death Penalty.* New York: Basic Books, 1979; Bedau, Hugo Adam. *Death Is Different.* Boston: Northeastern University Press, 1987.

15. For a discussion of the pharmacist's role see Brushwood, David B. "The Pharmacist and Execution by Lethal Injection." *U.S. Pharmacist,* September 1984, pp. 25–26, 28.

16. American Medical Association. Council on Ethical and Judicial Affairs. *Code of Medical Ethics: Current Opinions with Annotations, 2004–2005 Edition.* Chicago: American Medical Association, 2004, pp. 18–19.

17. American Society of Health-System Pharmacists. *Use of Drugs in Capital Punishment Policy (8410).* Bethesda, MD: American Society of Health-System Pharmacists, 2001.

Part III

Special Problem Areas

10

Abortion, Sterilization, and Contraception

One of the areas that has regularly generated controversy in health care ethics is the set of problems surrounding obstetrics: abortion, sterilization, and contraception. They raise all the general moral themes represented by the principles discussed in Part II but in a dramatic and often emotionally charged setting. Moreover, these issues of obstetrical ethics pose a different kind of question: to whom do the basic principles of biomedical ethics apply? We need to determine, for example, whether a principle such as avoiding killing applies to fetuses or only humans after they are born. If it applies to fetuses, then we need to determine whether it applies to all fetuses or only those with certain properties, such as consciousness, the ability to move in a way perceived by the pregnant woman (quickening), or the ability to survive independently outside the womb. These issues also present a complex overlay of religious and philosophical notions about the duties and expectations of marriage, the role of natural law (a theory that grounds moral obligation in the ends for which beings were created), and the role of the state in controlling intimate, personal choices. The first group of cases examines the ethics of abortion and the role of the pharmacist in abortions performed in a health care institution.

Abortion

Perhaps the most controversial and intractable issue in health care ethics is abortion.[1] The underlying issue is what moral status and moral claims should be attributed to embryos and fetuses after conception has taken place and prior to birth. Do the normal moral principles, such as beneficence and avoiding killing, apply and, if not, why not?

A major part of what is at stake is the moral standing of the early embryo and the fetus that it becomes. If the embryo or fetus is considered nothing more than a part of the pregnant woman's body, then there is little reason to doubt that she can do whatever she pleases with it, including removing it. However, if it is considered to have the status of an independent human being with moral standing, then the full range of principles we have been examining in this volume would apply to actions taken toward it. Not only would there be a prima facie duty to benefit and avoid harm, there would also be a duty to keep promises made, to provide a just share of resources, and to avoid killing.

It is true that some who are more liberal on abortion still grant the full standing of the fetus. They might argue that the pregnant woman's moral claims are enough to override the fetus's claim. Some argue that one can recognize the full moral standing of the embryo as early as implantation and still recognize that the moral standing of the pregnant woman could force an awful choice between the two in some circumstances. This is particularly true in cases such as rape, in which the woman has in no way consented to taking the risk to become pregnant.

Holders of the most conservative position believe that the embryo as well as the fetus have the full standing of other human beings from the moment of conception. The embryo already has whatever is necessary to give it such standing. That might be the unique genetic composition or the genetic potential to develop certain features thought necessary to be treated as having this full standing. These features might be certain capacities for brain function or circulation and respiration.

Increasingly, controversy is emerging over exactly what gives this standing. For example, some have suggested that the genetic code may not actually be fixed exactly at the moment of conception but may be capable of variation for some days thereafter. One Catholic bioethicist has suggested that the development of the so-called primitive streak signals the point at which a unique individual is established.[2] Others who are traditionally conservative have identified the latest point at which twinning can take place.[3] Still others may emphasize the development of more complex brain functions but hold that what is critical is the potential for these functions as signaled by the presence of the genetic information necessary for their expression.

Others who are more liberal on the ethics of abortion believe that some other functions, such as neurological integration, quickening, or the development of capacity for consciousness, must actually have appeared before the fetus has full moral standing. Of course, no one denies that from the moment of conception the embryo is made up of human cells. In that sense the tissues are "human." What is at stake is whether those tissues have moral claims against the rest of the human community. Some who hold these more liberal views would readily acknowledge that there is some intermediate or lesser claim prior to the appearance of the feature they consider critical for full standing. Just as one might have an ethical duty to show respect for a human corpse after the death of an individual, so there might be a similar obligation to treat early embryos and fetuses with a certain degree of respect. What is the matter of real controversy is whether full equality of moral claims comes from the moment of conception or at some later time. In theory one might identify that moment even after birth. Some extreme commentators hold, for example, that a newborn infant still lacks the key feature (such as the ability to reason or use language) that would give it a full claim against the human community. Most, however, recognize that at least by birth this full moral standing is present. The real controversy is whether it arises at conception or some later time and precisely what is responsible for this standing.

Different reasons given for abortion raise these issues in different ways. For example, if someone proposed to abort a fetus because of a genetic abnormality, at stake would be whether the key genetic characteristics are nevertheless present. Abortions proposed for other reasons, such as the health of the pregnant woman, rape, or socioeconomic issues, would require some argument supporting the abortion even though the fetus presumably is genetically intact. The following cases all look at abortions for commonly proposed reasons.

Abortion for Medical Problems of the Fetus

One of the most commonly offered reasons for abortion is that the fetus has some genetic or other medical abnormality that justifies the abortion. This can happen on two different grounds. First, in some extreme cases the fetus might not be medically capable of surviving. A fetus prenatally diagnosed with anencephaly (absence of all or major portions of the brain) is one example. More often, the fetus unarguably has the capacity to survive, at least for some time, but still has enough of a medical problem that some might consider abortion justifiable. What is striking here is that the parents may, in general, be eager for a child. If they abort they will be deciding that this child is so compromised that the medical problem warrants the abortion. Pharmacy personnel working in facilities that do abortions face the question of whether they will cooperate in such abortions. The following case illustrates the problem.

CASE 10-1   Abortion for Teratogenic Indications

Ariel Watson had been taking isotretinoin for nodular acne for 6 months before her marriage. Ms. Watson met the criteria for isotretinoin use since she was unresponsive to standard therapy. Because she was of childbearing age, she was also enrolled in the iPledge program, which has the goal of preventing pregnancies in females taking isotretinoin and to prevent pregnant females from taking isotrentinoin. The iPledge program requires female patients who can get pregnant to take birth control for at least 1 month before, during, and 1 month after stopping treatment. Ms. Watson was extensively counseled about the side effects of the drug particularly to avoid pregnancy. However, at the time, Ms. Watson wasn't sexually active so she half-heartedly listened to the list of deleterious effects that the drug could have on the fetus. She understood that she had to have negative pregnancy tests before, during, and after treatment. She signed the Patient Information/Informed Consent form indicating that she had received oral and written warnings of the hazards of taking the drug during pregnancy and would comply with the recommended two forms of contraception and pregnancy tests. She complied with the monthly urine tests to determine whether she was pregnant before she got her prescription refilled.

CASE 10-1 *Continued.*

Victor Radlauer, Pharm.D., knew Ms. Watson well because she got her refills for isotretinoin at his ambulatory clinic pharmacy that is registered with the iPledge program. Dr. Radlauer remembered that Ms. Watson had gotten married about four months ago. She came into the pharmacy today, about a week early, for her refill. When Ms. Watson got to the head of the line she softly stated to Dr. Radlauer, "I really need to talk to you. I have some questions about the drug I take for my acne. Something has come up. Can we talk some place private?" Dr. Radlauer suggested that they meet in the counseling room in the pharmacy.

Ms. Watson stated, "My husband and I have been using two forms of birth control, but I guess they aren't the right ones because I think I am pregnant. I took a home pregnancy test today, and it is positive. I know you and my doctor told me that the medicine could have an effect on the baby. How serious can this be?" Dr. Radlauer explained that this was indeed serious. Ms. Watson responded, "I don't think I could continue this pregnancy if there is something really wrong with the baby."

Dr. Radlauer is opposed to abortion in most cases. Yet he also believes there are some cases of genetic deficit, such as Tay-Sachs, or anomalies like anencephaly, that justify an abortion since they result in certain death for the infant. He believes that if Ms. Watson is told the truth about the birth defects that have been documented, such as abnormalities of the face, eyes, ears, skull, thymus, heart, and central nervous system, she will abort the fetus. At a minimum, he knew he needed to inform her to stop taking the drug immediately.

Commentary

At least two questions are raised by this case. The first is substantive: is it legitimate to abort a fetus because it has been exposed to a teratogen that could cause a serious genetic or other anatomical afflictions? The second is more procedural: what role should Dr. Radlauer play in providing information to Ms. Watson? Clearly the two are linked, but separate, issues.

Serious genetic disorder is one of the reasons for abortion that has been found plausible even among those who object to abortion for more vague social and psychological reasons. The other "hard core" reasons include rape, which will be discussed in Case and incest as well as the saving the life of the pregnant woman, which will be the subject of Case 10-3.

Isotretinoin could cause a potentially serious teratogenic affliction. Ms. Watson's decision is made more difficult by the fact that she has a vague understanding about what the possible effects of isotretinoin could be but does not know how the drug has affected the fetus if she is indeed pregnant. Yet terminating the pregnancy would involve active and direct killing, something those who oppose abortion would find unacceptable. Even if they accept the moral legitimacy of forgoing life support (as discussed in the cases in Chapter 9), they would not agree to active, direct killing even if it would spare the child certain suffering before it died. Only if ending this pregnancy were somehow morally different from killing a postnatal human, would those who object to mercy killing agree to abortion? What reasons, if any, can be given for this difference?

Even though she and her husband were not intending a pregnancy, Ms. Watson appears to be willing to carry her fetus to term unless there is something "really wrong." However, she is apparently open to abortion, at least in extreme cases of fetal deformity. How should she go about assessing possible problems she might find through genetic testing or sonograms? The easiest case to justify is probably the one that is incompatible with life. Especially if the baby were destined to suffer throughout a short existence. Teratogens in some cases cause physical deformities—such as the absence of limbs seen with the drug thalidomide. Does physical deformity per se justify abortion? If so, how serious would the deformity have to be? What about mental deficit? Does the mere fact that a child can be expected to have some physical or mental deficit provide a basis for aborting a fetus that Ms. Watson would otherwise carry to term?

Dr. Radlauer must first decide whether he considers the abortion plausible. Here his decision is similar to Ms. Watson's except it's not whether to undergo the actual abortion but what his role should be in providing information to his patient Then he has to address the difficult question of determining the extent of his cooperation in a project that he believes could have moral implications that may be unacceptable to him. Since the iPledge program obligates pharmacists to be involved in in-depth counseling on what might happen in the case of pregnancy, he should have considered these issues when agreeing to his employment. These issues should be faced in advance. He must either be willing to fulfill the duties of his employment (including this counseling) or make arrangements in advance for someone who can cover for him.

Normally, the pharmacist has duties of pharmaceutical care that require educating the patient with information that is likely to be meaningful to her in deciding about her situation. It might imply that Dr. Radlauer should give Ms. Watson relevant facts even if he believes it would be wrong for her to abort in this situation. However, there are some types of information that would be wrong to provide to a patient. If Ms. Watson were to carry a deformed child to term and then ask Dr. Radlauer whether certain overdoses might be lethal, just about everyone would agree it would be morally wrong—not to mention illegal—for the pharmacist to knowingly provide information where the intention was to kill the child. Is the only difference in the present case that abortion is legal while killing the postnatal child is not? Is the pharmacist's role here to provide any possibly relevant information even if he is convinced that great harm will result?

In effect, Dr. Radlauer is facing a situation in which he might try to invoke a claim to a right of conscientious objection to performing a duty normally implied by his professional role, i.e., the duty to provide counseling and education about the risks and benefits of alternative procedures that might be available to the patient. If Dr. Radlauer tries to refuse to provide counseling on the grounds it violates his conscience, he would, at minimum, need to meet certain standard criteria for ethically justifiable conscientious objection. This would include what is referred to as the criterion of publicity. That means he must be willing to state publicly what he is doing and what the moral reasons are for his action. He must also ground his action in deeply held authentic elements of his character. He must be willing to take the consequences of his action. In this case that could even include sanction by his employer or by the state licensing board.

Conscientious objection by a health professional raises unique problems beyond those involved in all actions of conscience. Professional roles, including that of pharmacist, are publicly sanctioned roles that create fiduciary obligations to patients. Patients cannot be expected to know when a pharmacist is withholding information unless, at minimum, the professional informs them. In some cases, a professional may even be obliged to provide services that are a normal part of the role even when they violate conscience. For example, the courts have repeatedly ordered physicians to provide life-prolonging treatments to patients who want them, even if the physician insists that it violates his or her conscience to do so.[4] There is considerable controversy over whether pharmacists can legally refuse to provide information that would likely lead to abortion.[5]

One approach would be to have Dr. Radlauer simply transfer the patient to a pharmacist willing to assist, but if he is morally opposed to the abortion, he may also object to helping her find a colleague of his willing to assist. If Dr. Radlauer is unable to resolve his problem by transferring the patient and providing such information that is seen to be an essential part of pharmaceutical care, he may be required to provide the information if he is to keep his state-sanctioned license.

Abortion Following Sexual Assault

Another major reason offered for abortion is that the pregnant woman was raped and, therefore, did not consent to the risk of getting pregnant. In such a case, however, as contrasted to the previous one, the fetus presumably is perfectly normal or at least not at significant medical risk. If the fetus is aborted, it is in order to serve the psychological well-being of the pregnant woman. Does the fact that the woman was exposed to pregnancy against her will justify aborting a presumably healthy fetus?

CASE 10-2   Postcoital Contraception of Abortion: Moral Choices Following
             a Rape

Virginia Gasson, Pharm.D., was covering the satellite pharmacy for the Green Valley Hospital's emergency department on the weekend with the assistance of a pharmacy technician. Dr. Gasson generally worked in the inpatient, oncology pharmacy of the hospital, but she often worked on call on weekends to earn extra money to pay back her student loans. Dr. Gasson had not worked in the emergency department before. Pharmacists in the emergency department were expected to not only fill prescriptions and counsel ambulatory patients, but also to spend time with patients and their families in the examination rooms, counseling them about their medications prior to discharge.

Dr. Gasson was returning to the pharmacy from the emergency room when the emergency medical technicians brought in a young woman who appeared to be the victim of some type of assault. Dr. Gasson shuddered in sympathy and continued to the pharmacy to complete the additional prescriptions that she was sure had stacked up in her absence. Dr. Gasson did not think about the young woman again until she received the physician assistant (PA)'s order sheet and medical summary for the patient. The young woman, 21-year-old Anna Witt, had been sexually assaulted and beaten while on her morning run.

CASE 10-2 *Continued.*

The PA had ordered a nonsteroidal anti-inflammatory agent (NSAID) for pain relief, an antibiotic as prophylactic treatment for a possible sexually transmitted disease, a 28-day course of HAART (highly active retroviral therapy), and Plan B. The PA wrote that he wanted the pharmacist "... to counsel the patient about the necessity of taking Plan B as ordered as well as the 3-drug combination to prevent HIV+.

Dr. Gasson realized that the PA had ordered Plan B because Ms. Witt was at risk of becoming pregnant. Dr. Gasson knew there was controversy about how the so-called morning-after pills work, but she believes their main mechanism is to modify the endometrium so as to disrupt the implantation of the ovum. Dr. Gasson's religious beliefs are quite strong regarding the sacredness of life, which she believes begins at the time of fertilization of the ovum, i.e., at conception. Any action that causes the endometrial wall to become hostile to implantation resulting in the premature, artificially induced expulsion of the newly conceived embryo, according to Dr. Gasson, is abortifacient and therefore prohibited.

Dr. Gasson took the medication orders back to the prescribing PA, Roger McCrystal, to explain to him that she could not dispense Plan B. Mr. McCrystal explained that the drug must be administered within 72 hours in order to be effective, and he did not see any reason for the patient to go elsewhere for the drug. Mr. McCrystal stated that he believed Ms. Witt was a competent adult and that she had told him she wanted to protect herself against pregnancy. "You have a duty to dispense the drug and counsel her in an unbiased manner on its appropriate use and potential side effects, Dr. Gasson," Mr. McCrystal stated. Dr. Gasson stood her ground and refused to dispense the medication. Mr. McCrystal replied, "This hospital has no religious affiliation. The pharmacy's policy is to fill all valid prescriptions."

Commentary

In contrast to the previous case, the medical status of the fetus does not provide any moral basis for aborting this potential pregnancy. Two reasons might be given. First, while Ms. Witt has no explicit physical health problems that lead her directly to seek to terminate any possible pregnancy, she might have mental health concerns. Surely, the trauma of the rape can be psychologically agonizing. Having the reminder of that horrid event during the rest of Ms. Witt's life could add to that trauma.

But if the woman's mental health is the basis for the abortion, Ms. Witt and Dr. Gasson would need more information before reaching a decision about how to respond. They would have to have some understanding about just how much mental trauma would be necessary to justify an abortion. Presumably any unwanted pregnancy is traumatic. If just any mental disturbance justified the abortion, then any woman who is upset about a pregnancy would be justified on these grounds. Case 10-5 later in this chapter looks at abortion for social and economic reasons. Is there a significant difference between abortion for the mental stress of a pregnancy following rape, on the one hand, and abortion for the stress caused by social and economic reasons or for a woman who simply does not want to be pregnant, on the other? If the reasoning is based on mental health, is there some minimal level of psychological trauma that is necessary to make the abortion morally justified? For example, would a real risk of suicide be necessary as some conservatives on abortion would claim, and if so, what level of risk would be appropriate? Or would any mental health risk be sufficient, as more liberally inclined commentators would suggest? Is there some level of mental suffering that would convince Dr. Gasson that Ms. Witt's use of the medication would be tolerable? Would adoption help abate some of this trauma, making the abortion less defensible?

Abortion following rape seems to command more sympathy than other cases involving similar levels of mental trauma. Could it be that there is some other reason beyond the psychological stress standing behind such intuitions? Some have argued that the morally special feature of rape is that in no conceivable way was the woman agreeing to take the risk of getting pregnant. Some philosophers have suggested that even if the fetus has the right to life in some strong sense, a woman should not be made to carry a pregnancy to term if she did not consent to the behavior that led to the pregnancy.[6] If it were technically possible, this could lead to the position that the fetus should be removed from the woman and incubated independently. Until such a procedure is technically possible, defenders of abortion following rape say that the woman has a right to remove the "intruding" fetus even if doing so results in the death of the fetus.

More conservative critics of abortion reject this reasoning and point out that the end result is what, to them, is evil, the killing of the fetus. In the previous chapter, we discussed the Catholic doctrine of indirect or double-effect killing. This doctrine tolerates an evil if that evil is not intended, even if the evil is foreseen. They consider that this could justify removing a cancerous uterus even if the woman with the cancer happens to be pregnant as long as the death of the fetus is not the purpose of the removal of the uterus and the abortion is not a means to the desired end (which it would not be).

By contrast, if the woman claimed that she simply desired to be able to lead her life nonpregnant as she was prior to the rape, the abortion would be the means to her desired end and, according to Catholics and others who rely on the principle of indirect or double effect, the abortion would not be justified.

There is another issue in this case. Regardless of whether Ms. Witt decides the abortion is justified, Dr. Gasson also faces an important moral choice. Discussing the abortion option is not, and never has been, prohibited, but it would in this case violate Dr. Gasson's conscientiously held convictions. Insofar as the informed consent doctrine requires presenting the alternatives that the patient would reasonably want to know about, there is good reason to believe that discussion of the abortion option is required morally and legally as part of the consent process. If the medication prescribed for Ms. Witt functions as an abortifacient, either Dr. Gasson or someone else would have the obligation to inform the patient about the treatment alternatives.

Nevertheless, there are some procedures that would be such a dramatic violation of the conscience of the health provider that he or she would not be expected to discuss them and, in fact, might be expected to refuse to discuss them. For example, in some jurisdictions suicide is not illegal, and it could be considered a possible option for someone diagnosed as having a malignancy, yet it seems obvious that no health professional is required or expected to discuss the suicide option as part of the consent process for the treatment of the cancer. Likewise, most analysts of professional ethics hold that a provider is usually not required to be a party to a procedure that violates his or her conscience.

In some situations the problem might be resolved by having the pharmacist ask a colleague to take on the task. There are two problems with that strategy, however. First, Dr. Gasson is providing weekend coverage. Apparently, the only other person with her is a technician. Delaying until regular staff return would not meet Ms. Witt's needs. Would it be reasonable for her to ask Mr. McCrystal to do the counseling? If so, could he also dispense the medication?

This suggests a second problem with the strategy of transferring responsibility to a colleague. If Dr. Gasson really believes that the use of the drug would constitute murder of the embryonic human being, does it make sense morally for her to refer to someone else? Assuming she concludes that she cannot dispense or counsel and that she cannot refer, what is she to do?

Abortion to Save the Life of the Pregnant Woman

In the previous case we considered whether a rape victim would be justified in terminating a pregnancy if she were so distraught that she was suicidal. That is a special case of the general problem of whether abortion is justified when the life of the pregnant woman is in jeopardy. That case does not happen as often in the era of advanced obstetrical care, but it does still occur, as, for example, in the case of a woman who has a history of a ruptured uterus and is pregnant again and whose thin uterine wall is likely to rupture. Even some ethics commentators known to be strongly opposed to abortion have been challenged to acknowledge an exception in such cases. One example of such as case is a pregnant woman with systemic lupus erythematosus (SLE).

CASE 10-3   Abortion to Save a Pregnant Woman's Life

At midnight, a 19-year-old primigravida (woman who is pregnant for the first time), Emelina Peña, at 14 weeks, was seen in a general hospital emergency room with complaints of dizziness, decreased urine output, and difficulty breathing. Ms. Peña was accompanied by her husband, Manuel, who reported that his wife had a history of systemic lupus erythematosus. Before her pregnancy, Ms. Peña had been hospitalized because of cardiac involvement and pleural effusion. She had been on high-dose corticosteroids prior to her pregnancy to control rheumatic flares. She had discontinued all of her medications when she found out she was pregnant. She had also avoided seeing her physician because, as she told her husband, "He will want me to be on those drugs, and that is no good for the baby." The past few days, Ms. Peña had become sicker and sicker, so her husband decided to bring her to the emergency room. The ER physician diagnosed possible pericarditis, serious hypertension, and pending renal failure.

Perry Sledge, Pharm.D., was the clinical pharmacist for the intensive care units of the hospital. Dr. Sledge knew there was an SLE patient in the unit when the first order

CASE 10-3 *Continued.*

appeared for high-dose glucocorticoids in the pharmacy. When Dr. Sledge delivered the medications to the unit, Roger Bishop, M.D., the obstetrician on call, asked him to join the rest of the team for a family conference regarding Ms. Peña's case. Dr. Bishop began the conference by stating, "The best treatment for your wife is delivery of the baby. At this stage of gestation, the baby will not survive. If we treat your wife with the proper medications to control her numerous systemic problems, the baby will most certainly be irreversibly harmed anyway." Mr. Peña responded, "So there is no way to save my Emelina and the baby?" Dr. Bishop replied, "I believe that the delivery of the baby is the only way to guarantee your wife's life." Dr. Sledge was extremely uncomfortable with what Dr. Bishop told Mr. Peña. Dr. Sledge was opposed to abortion, but he knew that Ms. Peña could die from renal failure if a caesarean section was not performed soon.

Commentary

The plan proposed by Dr. Bishop is to sacrifice the fetus in order to save the pregnant woman. This would constitute a directly intended killing of the fetus, something that we saw in Chapter 9 was unacceptable to many in both the religious and secular worlds. The killing would be the means of accomplishing an admittedly good end of saving the pregnant woman, but as a means to a good end, the doctrine of double effect always considers the means intended. According to the double-effect doctrine, intended killing is morally unacceptable. If one believes, as Dr. Sledge apparently does, that intentional termination of the fetus's life is morally wrong, the proposed termination of the pregnancy becomes controversial. The most militant opponents of intended abortion hold that such abortion is always unacceptable, even if it is necessary to save the pregnant woman's life. Holders of this view claim that if failing to abort leads to the woman's death, this is nevertheless not a "killing." Rather it is thought of as letting an evil occur. The evil is foreseen but not directly intended, a difference that holders of the double-effect doctrine consider crucial. Those who take the doctrine of double effect seriously may justify letting both die, if necessary, on the grounds that allowing a death—even two deaths—to occur is not the same as intentionally causing a death. They hold firmly to the view that what is wrong is not the death per se, but intentional human action that causes the death.

Some might argue that the intention is to save the mother's life, not kill the fetus. That reasoning is unacceptable, however, to proponents of the doctrine of double effect. They claim that if one intends a good end (such as saving the woman's life), one also intends all actions taken to accomplish that end. The abortion is considered a means to save the woman. In this case, they insist that one necessarily intends the fetus's death if the abortion is intended to save the woman. The only case in which an action that caused a fetus's death would be acceptable, according to strict proponents of the doctrine, would be situations such as removal of a cancerous uterus of a pregnant woman. Here they claim that the hysterectomy is the normal treatment of the cancer and that the killing of the fetus occurs only secondary to the hysterectomy, not as a means of treating the cancer. This is seen by the fact that the hysterectomy is exactly the procedure one would use for uterine cancer even if the woman were not pregnant. By contrast, in Ms. Peña's case, what Dr. Bishop proposes makes no sense if she is not pregnant. Killing the fetus is, according to defenders of the doctrine, a direct means to the good end and is therefore intended and morally unacceptable.

Of course, those who are liberal on abortion would not be as troubled by the plan of sacrificing the fetus to save the pregnant woman. They are willing to accept abortion for much lesser reasons. They might see the ending of the fetus's life as tragic but morally tolerable to serve a worthy purpose. Saving a woman's life would certainly in their eyes be a particularly worthy purpose.

The most interesting position is the intermediate one held by those who generally are opposed to abortion but are troubled by the choice of the death of the pregnant woman *and* the fetus, when termination of the pregnancy could save at least one. Not all who are generally opposed to abortion and who usually take the doctrine of double effect seriously will go to the wall in the kind of case presented here. They may view the case as a choice between one death and two and conclude that aborting to save the life of the pregnant woman is the one exception to the abortion prohibition.

Dr. Sledge apparently opposes the abortion. One plan he could consider would be to point out to Dr. Bishop and Ms. Peña that with aggressive treatment there is a chance that both the fetus and Ms. Peña could survive or at least that the pregnancy could be maintained until the fetus was viable, at approximately 25 weeks gestation. He would have to disclose that the results of such attempts are not promising, but this option seems not to have been presented by Dr. Bishop to Ms. and Mr. Peña. Assuming Dr. Sledge concludes that abortion in this circumstance would be unacceptable, what are his options beyond making sure that the option of attempting to save both the pregnant woman and the fetus needs to be presented?

Abortion and the Mentally Incapacitated Woman

Another difficult situation in which abortion might be considered involves women who become pregnant but are not mentally competent to consent to sex. In some ways the situation is like the rape. The pregnancy is not the result of a consensual act. In the case of the mentally incapacitated woman, however, she may not have resisted the sexual encounter. In fact, she may have voiced an approval, albeit one that may not be truly voluntary.

This scenario poses another problem, however. If the woman is incompetent, she may not be capable of raising the child. Thus both the woman and the child may be at risk.

That suggests still another difference. In the case of rape, the victim is capable of making her own choices about terminating the pregnancy while in the case of the woman with severely diminished mental capacity, someone else will have to make the choice for her. In the following case, a health care team, including a pharmacist, confront the problem of whether to push for terminating a pregnancy in one of their incompetent patients.

CASE 10-4   Abortion for the Mentally Incapacitated Patient

The members of the community mental health team for the county's independent living facilities or group homes gathered monthly to review the treatment plans and progress of the various residents. The main topic of concern this month was the status of one of the female residents, Leigh Shockley, a 37-year-old with a long history of mental illness who had become pregnant. She was diagnosed more than 20 years ago with chronic, paranoid schizophrenia. Although she was presently living in a group home under moderate supervision, she had a history of long periods of institutionalization. Ms. Shockley either did not know or would not tell who the father was.

The psychiatrist on the team, Dr. Cyril Bell, spoke first, remarking, "You know, there was a time when sterilization was a prerequisite to successful placement in a community-based mental health setting. Looks like that policy would have prevented our present problem with Ms. Shockley."

Paul Starkman, Pharm.D., the pharmacist member of the team, was fully convinced that Ms. Shockley would not be capable of responsible motherhood. Dr. Starkman had worked with Ms. Shockley several times in the past trying to help her independently take her medications. To date, Dr. Starkman had been unsuccessful. Ms. Shockley remained essentially noncompliant. Unless the nurse in the group home gave her the drugs, she "forgot" to take them.

Dr. Starkman expressed his strong reservations about Ms. Shockley's capacity, "I am concerned that the experience of pregnancy, not to mention the experience of labor and delivery, will be too much for Ms. Shockley. I think it is cruel to put her through this whole process when we all know she will have to give the child up for adoption after it is born. How would she ever be able to care for a baby when she cannot even care for herself? Furthermore, there is an increased possibility of fetal defects because of the medications she currently takes and her age. Considering all of these factors, I believe that an abortion should be performed."

Dr. Bell responded, "I think that Ms. Shockley is capable, at least some of the time. She told me very clearly that she understands that she is pregnant and that she wants to keep the baby. Of course in the next breath, she accused one of the other residents of tampering with her food. We would have to work through the legal process of declaring her incompetent and appointing a guardian if we wanted to perform an abortion even though she will not give consent. Since you feel so strongly that an abortion is the best option, would you like to persuade her, Dr. Starkman?"

Commentary

Ms. Shockley is clearly suffering from a serious mental problem. Not all mentally ill persons are incompetent to nurture their children or to make health-care decisions, however. Should Dr. Starkman and Dr. Bell treat Ms. Shockley as mentally incompetent or as one who, though compromised, is capable of making her own choices? What difference would it make?

The suggestion of Dr. Bell that Dr. Starkman try to persuade Ms. Shockley to consent to the abortion seems to imply that he believes her to be competent to make her own choices. Can a case be made that her decision should be the guiding one here? If so, would the abortion be for the welfare of the child, who might suffer if he or she comes into a world without adequate parenting, or should it be for the welfare of the pregnant woman? Should this be treated as a case of a fetus with a potential genetic anomaly inherited from its mother, or of a case posing questions about the environment in which the child will be raised. Does either provide a basis for terminating this pregnancy?

Dr. Starkman seems less persuaded that Ms. Shockley is competent to make the abortion decision herself. Assuming he is correct, is there someone else with the authority to decide that this pregnancy should be stopped? Would a health professional have such authority? Would a legal guardian have to be appointed, and if so, would that person have such authority? Would a judge properly be able to make such a choice?

Abortion for Socioeconomic Reasons

The most controversial abortion cases are also the most frequent. They are abortions desired by women who simply do not want to be pregnant—at least at the present time and under the current circumstances. Either the woman is not ready to have children or cannot afford to care for them. These abortions, illustrated in the following case, are often referred to as abortions for socioeconomic reasons.

CASE 10-5   Abortion for Socioeconomic Reasons

Riley Dansky, Pharm.D., worked in the drug information center of a large medical center that included a 500-bed hospital and a multiservice ambulatory clinic. Ever since the medical center's institutional review board had approved a clinical study of single intramuscular dose (50 mg/m2) methotrexate followed a few days later by 800 micro gm of intravaginal misoprostol for the medical termination of early pregnancy, Dr. Dansky had received numerous questions from obstetricians with questions about effectiveness, side effects, and the pharmacology of the two drugs. The call from Alicia Erden, MD, a family practitioner with a large obstetrical practice, was also about the methotrexate/misoprostol combination. Dr. Erden asked a few questions about the pharmacology, dosing, and toxicity of methotrexate. Dr. Dansky wanted to make certain that he provided the information Dr. Erden needed, so he asked a few clarifying questions. "Women who are the best candidates for medical abortions should be between the ages of 19 and 40 and within the first 60 days of pregnancy or less. Does your patient fit within these parameters?"

Dr. Erden replied, "Yes. She's a 28-year-old, single mother of two children who are both in grade school. She's just barely making enough money to support her family, and she's trying to go to night school to help get promoted to a better paying job. She just can't afford another baby right now. She's a large woman, tall and heavy set, so I need your advice about the proper dose."

Dr. Dansky hadn't asked for all of this personal information about the patient, but now that he had received it, he was troubled by what he learned. He believed that abortion, surgical or chemical, was justified to protect the mother's health in cases of severe diabetes or hypertension, for example, or because the fetus had a genetic anomaly that

CASE 10-5 *Continued.*

would result in certain death. In the case of Dr. Erden's patient, however, there was nothing wrong with the pregnant woman's or the fetus's health. The healthy fetus was being aborted because of lack of finances. Dr. Dansky had not given this reason for abortion much thought, but now he was being asked to support such an abortion, at least indirectly, by providing information that would guarantee the successful termination of the pregnancy.

Commentary

If the fetus of Dr. Erden's patient is considered to have the same moral standing as a postnatal human, use of the drugs to produce an abortion would be indefensible. This can be seen by how society would react if a mother proposed to kill one of her existing children because of her financial situation. Almost certainly she would not even consider such an idea, and if she acted on the thought, she would be guilty of homicide. That she was economically desperate would not work as a justification.

Likewise, the case would pose no problem if someone believed that a fetus at this stage of development had no moral standing whatsoever. Dr. Dansky seems to have adopted an intermediary position typical of many who have moderate views on abortion. He is willing to support abortion for serious reasons, such as the health of the pregnant woman or serious genetic anomaly. This strongly suggests that Dr. Dansky admits that fetuses have some moral standing but not the same standing as that of postnatal children.

Many who hold this view end up trading off the interests of the fetus for the interests of the pregnant woman and others who also have an interest in the situation (such as her other children). This could imply that the more serious the interest of the woman, the more justifiable the abortion. However, they may also view moral standing as increasing with fetal development, meaning that moderate interests of the woman could justify abortion in the earliest days of the pregnancy while only more serious interests would be sufficient in later stages of pregnancy. Is this mode of reasoning an acceptable one for Dr. Dansky to adopt?

Assuming this approach is acceptable in principle, what role should the pregnant woman's finances play in making these decisions? There seems to be something questionable about forcing a low-income woman to make a choice between her fetus and the interests of her other children based on finances. Some would argue that society should never put women in such a position, but assuming that it does, should the woman be able to base her abortion decision on these economic factors?

Sterilization

Another intervention that has traditionally raised moral controversy in biomedical ethics is sterilization. Designed to permanently prohibit fertility, it has run afoul of

Catholics and others who apply natural law reasoning to matters of medical morality.[7] They hold that there are certain "natural ends" of human beings that are associated with certain bodily organs and tissues. One of these natural ends of the human is said to be procreation and that any directly intended interference with this function violates the moral law.

Others, who may not share this natural law reasoning, also encounter moral problems related to sterilization. Other women have reported finding it extremely difficult to convince physicians to sterilize them, especially if they are not considered too old for childbearing or had not already given birth to a number of children.[8] Low-income women have reported being pressured by health care professionals to consent to being sterilized out of a paternalistic concern by the providers that pregnancy would not be good for either the woman or her offspring, as in the following case.

CASE 10-6   Sterilization of an Economically Deprived Woman

It was a busy afternoon in Center Pharmacy, a community pharmacy in a low-income area of a large metropolitan city. Paul Louie, Pharm.D., the owner of Center Pharmacy, was focusing on patient counseling this afternoon rather than filling prescriptions. Although Center Pharmacy filled numerous prescriptions, Dr. Louie attempted to counsel each patient. In fact, he was so serious about this obligation that he had remodeled the pharmacy to include a "counseling booth." Out of the corner of his eye, he noticed that Sona Simms had entered the pharmacy. Dr. Louie had counseled Ms. Simms, who was 19 years old and unmarried, on her prescriptions for prenatal vitamins for her first pregnancy and various prescriptions for her son, Nathan, since his birth 2 years ago. Ms. Simms was unusual in that she had completed high school in spite of her pregnancy. Dr. Louie knew that Ms. Simms had struggled to find employment without success. Her grandmother helped look after Nathan.

After Ms. Simms received her prescription from the technician, she waited to talk with Dr. Louie. Dr. Louie noted that her prescription was for prenatal vitamins. Ms. Simms sighed as she caught the look of surprise and disappointment on Dr. Louie's face. "I know. I didn't plan on being pregnant. Seems my doctor, Dr. Mullen, doesn't think I should get pregnant again either. Dr. Mullen spent a lot of time today really pushing me to have my tubes tied after I deliver this baby. He says he can take care of it at the same time that I deliver. He said two kids, no husband, and no job are bad enough, let alone the chance of bringing more babies into the world. God knows, I'm having trouble making ends meet, but I don't think I want to do this. If I have my tubes tied it means I'll be sterile, right?"

Dr. Louie affirmed that Ms. Simms was correct; she would indeed be sterile. Dr. Louie had serious moral reservations about all sterilization, preferring reversible methods. Dr. Louie wondered if he should say something to Ms. Simms's physician, Rodney Mullen, MD, one of the few obstetricians willing to work in the prenatal clinic several blocks from Center Pharmacy. Dr. Louie wonders if this is standard operating procedure for Dr. Mullen with all of his low-income, single, pregnant patients. What should he say to Ms. Simms? Dr. Louie is not only concerned about his own moral objections to sterilization, but also his belief that Ms. Simms is being coerced into a procedure rather than freely giving her consent.

Commentary

This case presents a complex combination of religious, medical, and personal issues for both Dr. Louie and Ms. Simms. Focus first on the ethical issues about sterilization. What is the reason for Dr. Louie's resistance to the sterilization? One possibility is that he opposes all sterilizations as a violation of the moral natural law. Surely, sterilization will permanently disrupt the reproductive function, considered by many, including many Catholics, to be a primary end of marriage.

Nothing in the case indicated that Dr. Louie was Catholic. But there are other reasons why some people have traditionally objected to sterilizations. Especially among Protestant and liberal, secular thinkers there is a belief that keeping one's options open is a good thing. Permanent loss of fertility has been seen as foreclosing options. Such objectors have a strong preference for temporary forms of birth control. Would the advantage of keeping options open justify Dr. Louie's resistance to the sterilization in this case?

Dr. Mullen, however, is also thinking about Ms. Simms's future. He appears to think that she would have a brighter one if she had no more children. Sterilization of young, unmarried females is controversial. In fact, often they have difficulty convincing physicians to perform the procedure because physicians, reasoning the way Dr. Louie does, like options to be kept open. But Dr. Mullen's attitude is different. He appears to think that, in this case, the harms of any future pregnancy, no matter what the circumstances, will outweigh the benefits.

Ms. Simms appears to have her own reasons that may not conform to either Dr. Louie's or Dr. Mullen's reasoning. Young women from low-income families often place very high value on their fertility. They may not be as future-oriented as either Dr. Louie or Dr. Mullen. They may see their identity and their future happiness as tied to procreation in ways that neither the middle-class male physician nor the middle-class male pharmacist can understand. Does that suggest that both the pharmacist and the physician should stay out of Ms. Simms's decision-making? Does the convergence of Dr. Louie's thinking with that of Ms. Simms justify his support for her point of view? What are Dr. Louie's options?

Contraception

The third area of moral concern related to fertility and birth is contraception. Until the 1930s most of the major religious traditions had moral objections to efforts to control fertility through contraception. The techniques that were available were not very reliable, and such efforts were seen as infringing on the traditional "duties of marriage" as well as furthering promiscuity in sexual relations.

In 1930, the Lambeth Conference signaled the willingness of the Anglican tradition (Episcopalians in the United States) to open the door cautiously to some fertility control. The other Protestant traditions soon followed,[9] but Catholic moral theology reinforced its traditional view that all sexual acts had to be open to the possibility of procreation as well as express the unity of marriage.[10] The mainstream of Catholic thought acknowledged that the rhythm method of fertility control, which was considered "natural," might be acceptable, but no barrier methods were considered tolerable because they interfered with the natural ends of marriage.

By the 1960s, some Catholics were beginning to consider such strong prohibitions as unnecessary and were becoming more open to the use of the new oral contraceptives.[11] The majority of a Papal Commission considered such an opening acceptable, but with the issuance of the papal encyclical *Humane Vitae* in 1968, a condemnation of all except so-called natural methods was reaffirmed.[12] Similar disputes arose within the Jewish tradition, with its commitment to the duty to procreate seen as being in conflict with the more liberal stance of recognizing self-determination regarding fertility.[13]

There is increasing evidence that all people have underlying value commitments that influence their medical decisions. These value commitments often are manifested in decisions about birth control, and even those who attempt to be fair and neutral may find themselves using language that reflects those value commitments.[14] As seen in the next case, pharmaceutical care providers may find themselves in positions in which their often hidden values may come into play as they teach or counsel about fertility control.

CASE 10-7   Biased Counseling: Teaching About Birth Control

Although Peggy Walters, a third-year doctor of pharmacy student, had only worked at the University Student Health Service Pharmacy for 2 weeks, she had already noticed a great deal of difference in the counseling practices of 2 of the pharmacists on staff regarding the use of oral contraceptives. Grace Dossey, Pharm.D., is single-minded in her beliefs about preventing pregnancies in young, unmarried women. Dr. Dossey told Ms. Walters, "Approximately 1 million adolescents become pregnant each year. Unintended pregnancies continue to occur, despite the availability of highly effective contraceptives. I believe it is vital that pharmacists encourage contraceptive methods, especially oral contraceptives. We have to do everything we can to prevent these young women from getting pregnant since it is unlikely they will be good parents."

Ms. Walters had seen Dr. Dossey aggressively "sell" contraception to almost every student she saw, whether they were picking up a prescription for contraceptives or not. Whenever she spoke with patients, Dr. Dossey emphasizes the health benefits of taking oral contraceptives, such as fewer menstrual cramps, decreased incidence of fibrocystic breast disease, and protective effects against ovarian and endometrial cancer.

The opinions of Timothy Sagbah, Pharm.D., the other pharmacist in the Student Health Pharmacy with strong views about contraception, could not be more opposite from those of Dr. Dossey. Dr. Sagbah, a devote Catholic, participates in the university's Celebrate Life organization that routinely and peacefully protests at a local abortion clinic. Dr. Sagbah makes every effort to convince female students who present a prescription for oral contraceptives to think again. Dr. Sagbah so emphasizes the health dangers of oral contraceptives, such as headaches, depression, cardiovascular problems, and breast cancer, that he often is successful in dissuading patients from getting the prescription filled. However, Ms. Walters has heard Dr. Sagbah tell patients, if he was unsuccessful in convincing them, that he would not fill the prescription because he believes that oral

CASE 10-7 *Continued.*

contraceptives act as an endometrial abortifacient and he opposes abortion. If the student persists in getting the prescription filled, Dr. Sagbah leaves the prescription for another pharmacist to fill the next day.

Ms. Walters does not think counseling should incorporate explicit moral dimensions. Furthermore, students who use the Student Health Service Pharmacy have no choice about who will be on duty, Dr. Dossey or Dr. Sagbah, when they get their prescriptions filled. Ms. Walters believes that pharmacists have a duty to provide unbiased, factual information on contraceptive methods, in a comfortable environment. She is convinced that neither Dr. Dossey nor Dr. Sagbah is fulfilling this duty.

Commentary

Those who are more accepting of birth control are likely to accuse Dr. Sagbah of being biased in his presentation. However, those who are critical will make similar accusations against Dr. Dossey. Many may find themselves sympathetic with Ms. Walters' desire to be more neutral and stick to the facts in a value-free manner.

This matter of value-neutrality, however, is rather complex. Everything that Dr. Sagbah and Dr. Dossey said appears to have a basis in fact. It was not that the two pharmacists were purposely saying untrue things about birth control. In fact, what they said could be supported by good scientific data. Yet each had selected the data presented.

Ms. Walters would like to avoid such biased selection of facts, but she may be in a position that is not as different from her supervisors as she might expect. Any health educator has a virtually infinite array of medical information at hand. He or she must select those data that seem most relevant and important. Those selections must be made on the basis of one's beliefs and values about what is important. Every communication with a patient, at least to some extent, will be shaped in this way.

Assuming Dr. Sagbah strongly believes, based on his knowledge of the data and his sense of what is important, that artificial methods of birth control cause problems that are not worth the risks, how should he communicate his understanding to the patient? Similarly, Dr. Dossey has strong feelings that oral contraceptives and other methods that some call artificial have benefits that far exceed the risks. She is in a position that is more similar to Dr. Sagbah's than many people realize. They both have to choose from an array of possible facts worth communicating. Neither will be able to tell "all the facts." There are too many, and some are trivial. Neither pharmacist will be able to stick to just the facts. They will have to make evaluative judgments about which facts to present and how much emphasis to place on them. They will also have to decide whether filling the prescription conflicts with their view and, if so, whether they would be willing to fill it.

Moreover, those who like Ms. Walters have values that are somewhere in between will have to select from an enormous number of pharmacological studies, the package of facts they consider important. They will have to decide whether to willingly fill the prescription or, if they determine that it would violate their conscience, refuse to do so, yielding to a colleague even if it inconveniences the patient.

Trying to be value neutral in communicating with patients is more complicated than it sounds. Words with shades of meaning will have to be communicated. Moreover, some health care providers may believe that some options are inherently so immoral that they simply cannot be presented in a cold, hard, value-neutral manner. Infanticide as a method of controlling family size has been practiced in some cultures, and it is not unheard of in contemporary Western culture. Yet no health care provider should ever list among the methods available for limiting family size killing the child after birth. Only those methods that are morally and legally plausible should be presented.

The other major issue for the pharmacy care provider is whether she should simply refuse to participate in services for patients that violate her conscience. If so, will that not leave the educational task for matters like abortion, sterilization, and birth control to those who have not disqualified themselves, making the group systematically skewed toward a more accepting position? This problem of whether pharmacists may conscientiously object to dispensing medications about which they have moral objections is the focus of Case 10-2 in this chapter.

CASE 10-8   Transdermal Contraceptive Patches

When Lloyd Howe, Pharm.D., was elected to the Haworth School Board he had no idea that he would be called upon to offer professional advice from a pharmacy perspective. Mr. Howe found himself at the center of a debate regarding a proposal to allow the use of transdermal contraceptive patches in the high school with the county's highest percentage of pregnant and parenting teens. The proposal was brought to the school board by interested parents and students. The proposal also had the support of the County Health Department. Although transdermal contraceptive patches were available in the County Health Department's Family Planning Clinics, the proposal was to make the patches available at little to no cost in the school-based health center without the requirement of parental consent. Those who proposed the plan were convinced that the use of the patches was covered under state law permitting dispensing of contraceptives to minors without parental consent. When the proposal was initially brought to the school board, the chairperson asked Dr. Howe to provide answers to several technical pharmaceutical questions, such as: What are the actions of the patches? What are the short- and long-term adverse effects? Are there any age limits on its use? How compliant are adolescent girls with the patch? Dr. Howe agreed to provide the answers at the next school board meeting that would also be the setting for a public hearing on the proposal.

The following week, Dr. Howe stood before the standing-room-only crowd at the public hearing and stated, "Transdermal contraceptive patches deliver 150 microg norelgestromin and 20 microg ethinyl estradiol daily. The contraceptive patch offers once weekly dosing, and several studies involving adolescents indicate a good level of compliance and no pregnancies during the study period.[15] I believe that the contraceptive patches are best for women who are in a stable, monogamous relationship, as there is the possibility for an increased risk of sexually transmitted diseases with the patch, since

CASE 10-8 *Continued.*

users are less likely to use condoms. The most common side effect is irritation at the sight. There are generally few side effects among adolescents. The patches have been used safely with adolescents as long as there is intensive counseling before and after receiving the patches."

The chairperson thanked Dr. Howe for his remarks and then opened the floor for comments. Dr. Howe lost track of the number of people who passionately spoke for or against the proposal, but some comments really stood out in his mind. A local minister stated, "I believe that contraception is immoral and should not be used by anyone, let alone a minor who cannot give valid consent for such a procedure."

A mother asked, "If I have to give my permission for my daughter to go on a field trip, why shouldn't I be asked my permission for something as important as contraception— whatever form it takes?"

A student countered this comment with the following, "Any teen old enough to get pregnant is old enough to make decisions about contraception."

A mother of a minority student argued, "I'm afraid that my daughter will be pushed into using these patches against her will."

A school nurse stated, "We are trying to keep these girls from getting pregnant until they are out of high school. It is a fact that adolescents who have given birth are at higher risk of becoming pregnant than are other adolescents."

A community activist got a round of applause when he stated, "I am a taxpayer, and I support all of these children who are the outcome of teenage pregnancies. Since I have to pay for this, I think I should have a say in whether children will be conceived by teenagers when there is a simple, effective method to prevent pregnancy.

After the lengthy and emotional hearing Dr. Howe realized that the drug information he had provided might be helpful in answering questions about the therapeutic use of transdermal contraceptive patches but that it was not sufficient to help the school board make a decision that involved the issues of personal autonomy, instruments of social control, discrimination, and moral beliefs about contraception in general.

Commentary

It is tempting to say that Dr. Howe should divide his involvement into two roles. He might first be seen as playing the role of pharmacy educator by providing the pharmacological facts about contraceptive patches. That seems to be the role he was playing when he addressed the meeting. But he will soon be forced to cast a vote on the proposal to establish the contraceptive patch program. At that point he might think of himself as a school board member making a public policy choice just like the other members of the board.

The problem here, however, is whether this role division is possible. He may realize that, as in the previous case, what a pharmacist counsels necessarily involves value choices in the selection of data to be presented as well as in the choice of words, the latter possibly conveying evaluative judgments that cannot be seen as "purely factual." For example, what does it mean when Dr. Howe said that the contraceptive patches are best for women who are in a stable, monogamous relationship. Is it a "fact" from the pharmacological literature that it should be used for women in a stable, monogamous relationship but not for those in unstable relations? That seems obviously to go beyond providing just the facts. There may be more subtle value judgments as well. For example, his claim that "the patches have been used safely with adolescents" is more complicated than it appears. The pharmacological studies on which that claim is based probably conveyed that this statement could be made with some statistical degree of certainty. Does Dr. Howe mean it is 100% certain that all adolescents who rely on the contraceptive patch will not have problems with safety, or, based on the data, can this statement only be made with a tolerable level of certainty? Is Dr. Howe also saying that the risks are justified given the envisioned benefits? Is there any way that Dr. Howe can avoid transmitting his authority as a pharmacological expert, thereby influencing the opinions of those at the meeting and the votes of the other members of the school board? Should that be Dr. Howe's goal?

The issues of this chapter, which traditionally arose in the context of abortion, sterilization, and contraception, are increasingly being seen in newer problems related to genetics and birth technologies designed to enhance fertility. The cases in the next chapter present some of the moral controversies related to these new technologies.

Notes

1. For further discussion of the ethics of abortion see Callahan, Daniel. *Abortion: Law, Choice, and Morality.* New York: Macmillan, 1970; Feinberg, Joel, Editor. *The Problem of Abortion.* Belmont, CA: Wadsworth Publishing Co., 1973; Bayles, Michael D. *Reproductive Ethics.* Englewood Cliffs, NJ: Prentice-Hall, 1984; Noonan, John T. *The Morality of Abortion: Legal and Historical Perspectives.* Cambridge, MA.: Harvard University Press, 1970; and Dworkin, Ronald. *Life's Dominion: An Argument about Abortion, Euthanasia, and Individual Freedom.* New York: Vintage Books, 1994.

2. McCormick, Richard A. "Who or What Is the Preembryo?" *Kennedy Institute of Ethics Journal* 1 (1991): 1–15, esp. 4, 9, 11–12.

3. Hellegers, A. "Fetal Development." *Theological Studies* 31 (March 1970): 3–9.

4. *In the Matter of Baby K,* 832 F.Supp. 1022 (E.D. Va. 1993); Veatch, Robert M., and Carol Mason Spicer. "Medically Futile Care: The Role of the Physician in Setting Limits." *American Journal of Law and Medicine* 18, nos. 1 and 2 (1992): 15–36.

5. Weinstein, Bruce D. "Do Pharmacists Have a Right to Refuse to Fill Prescriptions for Abortifacient Drugs?" *Law, Medicine, and Health Care* 20 (Fall 1992): 220–223; Brushwood, David B. "Conscientious Objection and Abortifacient Drugs." *Clinical Therapeutics* 15 (January-February 1993): 204–212; Brushwood, David B. "Must a Catholic Hospital Inform a Rape Victim of the Availability of the 'Morning-after Pill'?" *American Journal of Hospital Pharmacy* 47, no. 2 (1990): 395–396; Cantor, J., and K. Baum. "The Limits of Conscientious Objection—May Pharmacists Refuse to Fill Prescriptions for Emergency Contraception?" *New England Journal of Medicine* 351 (2004): 2008–2012.

6. Thomson, Judith Jarvis. "A Defense of Abortion." *Philosophy and Public Affairs* 1, no. 1 (1971): 47–66.

7. Ashley, Benedict M., and Kevin D. O'Rourke. *Healthcare Ethics: A Theological Analysis.* Third Edition. St. Louis, MO: Catholic Health Association of the United States, 1989.

8. Scrimshaw, Susan C., and Bernard Pasquariella. "Obstacles to Sterilization in One Community." *Family Planning Perspectives* 2 (1970): 40–42.

9. Fagley, Richard M. *The Population Explosion and Christian Responsibility.* New York: Oxford University Press, 1960.

10. Noonan, John T. *Contraception: A History of Its Treatment by the Catholic Theologians and Canonists.* Cambridge, MA: Harvard University Press, 1966.

11. Callahan, Daniel, Editor. *The Catholic Case for Contraception.* New York: Macmillan, 1969.

12. Pope Paul VI. "Encyclical Letter on the Regulation of Births (July 25, 1968)." In *Medical Ethics: Sources of Catholic Teachings.* Kevin D. O'Rourke and Philip Boyle, Editors. St. Louis, MO: Catholic Health Association of the United States, 1989, pp. 85–91.

13. Feldman, David M. *Birth Control in Jewish Law.* New York: New York University Press, 1968.

14. Veatch, Robert M. *Value-Freedom in Science and Technology.* Missoula, MT: Scholars Press, 1976.

15. Rubinstein, M. L., B. L. Halpern-Felsher, and C. E. Irwin, Jr. "An Evaluation of the Use of the Transdermal Contraceptive Patch in Adolescents." *Journal of Adolescent Health* 34, no. 5 (2004): 395–401.

11

Genetics, Birth, and the Biological Revolution

In addition to the moral problems related to contraception, sterilization, and abortion, which were addressed in Chapter 10, newer, more complex ethical questions are emerging in connection with the processes of conception, prenatal development, and birth.[1] Some of these issues are related to the increasing importance of the science of genetics. For many years we have had a vague idea that certain diseases were inherited, but only recently have we had the precise knowledge and ability to determine the chances that a disease will be transmitted and to counsel the prospective parents about intervention alternatives. At first, it may not appear that pharmacists often encounter these issues, but, especially in the hospital setting where pharmacists may serve on ethics committees or in the capacity of supplying relevant medications, these issues can be very much on the pharmacist's agenda. For example, a pharmacist may be involved in dispensing an abortifacient drug whose use is based on judgments derived from genetic counseling. Even if the pharmacist is not directly involved in these issues, a brief examination of the cases involving the biological revolution will help complete the exploration of ethics in the health professions.

The first level of these issues involves counseling that requires assessing and informing parents whether a condition is inherited and, if so, how. It may now involve prenatal sampling of amniotic fluid or chorionic villi blood sampling that permit either chromosomal or biochemical determinations of whether a fetus already gestating is afflicted with a disease.[2] Other efforts are oriented toward genetic screening of larger populations at risk for such conditions as Tay-Sachs disease so that individuals can be informed about whether they are at risk for passing the affliction onto their child and, if they are, what the chances are of a child being affected.[3]

When one shifts to mass screening, additional moral problems—confidentiality, record keeping, statistical morality—come into play.

More recently, the technologies related to in vitro fertilization (IVF)—removing an egg from a woman and fertilizing it in the laboratory—have posed new and controversial problems.[4] IVF also requires hormonal agents to support the pregnancy. It is likely that pharmacists will become increasingly involved in providing answers to questions about appropriate pharmacotherapy regarding IVF and other types of infertility treatment. Pharmacists have found themselves in positions in which they are asked to consult on the ethics of efforts to manipulate human embryos, store them, freeze them, and even discard those not needed.

Once the technology to fertilize human eggs outside the woman's body is available, there will be no technical necessity to return the fertilized egg to the woman from whom it was taken. Surrogate motherhood involves reimplanting the fertilized egg into some other woman either so that she may bear the child and continue to be its social mother after the birth or so that she may bear the child in order to return him or her for parenting to the woman who supplied the egg.[5] In theory, the egg could be obtained from one woman, gestated and delivered by a second, and parented by a third.

Still newer and more controversial is what is referred to as gene therapy or genetic engineering.[6] Efforts are underway to modify the actual genetic codes of patients suffering from genetic diseases. This has already been attempted to treat some conditions, such as the enzyme deficiency adenosine deaminase (ADA) deficiency, and research is rapidly developing similar technologies to treat other conditions. Initial attempts at the use of this technology have been made to treat HIV.[7]

The first efforts are designed to modify somatic cells (so that only the treated individual and not his or her offspring will have the genetic material changed). Eventually, similar technologies will probably be used to modify reproductive cells (so that the genetic change will be transmitted to the offspring).

Ethical problems arise at many levels with these birth technologies. Perhaps the most fundamental issue is whether tampering with genetic and birth processes is "playing God" in an unacceptable way. Such technologies have the potential to change the nature of the human species.[8] While the species undoubtedly is already undergoing change, changes to date have been in a much slower, unplanned evolutionary fashion. The technologies under development have the potential for much more rapid change in the genetic character of the species as well as in basic biological processes, such as reproduction. The first question raised is thus whether such efforts reach beyond what humans should be permitted to do.

Even if one accepts the idea in principle of producing such fundamental changes, there will remain controversy over just which changes are ethically acceptable. This will, in turn, require judgments about what conditions in our species are unacceptable. Everyone might agree that a terrible disease like Lesch-Nyhan syndrome—condemning an infant to a dreadfully painful life lasting no longer than a few months—is a condition worth changing if we can; however, the same technologies are likely to permit us to intervene to modify conditions less obviously unacceptable. Color blindness, for example, might be amenable to some of these technologies. Even conceiving an embryo of an undesired sex can be determined prenatally and is, in principle, subject to interventions. The question is, "Does such a condition justify genetic intervention?"

Many other moral problems arise with these technologies: problems of identifying unexpected paternity, notifying other family members of the diagnosis of a genetic anomaly, and conflicts among parties over custody of a child. The cases in this chapter raise many of these issues.

Genetic Counseling

Increasingly pharmacy professionals working in hospitals will be involved in communicating with patients who are being counseled about the statistical risk of conceiving a child with a genetic anomaly.[9] This could involve a condition already present in a child, a parent, or some other member of the family. Or it could involve concern about a new genetic problem, such as the risk of an older woman conceiving a child with trisomy 21 (Down syndrome). The following case shows how pharmacy personnel are involved in ethical problems of genetic counseling.

CASE 11-1   Genetic Counseling: Explaining Ambiguous Results

When the University Medical Center made the decision to offer comprehensive genetic screening and counseling, the administration also established a working group composed of members of the institutional ethics committee to review policy and procedures in detail and make recommendations to the medical staff involved in this special area of practice. Regina Maser, Pharm.D., had been appointed to the working group because the chairperson believed that the completion of the Human Genome Project in 2006 had substantial implications for pharmacy practice with the development of many biotechnology-derived drug products. Even though the issues that came before the working group did not involve the use of drugs directly, Dr. Maser was very knowledgeable about advances in somatic gene therapy and participated actively in the working group's deliberations regarding the ethical, legal, and social consequences of screening, counseling, and treatment issues.

Early in its development, the working group adopted the following purposes for prenatal genetic counseling and screening: (1) to relieve the burden of uncertainty in cases in which genetic disease was a reasonable probability and (2) to clarify courses of action open to the parent(s).

The case presently facing the working group did not appear to fall into the typical prenatal counseling cases they had commonly reviewed. A 35-year-old married woman, pregnant for the first time, had undergone a chorionic villus sampling indicating that the fetus had an apparently balanced de novo translocation in 5% of the cells. This is confirmed with amniocentesis. Level III ultrasound is negative. The woman has declined percutaneous umbilical blood sampling (PUBS) because she considers the risk of the procedure too high. There is disagreement among the medical geneticists responsible for the analysis as to the meaning of the test results.

In this case, there is a possible risk of mental retardation. Given the present state of knowledge, there is no way of resolving this disagreement scientifically within the legal

CASE 11-1 *Continued.*

time limit of termination of pregnancy, because the results of repeat tests will not be available until after 24-weeks gestational age. Dr. Maser empathizes with the medical geneticist who is responsible for dealing with the prospective mother. The question is largely one of how the mother should be counseled about the results of the test. The working group must determine whether the mother should be given the ambiguous, potentially erroneous results of the genetic testing and if she should be informed of the disagreement among the professional colleagues concerning the analysis.

Note: This case is adapted from: Wertz, D. C., and J. F. Fletcher. *Genetics and Ethics in Global Perspective.* Dordrecht/Boston/London: Kluwer, 2004, p. 24.

Commentary

The moral problem faced in his case by Dr. Maser and the medical geneticist is related to the ethics of abortion discussed in the cases of the previous chapter. Of course, for someone who is morally opposed to all abortions no matter what, this case poses no special problem. The only plausible intervention would be an abortion. Those who are unabashedly opposed would have no clinical choices to make. But for those who will accept termination of pregnancy under some circumstances, this is a troublesome case. The possibility that the fetus has a genetic abnormality is a problem primarily because there is reason to believe that the pregnant woman may decide to abort the pregnancy. Even those who can accept the termination of pregnancies when a fetus is destined to die soon after birth are likely to be troubled if a normal fetus is aborted.

In calculating consequences of alternative courses of action, we saw in the cases of Chapter 4 that one approach is to determine the benefits and harms of each alternative and then to adjust that estimate based on the probability. That presumably would mean that, if in this case there is a 50% chance of a false positive, we would assume that the benefit of terminating the pregnancy would be 50% of that of avoiding the harm of producing a baby with mental retardation. However, the harm would be 50% of whatever harm is considered to be done by aborting a fetus with the condition plus 50% of whatever harm is considered to be done by aborting a normal fetus.

The issue here, however, is whether this statistical approach is morally valid. Some parents and counselors might reason that if a normal fetus is aborted a terrible wrong is done and that the wrong is not lessened at all by considering the probabilities. Many parents and counselors are willing to accept terminating pregnancies of fetuses diagnosed with great certainty to be afflicted with some terrible genetic condition incompatible with life; however, the diagnosis here only presents some degree of certainty. The only plausible way of justifying the possibility that they will terminate a normal pregnancy would seem to be discounting the harm by adjusting for the probability.

Dr. Maser and the genetic counselor will have to come to terms with the difficulties of making these statistical judgments in a case such as this. When they decide, they will face another issue that raises questions encountered in the discussion of truth telling and respect for autonomy. Once they understand the statistical probability of a false positive, which could lead to the termination of a normal pregnancy, they have to decide what to tell the woman or couple being counseled. The most obvious choice, if they are committed to respecting the autonomy of the pregnant woman, would be to explain to her what the possible outcomes are—including the possibility that the test may lead her to terminate a normal pregnancy. They may face a complicated task of explaining the statistics involved in the results, but that problem should not be very different from other consent settings, which we will explore in more detail in the cases of Chapter 15. If, however, they are more inclined toward the more paternalistic Hippocratic ethic, they will disclose only the information about the situation that they take to be beneficial for the "patient." That, of course, requires that they determine whether only the woman is the "patient" or whether the father of the fetus as well as the fetus also are considered "patients" as well.

After resolving that issue, they may be challenged still further to decide how much to reveal of their own views about what is morally correct. If they are directive in their counseling, they will urge her to follow the course they think is morally preferable, but if they prefer a nondirective strategy—an approach currently favored by many genetic counselors, particularly in the United States—they will keep their own conclusions to themselves in trying to help the decision-maker reach her own conclusion.[10]

One problem with nondirective counseling is that contemporary philosophers of science are now questioning whether counselors have the capacity to present "just the facts." Critics claim it is inevitable that information will carry subtle value messages no matter how hard the counselor tries to give "value-free" facts. They claim that no human has the capacity to completely hide all subtle, unintended messages in tone, word selection, and body language. Some go even further to claim that value-free communication of facts is impossible, in principle. They say that values necessarily must be used in selecting the information to transmit. Since it is impossible to tell the patient "everything," only the "important" or "meaningful" information will be transmitted, and that, necessarily, requires some evaluation by the counselor. In this case the counselor will have to decide how many effects of the genetic abnormality to disclose, whether to give an account of the psychological risks to the pregnant woman and others and, if so, how great the risks are and whether to go into the moral issues the woman might want to consider as well as the medical and psychological effects. If Dr. Maser ends up proposing a nondirective approach to counseling, how should she propose to the geneticist to address these issues?

CASE 11-2   Disclosure of Unanticipated Findings

At the same University Medical Center discussed in the previous case, the working group on genetic screening and counseling was reconvened to discuss another case that involved an ethical issue that was not covered under any of the previously established guidelines. The case in question involves the evaluation of a daughter with an autosomal recessive disorder for which carrier testing is possible and accurate. In the process of testing the child's relatives for genetic counseling, the attending physician discovered that the mother and one other sibling are carriers, whereas the husband is not, which means that, barring an extremely rare spontaneous mutation, the husband is not the father of the child. As far as the physician knows, the husband believes he is the child's biological father. Should this inadvertent finding be revealed? If so, to whom?

Dr. Maser, the pharmacy member of the working group, thought that the implications of the case reached far beyond what this family should or should not be told. It seemed to Dr. Maser that unanticipated findings would probably occur with greater frequency as more papers were published using the findings from the Human Genome Project.

Commentary

Like the previous case, this situation involves problems of what to disclose and how directive the counselor ought to be. It is the nature of medical testing, especially genetic testing, that gratuitous findings may surface in unexpected settings. There is some small possibility that the appearance of the gene in the daughter has an innocent explanation. Spontaneous mutations do occur, and samples get mixed up in the lab. It is very likely, however, that this girl carries two copies of the gene for the disease and that she got one of them from someone other than the man she believes to be her father. Even those who are very committed to truth telling must recognize that enormous harm can come from disclosing a piece of information about which there seems to be little one can do at this point. Those oriented to deciding ethical questions based on the consequences are likely to be inclined not to say anything. However, defenders of disclosure may appeal to consequences as well as the inherent rights of people to information.

Among the reasons why it could be important for the young woman to know who her biological father is, she may need further genetic information from him at some point in her life. If she thinks the man she believes to be her father is the carrier of one disease, she might unnecessarily be concerned that he is the carrier of others. She might some day unnecessarily limit possible partners based on information about him. Moreover, she might have a need for genetic information about her actual biological father. In a future involving genetic engineering, it may be important to know one's biological parents for the purpose of further testing, for manipulating genetic material, or for providing information for siblings. While the psychological trauma resulting from the disclosure could be severe, it could be even worse if the disclosure were to come from other, less carefully planned revelations—from an emotional outburst from gradual suspicion about physical characteristics. There are both principled moral reasons and practical consequentialist reasons why the information should be disclosed.

One strategy is to leave the choice up to the mother. While that would protect her confidentiality and her rights of nondisclosure, it at least presumes a decision to disclose to her—something that benevolently paternalistic counselors might resist. It also presumes that, if the mother does not choose to make the revelation, it is morally acceptable to go along. Some would argue that it is the child who has the right to the information, if not at this point in her life, at least someday. Placing the judgment in the mother's hands would deprive the daughter of any such rights. Under what circumstances, if any, could the counselor decide on his own not to disclose the information? Would having an institutional policy help in this case? If so, what should that policy be?

Genetic Screening

Sometimes genetic counseling arises in the context of community-based genetic screening programs. These differ from the previous cases in that the pharmacist would be involved in decisions about a mass or group screening rather than one-on-one counseling. These efforts often take place in churches or community programs in which the professional staff really has no ongoing contact with the people being screened. Sometimes these programs have racial or ethnic implications that further complicate the counseling. For example, proposals to screen for sickle-cell anemia, a blood disease affecting primarily persons of African origin, raises issues of whether the purpose is to discourage fertility among this group.

One major effort has been directed toward Tay-Sachs within the Jewish community. Tay-Sachs is a devastating disease that leads quickly to complete loss of bodily functions and death within a few months, but it is an autosomal recessive disorder so that carriers of the disease lead perfectly normal lives. The primary purposes of the screening are to discourage fertility when two people who each have the recessive gene marry or to identify and abort fetuses with the actual disease. Both discouraging fertility and facilitating abortion are morally controversial within the Jewish community.

CASE 11-3   Genetic Screening to Reduce Tay-Sachs Disease

As the members of the planning group for voluntary screening for Tay-Sachs heterozygotes gathered in the synagogue community center, Helen Cohen, Pharm.D., reviewed the information she had been given at the group's first meeting by the medical geneticist who served as technical consultant to the group. Dr. Cohen had been asked to serve on the planning group that was exploring the possibility of setting up a screening program for Tay-Sachs, since a large number of the members of the Orthodox congregation of which Dr. Cohen was a member were of Ashkenazi Jewish descent.[11] Tay-Sachs occurs with a frequency of about 1 in every 3,000 persons of Ashkenazi descent. Dr. Cohen reread the material describing the etiology and course of the disease, "Tay-Sachs disease results from the absence of hexosaminidase A, an enzyme that is part of the catabolic pathway for membrane lipids known as gangliosides. The absence of hexosaminidase A results in a buildup of gangliosides in the brain causing neurological deterioration and eventual death. Tay-Sachs infants begin to show abnormal motor responses early; although they may

CASE 11-3 *Continued.*

crawl and sit, they rarely become able to walk. Blindness occurs by 1 year of age. After 18 months, seizures, generalized paralysis, and progressive deafness develop. The child usually dies by the age of 4 or 5. There is no treatment."[12]

The voluntary screening program planning group had been organized by the rabbi after several families in the congregation had suffered the loss of a Tay-Sachs infant. Dr. Cohen believes that she was appointed to the planning group because of her clinical knowledge. However, that knowledge is in conflict with her personal, religious beliefs. Couples in which both are heterozygotes have a 25% chance of the fetus being affected with Tay-Sachs disease for each pregnancy. They also have a 50% chance of a fetus who, like them, will be a carrier as well as a 25% chance of having a fetus without any copies of the Tay-Sachs gene. Heterozygote couples can choose to refrain from conceiving children or take the chance and have the fetus measured for enzyme activity, a relatively straightforward biochemical assay. Affected fetuses are almost always intentionally aborted because of the hopelessness of the disease. Dr. Cohen believes it is religiously important for Jews to bear children. She also believes that abortion is essentially murder. She is deeply concerned that the mass screening program that the planning group is contemplating for "expectant fathers" will lead to a decrease in the number of children born to Jewish couples. Should she oppose the screening on these grounds?

Commentary

Part of Dr. Cohen's ethical dilemma arises from what appears to be moral tension within the synagogue. While traditional Orthodox Judaism is deeply committed to creation of new lives and is strongly opposed to abortion, another strand of thought in the Jewish community—more secularized and liberal—believes in the value of limiting fertility even through the practice of abortion. Particularly when the birth will be of an infant who is destined to suffer a short, seriously debilitated life, abortion is an option that many people of Jewish faith take seriously.

Dr. Cohen's congregation seems open enough to these practices that it wants to support a Tay-Sachs screening program. Part of the problem may stem from the goal of discouraging engaged couples from procreating. This could come in the form of either discouraging marriage or discouraging childbearing within marriage. Neither is necessary to avoid giving birth to offspring afflicted with the disease provided one is willing to test and abort afflicted fetuses.

One argument sometimes given against this is that, with such an approach, two-thirds of the children born of parents who both are carriers will themselves be carriers. This would eventually increase the frequency of the gene in the population. Critics argue, however, that it will take a long time to affect the gene pool significantly and that the science of genetics is moving so rapidly that other technologies may be available to deal with that problem. Particularly if prenatal screening is available to identify fetuses with the actual disease, they believe that the slight increase in gene frequency is worth it if it would give couples a chance to bear children who are not afflicted with the disease.

There is some support for screening programs as a means of providing advance warning in order to give time for psychological, social, and medical preparation even for couples who would continue with a pregnancy of an afflicted fetus. If that is a reason for the screening, then Dr. Cohen might find reason to support it, even if she opposes abortion and discouraging childbearing. Assuming Dr. Cohen realizes that many couples will actually use the screening to limit fertility or to abort afflicted fetuses, is the possibility that some people will simply use the information for advance preparation a reason for Dr. Cohen to support the program, or is that merely a rationalization?

In Vitro Fertilization

Some of the most exotic and controversial developments in biomedical ethics involve our newfound capacity to manipulate the human egg and sperm cells in the laboratory in ways that permit the actual creation of human life in the test tube.[13] These technologies were originally designed to help couples overcome certain kinds of female infertility, such as blockage of the oviduct, to bypass the cause of infertility. They involve removal of one or more egg cells from the ovary followed by fertilization mechanically in the clinic.

Some of these ethical problems have actually been around for a long time, as newer technologies replicate what has long been accomplished through artificial insemination. They all raise the issues discussed earlier in this chapter of whether it is unethical to mechanically mimic the reproductive process. Some, especially within the Roman Catholic tradition, consider such manipulations "artificial," which is taken to mean "immoral."[14] Others see the moral issues not so much in the physical manipulation of the gametes per se, but in the risks of injury that are involved. Still others are concerned primarily about the more exotic uses of these technologies, which would permit conception of a child in ways that involve more than a married couple: first through artificial insemination by a donor and more recently through surrogate motherhood and schemes whereby a woman who wants to bear a child that was genetically hers could engage another woman to carry the fetus through the pregnancy. The following two cases illustrate how pharmacy professionals will be involved in such issues.

CASE 11-4   In Vitro Fertilization: Assessing a New Technology

---

It had only been a year since the Ethics Committee of the State University Medical Center approved the use of artificial insemination with a husband's sperm or with a donor. Now the Ethics Committee was being asked to explore in vitro fertilization (IVF) in married couples who were unable to conceive a child any other way. IVF was the next logical step in the progression of high-tech methods to help an infertile couple conceive a child that was connected to them biologically.

Collin Sobeira, Pharm.D., had been appointed to the Ethics Committee when the committee began its discussion of IVF because of his knowledge of IVF stimulation protocols. The protocols involve the use of 3 types of drugs to suppress luteinizing hormone surge and stimulate the development of follicles and eggs. Dr. Sobeira was aware that not

CASE 11-4 *Continued.*

all of the fertilized eggs were implanted in the mother's womb but assumed that several eggs were because the IVF procedure often resulted in multiple births. He had soothed his conscious about the enterprise by not asking too many specific questions about what happened to the fertilized eggs that were not implanted. As long as the line was drawn at IVF, Dr. Sobeira accepted it as an essentially moral enterprise.

He had recently been challenged, however, by Rosie Greenwood, RN, who represented nursing on the committee. Ms. Greenwood voiced strong opposition to approval of IVF at their institution. She said the problem began by assuming that the function of women in the society is to be bearers of children. She believed that women whose personal identity was so wrapped up in the traditional role of childbearer were missing many other opportunities in life. She thought women who were so desperate that they would try IVF needed counseling to consider other options: pursuit of careers as well as adoption if they really must place themselves in the maternal role. She thought it was irresponsible to spend enormous sums at some medical risk to the woman in order to bring another child into the world when there are so many children who cannot be placed for adoption. Moreover, Ms. Greenwood was worried about what she called the "slippery slope," the eventual use of the IVF technology for other, more controversial purposes, including compensation for ovum donors, paid surrogate motherhood, and bearing children outside of wedlock.

Dr. Sobeira wondered whether IVF really raised all these problems.

Commentary

Dr. Sobeira is in the middle of some of the most controversial and complex moral issues in health care today. Like artificial insemination for a previous generation, in vitro fertilization raises issues of whether it is unethical to manipulate the conception process and whether there is an artificiality about it that makes it unethical.

In vitro fertilization is more complex, however. Especially in the early days, there were serious questions of the risk to the offspring as well as to the woman. Now many of the basic safety issues appear to have been resolved, but other questions remain.

For technical reasons, it is standard to retrieve and fertilize several eggs at the same time, freezing extras for possible later implantation or cultivating several and selecting the most promising for implantation. The task of selecting and then discarding those not selected puts the health professional in an awesome position. Dr. Sobeira must consider whether there are moral problems raised by this selection-and-discard process.

Frozen eggs raise another set of issues. They could be discarded once a conception has taken place, or they could be used elsewhere, either for research or for implantation into another woman, such as one who is infertile because of damaged ovaries.

One of the results of the professionalization of pharmacy is a questioning of the traditional view that roles such as that of Dr. Sobeira are merely technical. He may not be able to limit his involvement to consultation on matters of hormones. Dr. Sobeira must decide whether he will take responsibility for the moral implications of the work he is doing in literally creating human life.

The challenge posed by Ms. Greenwood raises still another set of issues. Ms. Greenwood appears to doubt that IVF, even for married couples, is a morally appropriate use of technology. Whether she is concerned about the artificiality of reproduction in this fashion or the need to adopt rather than treat infertility technologically, she forces Dr. Sobeira to determine whether there are moral limits on the use of new birth technologies. She also presses the slippery slope problem. Assuming Dr. Sobeira satisfies himself that the use of IVF by infertile married couples is morally legitimate, should he at this time also be forced to take into account the fact that the same technology can be used for other, more controversial purposes, including conceptions outside of wedlock, selling ova, and surrogate motherhood? Must the morality of these uses of the technology be judged at the beginning of the use of the technology, or should Dr. Sobeira consider only the initial envisioned use for infertile couples within a marriage?

CASE 11-5   Embryo Biopsy

It was only a few months after the in vitro fertilization procedure was approved that Dr. Sobeira realized he would not be able to maintain his ignorance regarding the exact disposition of fertilized eggs. A proposal was presented to the Ethics Committee for discussion and approval of a new procedure that would expand on IVF. The procedure, referred to as embryo biopsy, allows for preimplantation genetic diagnosis of simple gene defects, such as Huntington's disease and cystic fibrosis (CF) in embryos.[15] For couples who already have a child with CF and are worried about passing the condition onto another, physicians could offer standard IVF protocol with the following additional steps. The sample used to infer genetic composition includes polar bodies removed on day 1 after fertilization and 1 or 2 blastomeres on day 3 of cleavage-stage embryo development (the 6- to 8-cell stage).[16] The embryos that do not have the defect would be implanted into the mother's womb, ensuring that the child or children would not have the gene or be able to pass the gene onto future children.

Dr. Sobeira had deep concerns about this proposal for embryo biopsy. He was concerned about how accurate the test was and the potential for misdiagnosis. Even though the prevention of cystic fibrosis seemed an admirable goal, he was also concerned about opening the door to separating fetuses we wish to develop from those we wish to discontinue. Additionally, a child with cystic fibrosis is not doomed to death in infancy. The median age for survival for CF patients is 36.8 years, and there is no intellectual or behavioral impairment. Gene therapy offers great promise for treatment.

Commentary

In addition to the moral issues raised by IVF in the previous case, now Dr. Sobeira must deal with another issue: qualitative judgment in choosing which embryos to implant and which to discard. The process of embryo biopsy and assessment also poses a potential additional risk to the implanted fetus that is beyond the risks of the IVF itself. In the previous cases, however, even though some embryos might be discarded, the selection process seemed to be more nearly random. No judgment was made based on actual genetic testing to determine which embryos were "better." In this case, though, selection will be a function of someone's judgment about the quality of the life to be lived.

Even though in the case of cystic fibrosis it seems that choosing between those embryos with and without the disease would be uncontroversial, the general idea of qualitative selection could be very controversial. The potential already exists to select embryos of a particular sex. Soon it could be possible to biopsy and select for traits most would consider trivial, such as hair color, height, or color blindness. Does permitting biopsy and selection to avoid cystic fibrosis start Dr. Sobeira down the road to qualitative evaluation and selection of embryos? Is that a road he should avoid?

Surrogate Motherhood

The very same technology that Dr. Sobeira was considering in Case 11-4 and Case 11-5 permits creation of life in the laboratory in ways that involve people who are not married couples. Once the egg is removed, it could be implanted into a woman who was not the source of the egg, either to have her function as a surrogate, carrying the fetus to term for the purpose of returning it to the woman who supplied the egg, or to gestate a child she will not only give birth to but maintain after birth as well. In the latter case, the woman receiving the fertilized egg, the host mother, might be sterile due to damaged ovaries but capable of maintaining a pregnancy. The egg could be fertilized by the host mother's husband's semen, or she might be the recipient of extra fertilized eggs produced by another couple. Such arrangements add further complexity, as is seen in the following case.

CASE 11-6   Surrogate Motherhood: Medical Miracle or Exploitation of
            Women?

The Women's Health Center offered an array of maternal/child health services, including family planning, contraception, abortion, prenatal care, genetic screening and pediatric advice. Marcella Tucker, Pharm.D., the center's pharmacy supervisor, believed that all of these services were important and should be available to all women. Now, however, she thought the center had gone too far. The management team was listening to a presentation about the possibility of adding a surrogate mother program to the center's list of services. According to the presentation, state law permitted individuals and couples to enter into surrogacy contracts. The law permitted compensation for gestational surrogacy. Even if the mother did not possess a uterus, but retained her ovaries, it was possible to be genetically linked to her baby. Surrogates would be used for a variety of purposes along a continuum. A surrogate might be artificially inseminated with the husband's sperm, carry the child through pregnancy and delivery, then give the baby to the woman who was the source of the egg. In the case of a woman who still had functional ovaries, eggs can be harvested, fertilized in vitro with her husband's sperm, and then implanted in the uterus of a surrogate for gestation and delivery. The Women's Center would assist in all phases of the surrogacy program. The potential for increased revenues from a select group of married couples who had exhausted other methods of conception was impressive.

CASE 11-6 *Continued.*

> Dr. Tucker could hardly contain herself until the presentation was finished. "Am I the only one here that thinks this whole program exploits desperate women? Even though the surrogates are paid what appears to be a large sum of money, it doesn't amount to much when you consider that being pregnant extends over 9 months and that there are always risks associated with pregnancy that should be factored in as well. Besides, this is a "woman-centered" health facility, and this proposed program is disrespectful to women in two ways: first, it makes infertile women think that if they spend enough and are persistent, technology will provide them with a baby; second, it takes advantage of poor women. My guess is that most of the women who would be willing to be surrogates will be poor, women of color. So the program is potentially racist too!" Dr. Tucker stopped to take a breath, surprised at her own passion about this topic.

Commentary

Surrogate motherhood raises all the ethical issues of the use of IVF for a couple within a marriage but adds additional problems to consider. Some surrogates are volunteers, often relatives of a woman who is unable to bear children herself. Sisters, mothers, and other relatives offer to bear a child as an act of familial kindness. Other surrogates may also act out of charity, but if they are strangers to the infertile couple, it seems only fair for the surrogate to be compensated, at least for medical expenses. Most assume that it is also reasonable to compensate for the time and inconvenience involved. Some states have considered a policy of prohibiting paid surrogacies while permitting those that are voluntary. Is that something Ms. Tucker should consider, or are her doubts more fundamental? Is it the act of surrogacy itself that is problematic?

One of the central concerns with surrogacy is the disruption of traditional patterns of marriage and family. Three separate functions are often identified: contribution of the genetic information, gestation, and nurturing. In most cases of childbirth, all three are provided by the same woman who is unquestionably the mother. In some cases of surrogacy, such as that of Mary Beth Whitehead, a woman engaged as a surrogate who initially committed to gestating an infant conceived in vitro by another couple but later discovered she could not agree to return the child she bore. The emotional experience of the pregnancy, to her surprise, led to bonding that she had not anticipated.[17] In such cases, should the surrogate be able to retain custody of the infant she bore, or is the initial promise to return the infant to the couple that conceived the child morally binding? Would it make a difference if the surrogate mother provided the egg for the in vitro conception rather than the woman who is initially planning to be the nurturing mother?

An underlying argument among those who are critical of surrogate motherhood is that women cannot be expected to anticipate the psychological and physiological effects of pregnancy and therefore should not be bound by contracts or promises made prior to the pregnancy. Even if a woman agrees in advance to give up the infant at the end of the pregnancy, according to these critics, she cannot be bound by such a commitment.

Defenders of surrogacy contracts, however, claim that, in effect, this reduces women to second-class status, that because of psychology and physiology unique to women, at least in this one area they cannot be permitted to make binding contracts the way male adults can. Dr. Tucker will have to evaluate these issues in deciding whether to support a surrogacy program in her center.

Genetic Engineering

The future of innovative genetic technologies lies in interventions intentionally undertaken to change the genetic code. Some of these changes will occur in human gene therapy.[18] If a gene is missing, for example a gene that is responsible for producing a necessary enzyme, incorporating that gene can, at least in theory, correct the deficiency. One such disease is adenosine deaminase (ADA) deficiency, the disease that causes severe combined immunodeficiency, such as that of children who have to grow up in "bubbles" in order to be protected from infection. Other efforts are attempts to use gene therapy to switch off the gene for Huntington's disease and to treat the blood disorder thalassaemia as well as cystic fibrosis, sickle-cell disease, HIV, and some cancers.[19]

Several technologies are potentially available to transmit genetic material. The use of viruses to pick up and transmit genetic material into cells is one such technology. For some diseases the transfer of recombined or recombinant DNA can take place outside the body by removing bone marrow, making the transfer in the laboratory, and then reimplanting the modified marrow. Among the issues raised by these new technologies are the potential risks of the processes themselves.[20] If the virus transfers the genetic material incorrectly or to the wrong cells, serious harm is possible. For patients with life-threatening illnesses, such as ADA deficiency, the risks may be worth it, but some recombinant DNA transfer will eventually be considered for more minor medical problems, and it is not only the sick patients who could be affected by the genetic changes.

The direct risks are not the only concerns raised by these technologies. Some changes that at first appear to be beneficial may later in life produce indirect effects that are unattractive. Some are concerned that the remaking of the human genetic code will change the underlying fabric of the culture. While it used to be assumed that the nature of the human being was permanently fixed, increasingly it has been seen as temporary and subject to human manipulation. We are remanufacturing ourselves.

The same technologies that permit adding a critical missing enzyme might permit adding genes that would produce additional substances. In a competitive world, genetic engineering may eventually permit improvement on the normal average functioning of humans such that users of the technologies get "unnatural" advantages. If everyone else begins to use the technologies to gain an advantage, nonusers will be at a disadvantage, much like an athlete competing against opponents on steroids.

Similar technologies permit modifying animal or plant species, in some cases making possible the production of new drugs and biological products. In the following case, a pharmacist confronts the ethical implications of genetically engineered pharmaceuticals.

CASE 11-7   Genetic Engineering

Harry Tannen, Pharm.D., was one of the clinical pharmacists for United Health Systems, a comprehensive managed care provider in the metropolitan area. He was asked to consult with 1-year-old Henry Nightingale's parents about his treatment options, especially concerning drug therapy.

Henry had been hospitalized many times since his birth. He was suffering from adenosine deaminase (ADA) deficiency, a rare enzyme deficiency resulting from the absence of the gene responsible for producing adenosine deaminase. The result is a condition sometimes called severe combined immunodeficiency (SCID). Children with this condition are severely immunocompromised. Treatment for some has consisted of spending their entire early life enclosed in a sterile environment, giving rise to the name "bubble boy."

Fortunately, Henry has been able to be treated with porcine ADA, which is produced commercially as Adagen, manufactured by Enzon, and he has done quite well.

Now it appears that the medical director at United Health Systems is urging Mr. and Mrs. Nightingale to enroll Henry as a candidate for a gene therapy trial in which he would be one of the first with ADA deficiency to receive the missing gene through the process of an autologous bone marrow transplant. His marrow would be removed, exposed to the missing ADA gene, and then reimplanted. The hope is that he would take up the gene and that his body would be able to manufacture at least some of the ADA needed. Also, as a participant in the experimental protocol, he would have the costs of the gene therapy covered by a grant to the investigators.

The experiment sounded exciting to Dr. Tannen. In addition to being a part of a truly revolutionary new technology, Henry would have a chance of being able to reduce his use of Adagen. Of course, from United Health System's point of view, any reduction in Adagen would constitute a savings.

The economics is not insignificant. The average wholesale price for a 1.5 ml vial is $2,900 @ 250$\mu$/ml. A vial contains 375 units. Dosing consists of weekly intramuscular injections according to the following schedule: 10μ/kg, 15μ/kg, and 20μ/kg for the first, second, and third doses, respectively. Maintenance doses are 20μ/kg/week, with incremental increases by 5μ/kg/week to a maximum dose of 30μ/kg. The average maintenance dose is 15μ/kg/week. Thus, since Henry weighed 21 pounds, or 9.5 kg, he needed approximately 142.5 units, which amounted to 1 full vial every 2 weeks at $2,900 a vial for a grand total of $5,800 per month!

Dr. Tannen was surprised when he spoke with Mr. and Mrs. Nightingale. They were not at all impressed with the experimental protocol. The idea of making their child one of the first in human history to receive gene therapy scared them. They were worried about the idea of changing their boy's genetic code. They feared that something could go wrong and that his genes could be changed in some terrible way. This was, after all, one of the first times that humans had purposely tried to manipulate genetic material. They even had some vague religious doubts about whether this was "playing God," something they thought they should not do. They seemed to feel that, as long as the Adagen was working, they should leave well enough alone.

Dr. Tannen was not sure whether it was his responsibility to advocate for the financial interests of United Health Systems, but his real concern was whether the potential benefits of the gene therapy justified the risks. He had never had to deal with these kinds of risks before and was not sure how to counsel the Nightingales.

Commentary

This case raises many kinds of ethical problems. It could be viewed as a case of cost containment in managed care. The role of the pharmacist in such issues was discussed in Chapter 5. It also could be viewed as a case of research on human subjects, the focus of the cases in Chapter 14. The specific issue addressed here is the ethics of genetic engineering. The attempt to insert the ADA gene is the first protocol in a truly revolutionary area of medical research—attempting to insert a missing gene in a human.[21]

The first problem that experimental gene therapy raises is one of the concerns expressed by Mr. and Mrs. Nightingale. Seemingly radically different from any previous medical research, this work does not just cure a disease; it purposely changes a human's genetic makeup, creating, genetically, a new person. This particular experiment seems quite innocent. The disease being treated is a bad one. Potentially fatal. All that is being added is a single gene that will substitute for one that ought to be present but instead is missing.

However, the viral vector technology being used to introduce the genetic material into Henry should not be specific to the ADA gene. Once these initial experiments are perfected, the same technique could be used to introduce many other genes into humans. Some uses are potentially controversial. For example, a gene that would change the production of a certain brain transmitter could be inserted for the purpose of making a patient more docile or more athletic or more of some other desired characteristic. While such efforts are not what United Health System's medical director has in mind, Henry's contribution to science would directly make possible all manner of future uses of the technique, some of which are bound to provoke debate. Does it make any sense for Mr. and Mrs. Nightingale to worry about whether it is ethical to be a party to such innovation?

The Nightingales' second concern is the risks of the procedure. From everything that is known about the procedure, it seems to be safe. The bone marrow transplant would be painful, but the long-term risks would be minor. The real fear is whether something could go wrong in the manipulation of the genetic material. The thought that some foreign gene could be inserted or that the ADA gene could be inserted in a manner that disrupts some other key genetic function is frightening, even if the chances of these risks materializing seem to be small. Assuming that United Health System is paying for the Adagen, are the Nightingales just being prudent if they choose to continue the more traditional treatment?

Notes

1. Cohen, Cynthia B. "Reproductive Technologies: Viii; Ethical Issues." In *Encyclopedia of Bioethics*. Third Edition. Stephen G. Post, Editor. New York: Macmillan, 2004, pp. 2298–2307; Hall, Mark A., Mary Anne Bobinski, and David Orentlicher. "Reproductive Rights and Genetic Technologies." In their *Health Care Law and Ethics*. Sixth Edition. New York: Aspect Publishers, 2003, pp. 663–781; Arras, John D. "Reproductive Technology." In *A Companion to Applied Ethics*. R. G. Frey and Christopher Heath Wellman, Editors. Malden, MA: Blackwell, 2003, pp. 342–355.

2. Murray, Robert F. "Genetic Counseling, Ethical Issues In." In Post, *Encyclopedia of Bioethics*, pp. 948–952; Matthews, Anne L. "Genetic Counseling." In *Encyclopedia of Ethical, Legal, Policy Issues in Biotechnology*. Thomas H. Murray and Maxwell J. Mehlman, Editors. 2 vols. New York: John Wiley & Sons; 2000, pp. 342–352; Wright, Rollin M., John A. Balint, Ian H. Porter, and Wayne N. Shelton. "Ethical Issues in Genetic Research, Testing, Counseling, and Therapy." In *Advances in Bioethics: Bioethics for Medical Education*. Rem B. Edwards and E. Edwards Bittar, Editors. Greenwich, CT: JAI; 1999: 171–213.

3. Ford, Norman M. "Ethical Aspects of Prenatal Screening and Diagnosis." In *Genetics and Ethics: An Interdisciplinary Study*. Gerard Magill, Editor. Saint Louis, MO: Saint Louis University Press, 2004, pp. 197–215; Juengst, Eric T. "Genetic Testing and Screening: Iii. Population Screening." In Post, *Encyclopedia of Bioethics*, pp. 1007–1016.

4. Bonnicksen, Andrea L. "Reproductive Technologies: Ix. In Vitro Fertilization and Embryo Transfer." In Post, *Encyclopedia of Bioethics*, pp. 2307–2311; Lin, Olivia. "Rehabilitating Bioethics: Recontextualizing in Vitro Fertilization Outside Contractual Autonomy." *Duke Law Journal* 54 (November 2004): 485–511; Schotsmans, Paul T. "In Vitro Fertilization and Ethics." In *Bioethics in a European Perspective*. Henk ten Have and Bert Gordijn, Editors. Boston, MA: Kluwer, 2001, pp. 295–308; Steinberg, Avraham. "In-Vitro Fertilization." In his *Encyclopedia of Jewish Medical Ethics: A Compilation of Jewish Medical Law on All Topics of Medical Interest*. Nanuet, NY: Feldheim Publishers; 2003, pp. 571–586.

5. Gostin, Larry, Editor. *Surrogate Motherhood: Politics and Privacy*. Bloomington: Indiana University Press, 1990; Lincoln, David H. "Surrogate Motherhood." In *Life and Death Responsibilities in Jewish Biomedical Ethics*. Aaron L. Mackler, Editor. New York: The Louis Finkelstein Institute, Jewish Theological Seminary of America, 2000, pp. 188–192; Tong, Rosemarie. "Surrogate Motherhood." In Frey and Wellman, *A Companion to Applied Ethics*, pp. 369–381.

6. Resnik, David B. "Genetic Engineering, Human." In Post, *Encyclopedia of Bioethics*, pp. 959–966; Brock, Dan W. "Genetic Engineering." In Frey and Wellman, *A Companion to Applied Ethics*, pp. 356–365; Gert, Bernard. "Genetic Engineering." In *Encyclopedia of Ethics*. Second Edition. Lawrence C. Becker and Charlotte B. Becker, Editors. New York: Routledge, 2001, pp. 602–606.

7. Levine, Bruce L., Laurent M. Humeau, Jean Boyer, Rob-Roy MacGregor, Tessio Rebello, Xiaobin Lu, Gwendolyn K. Binder, Vladimir Slepushkin, Franck Lemiale, John R. Mascola, Frederic D. Bushman, Boro Dropulic, and Carl H. June. "Gene Transfer in Humans Using a Conditionally Replicating Lentiviral Vector." *Proceedings of the National Academy of Sciences* 103 (November 14, 2006): 17372–17377.

8. Baillie, Harold W. "Genetic Engineering and Our Human Nature." In *Genetic Prospects: Essays on Biotechnology, Ethics, and Public Policy*. Verna V. Gehring, Editor. Lanham, MD: Rowman and Littlefield, 2003, pp. 43–50.

9. President's Commission for the Study of Ethical Problems in Medicine and Biomedical and Behavioral Research. *Screening and Counseling for Genetic Conditions: The Ethical, Social, and Legal Implications of Genetic Screening, Counseling, and Education Programs*. Washington, DC: U.S. Government Printing Office, 1983.

10. Fransen, M., R. Meertens, and C. Schrander-Stumpel. "Communication and Risk Presentation in Genetic Counseling: Development of a Checklist." *Patient Education and Counseling* 61, no. 1 (2006): 126–133.

11. Hashiloni-Dolev, Yael. "Between Mothers, Fetuses, and Society: Reproductive Genetics in the Israeli-Jewish Context." *Nashim: A Journal of Jewish Women's Studies and Gender Issues* 12 (Fall 2006): 129–150.

12. See www.nlm.nih.gov/medlineplus/ency/article/001417.htm for the most recent information on Tay-Sachs pathophysiology.

13. For the classic statement of the ethical issues see Ramsey, Paul. *Fabricated Man*. New Haven, CT: Yale University Press, 1970. For a recent discussion see President's Council on Bioethics. *Reproduction and Responsibility: The Regulation of New Biotechnologies*. Washington, DC: The Council, 2004.

14. Sacred Congregation for the Doctrine of the Faith. "Instruction on Respect for Human Life in Its Origin and on the Dignity of Procreation." *Origins*, March 19, 1987, pp. 698–711.

15. Verlinsky, Y., J. Cohen, S. Munne, L. Gianaroli, J. L. Simpson, and A. P. Ferrareti et al. "Over a Decade Experience with Preimplantation Genetic Diagnosis: A Multicenter Report." *Fertility and Sterility* 82 (2004): 292–294.

16. McArthur, S. J., D. Leigh, J. T., Marshall, K. A. de Boer, and R. P. Jansen. "Pregnancies and Live Births after Trophectoderm Biopsy and Preimplantation Genetic Testing of Human Blastocysts." *Fertility and Sterility* 84 (2005): 1628–1636.

17. *In re Baby M*. 109 N.J. 396, 537 A.2d 1277 (1988).

18. President's Council on Bioethics, *Reproduction and Responsibility*, pp. 105–119.

19. See http://www.ornl.gov/sci/techresources/Human_Genome/medicine/genetherapy.shtml#status (accessed November 7, 2006).

20. For additional information on the ethics of genetic engineering see Wivel, Nelson A., and LeRoy Walters. "Germ-Line Gene Modification and Disease Prevention: Some Medical and Ethical Perspectives." *Science*, October 22, 1993, pp. 533–538; Medical Research Council of Canada. *Guidelines for Research on Somatic Cell Gene Therapy in Humans*. Ottawa: Minister of Supply and Services, 1990; and Fletcher, John C., and W. French Anderson. "Germ-Line Gene Therapy: A New Stage of Debate." *Law, Medicine, & Health Care* 30 (Spring/Summer 1992): 26–39.

21. Anderson, W. French, R. Michael Blaese, and Kenneth Culver. "The ADA Human Gene Therapy Clinical Protocol." *Human Gene Therapy* 1 (1990): 331–362; Angier, Natalie. "Girl, 4, Becomes First Human to Receive Engineered Genes." *New York Times*, September 15, 1990, pp. 1, 9; Thompson, Larry. "The First Kids with New Genes." *Time.*, June 7, 1993, pp. 50–53.

12

Mental Health and Behavior Control

Psychiatry and other forms of study and modification of human behavior raise many ethical problems in the pharmacy profession.[1] When we say that many people *suffer* from behavior disorders, we imply that they are harmed or injured by these conditions. To the extent that pharmacists can assist in relieving that suffering or in modifying undesired behaviors, the traditional ethics of health care professions that focuses on doing what will benefit the patient requires attempting to intervene. At the same time, we may lack consensus on whether the condition is really one requiring intervention. In the case of organically based illnesses we can normally ask the patient or surrogate whether he or she wants help in attempting to change the condition. In the case of behavioral problems, however, there is often doubt whether the patient is capable of making an informed and rational choice. It is the consenting organ itself that may be "diseased." If we rely on surrogates, significant conflicts of interest may exist between the surrogate decision-maker and the patient. The behavior of the patient may not bother the patient but can create inconvenience or embarrassment to the surrogate. Some of the most difficult ethical problems in the health care professions can arise in mental health and the behavioral sciences. In this chapter we look at cases raising these problems.

The first problem in dealing with mental health is the concept of mental health itself.[2] Traditionally many mentally abnormal behaviors have been viewed as problems of religion or of criminality. Only in the twentieth century did we begin to view these behaviors within the medical model. In the first section of this chapter we look at a case that raises the issue of the concept of mental health and whether mental problems should be deemed as "deviant behavior choices" or as "medical problems."

In the second section we take up one of the classical ethical problems in the mental health professions—whether patients with mental health problems should be viewed as having sufficient autonomy to consent or to refuse to consent to treatment in the same way as for organic medical treatments. The third section deals with the conflicts of interests that arise between the mental health patient and other parties—other patients, families, work colleagues, or other members of the society. The problems here involve confidentiality, loyalty to the patient, and the tradeoffs between patient interests and those of the others potentially affected by the patient's behavior.

Finally, in the fourth section of this chapter we focus on examples of other behavior-controlling technologies—the use of electroconvulsive therapy (ECT) on a mentally depressed patient and the use of aversion therapy.

The Concept of Mental Health

Human behavior is complex. It has been interpreted over the centuries in many different ways.[3] In traditional religious worldviews, members of the community manifesting unusual or strange behaviors might be thought to be possessed by demons or under the influence of a magical spell. We can say that the behavior is interpreted as religiously influenced deviance. The same behavior in another culture, also in a religious framework, might be interpreted as being sinful—as a violation of the will of God. Although both are religious cultures, there is an important difference. While the view that sees such behavior as the result of demon possession or a magical spell might imply that the behavior is not the "fault" of the individual (who can be called a "victim"), the behavior of the sinner, so-called, usually is seen as somehow within the voluntary control of the actor.

In other cultures, the behavior may be seen as simply an unusual lifestyle choice and not carry any of the religious implications. Such behaviors may be interpreted as unusual but acceptable. However, they also may be seen as socially unacceptable and in need of control. Especially if they harm others, they may be interpreted within a criminal model in which the behavior is illegal and warranting social sanction.[4]

In still other interpretations the behavior is viewed in what is called a medical model. According to this now-dominant view, many unusual behaviors are believed to be caused by some medical condition. The convulsions we associate with epilepsy are now thought to have an organic medical cause, not the result of demon possession, the wrath of God, or sinful lifestyle. If a behavior is believed to have an organic cause, it still remains a question whether that behavior is acceptable or should be the target of efforts to change it. Most would agree that even though epilepsy has an organic cause, it nonetheless produces undesirable consequences for the person who has epilepsy. For other conditions, controversy rages over whether the behavior is merely unusual, but acceptable, or should be modified. Many people increasingly view homosexuality as having a biochemical or genetic cause. Some conclude that, once one assumes such a basis for the orientation, one should recognize that there is no reason to attempt to change the behavior. Others, while acknowledging the organic cause, still believe there is something wrong or dysfunctional or unpleasant about the behavior and, like epilepsy, try to use pharmacological or other medical means to try to change it. This latter group would consider the gay orientation as a "disease," whereas the former would not.

While we have fully medicalized some conditions that once were thought of in other terms, other behaviors are less clearly medical. Alcoholism, for instance, is believed by some to be a disease, while others continue to see it as a sin. Still others interpret it as nothing more than a lifestyle choice. The medicalization of human behavior has very important and controversial implications.[5] The choice of a model for interpretation of behavior does important work. It conveys an implied understanding of the source of the behavior, whether one is responsible for it, what experts or authorities should be consulted to deal with the behavior, and what interventions are to be used in attempting to modify the behavior.

The medical model in its pure form implies that there is an important medical (usually meaning organic) element in the cause of the behavior.[6] It often implies that the individual manifesting the behavior is not volitionally responsible for it and is thus exempted from blame. It also implies that a medical professional is an appropriate expert for dealing with the behavior if one wants to change it. Many of the most interesting and difficult ethical problems for those working in mental health arise at the point of classifying the patient's behavior as fitting in the medical model. The following case shows how pharmacists may find themselves dealing with patients whose classification as medical is controversial.

CASE 12-1   Mentally Ill or Just a Troublemaker? The Concept of Mental Illness

It had taken Candace Toma, Pharm.D., the better part of 6 days to complete the chart review of medication regimens on every inpatient of the Center for Mental Health, a private psychiatric hospital. Jared Pence, Pharm.D., supervisor of the hospital's pharmacy, told Dr. Toma that he knew of no better way to orient her than to have her review every record. Now that she was through, Dr. Pence asked Dr. Toma, "Any questions?"

"As a matter of fact, I do have a few questions," Dr. Toma responded, "and numerous concerns. First of all, it seems to me, after looking through the clinical records, that almost every patient is receiving some type of psychotropic medication. Some with Alzheimer's disease and closed head injuries are on a regimen that makes therapeutic sense. However, more than a third of the patients are on antipsychotic medication, but only a fraction of those carry a diagnosis of schizophrenia or psychosis. Patients who are labeled as "aggressive" are often given antipsychotics, yet there is little to no documentation of the presence of psychosis in these cases, just violent outbursts.

"Sedatives and hypnotics are being widely prescribed for unruly and elderly patients on a regularly scheduled basis, not prn, which is compatible with the concept of sedation as 'chemical restraint.'

"The use of psychotropic medications extends even to the children and adolescent unit, where young patients with behavior problems, such as socialized aggression, are on antidepressants and minor tranquilizers. I don't see that pharmacologic intervention is justified in all of these cases. I am willing to put aside those cases where it is justified and the best drug within the proper therapeutic class isn't being utilized. That is a different sort of problem and one I'm ready to tackle. The larger problem, it seems to me, is treating all of these patients as if they were 'ill' and using drugs as the main method to fix these ills. What do you think, Dr. Pence?"

Commentary

Candace Toma is pressing her supervisor to explain exactly what it takes for someone to be considered ill—or at least what it takes for someone to be put legitimately on medication. The patients that have aroused her concern clearly seem to be engaging in behaviors that are unacceptable, at least to the professional caregivers on the health care team. Are they ill, however? And is medication warranted?

The concepts of illness and disease are more complex than many people realize. Sometimes the term *disease* is used to refer strictly to objective manifestations while *illness* is used to refer to the psychological components of suffering, stress, and *dis*-ease. The problem arises, however, when we realize that some conditions that are very distressing have no discernable objective, organic cause. To make matters more complicated, even though they appear to have no objective, organic cause, they may nevertheless respond to medication, surgery, or other medical intervention.

Imagine two people who have identical behavioral manifestations that are dissatisfying to caregivers (and perhaps to the patient as well). In one case, the behavior may be related to a clear organic factor that seems like the cause; the patient may have epilepsy or a gene that produces a chemical abnormality that seems responsible for the behavior. In the other, the behavior cannot be related to any organic element that can be said to cause it. For example, the patient may simply be prone to violent, unexplained outbursts. If both behaviors are the same in all relevant aspects—both distress the onlookers and the patient to the same extent—and if both are equally amenable to modification by the use of medication, is there any moral reason why the patients do not have an equal claim on the medication? Does the fact that the behavior has an apparent organic cause in one case make the use of medication more acceptable?

Calling a condition medical may have important implications. If a person is seen as having a significant medical problem, he or she is less likely to be blamed for the behavior. He will be seen as a patient to be treated by a psychiatrist, occupational therapist, or social worker. Medication may be more easily justified. The causal force that makes the patient behave strangely will be seen as organic or psychological rather than a voluntary choice or as resulting from some external source.

A person's behavior will be seen as "medical" if its cause is some organic lesion or chemical imbalance, especially if the lesion or imbalance was not the result of what is taken to be a voluntary choice on the patient's part. If there is a brain lesion or a tumor causing abnormal hormonal secretions that cause the peculiar behavior, it is unreasonable to blame the person. Moreover, what the patient needs will be seen as within the medical realm. A health care professional who has specialized knowledge capable of addressing the problems will be seen as the appropriate expert.

Classifying the individual's behavior within the medical model will be seen by some not only as mistaken, but offensive. If, for example, the individual is interpreted as rebelling against an immorally oppressive society, someone who labels him or her as having a "disease" will be seen as ignoring the real cause of the behavior—behavior that could be interpreted as morally appropriate rebellion. If the patient is interpreted as being punished by God or as having inherited bad karma from a previous life, then the behavior will be seen in an entirely different causal framework. Persons may be held accountable for their actions: either praised for rejecting societal oppression or blamed for past deeds that condemned him or her to the present fate. Different kinds of expertise will be seen as appropriate: the clergy or the police perhaps. If the individual is seen as responding appropriately to an oppressive society, probably no professional expertise will be seen as needed at all. In fact, he or she could be viewed as a saint, or martyr, or hero. (Consider whether Gandhi, Malcolm X, Jesus, or Stalin could be classified as mentally ill by the staff of the Center for Mental Health.)

The issue raised by this case is what it takes for a person to be classified as a patient, that is, as someone in need of the services of health care professionals. One condition seems to be that something bad is happening. Only if the patient's behavior is interpreted as inappropriate and negative will he or she be seen as needing medication. But more than that is needed. The behavior usually must be seen also as having a significant organic (or psychological) component. If evil spirits, divine forces, or freely chosen lifestyles cause them to act the way they act, their behaviors will less likely be seen as fitting the medical model. If it is believed that a significant medical (organic-psychological) component is causing the behavior, then it is more likely that those with the appropriate medical or psychological expertise (including the pharmacist) will be seen as having something to offer. Finally, if the behavior is beyond these persons' control (even if perhaps he or she was in some way originally responsible for the events that led to it), it is less likely they will be seen as blameworthy.

Dr. Toma seems unconvinced that many of these people have conditions that fit squarely in the medical model. She seems to view them more as personal or social deviations from the usual behavioral patterns that do not call for medication. What, if anything justifies the widespread use of psychopharmacological agents in this setting? If the drugs can change the behavior in desirable ways, is that sufficient, or is something else required? If behavior adjustment through medication is for the benefit of the health care professional, i.e., makes a patient more compliant, less difficult to care for, is that an inappropriate use of the drug?

Mental Illness and Autonomous Behavior

Once it has been agreed that the patient's condition is appropriately classified as a medical or health problem and therefore the appropriate concern of those in the mental health profession, the next issue to be confronted is whether the patient can be sufficiently autonomous to consent or refuse consent for medical treatment.

As was shown in Chapter 6, autonomy is both a psychological and a moral concept. One is said to be *psychologically* autonomous if one has substantial capacity to form a life plan and make choices in accord with it. Individual actions are autonomous to the extent that they are made in accord with such a life plan. Seen in this light, it becomes apparent that no person and no personal action can be said to be totally autonomous. Individual actions can be more or less autonomous depending on the degree to which the individual generates a decision based on his or her life plan.

Autonomy is also a *moral* concept. Also as shown in Chapter 6, autonomy as a moral principle states that actions are morally right to the extent that they respect the autonomous choices of individuals. Thus informed consent as a moral requirement is grounded largely in the moral principle of autonomy.

In order for the moral principle of autonomy to come into play, however, the individual must be deemed to be a substantially autonomous agent. For many patients this decision is relatively easy. Minors generally are presumed not to have sufficient autonomy to make their own medical choices, except in special circumstance. In special cases minors may be found to be mature and granted both the moral and legal right to consent to treatment on their own.[7] Some adults are so severely retarded or comatose that it is obvious they also are not significantly autonomous agents. However, most adults are sufficiently autonomous that they will clearly be treated as autonomous for purposes of making medical decisions. Even some people who are seeking mental health services are autonomous. The courts have determined that it is possible that a patient might be committed for mental treatment and still be sufficiently autonomous that he or she is deemed mentally competent for the purposes of consenting to or refusing treatment.[8] This is particularly true for certain critical medical treatments, including ECT.[9]

While autonomy is a moral and psychological category, competence is a legal category. Only a court can make a legal finding that a patient is incompetent to consent or refuse consent for treatment.

Nevertheless, a significant number of patients receiving mental health services present serious problems at the edges of autonomy. For these cases autonomy must be viewed as a threshold concept.[10] A patient must be deemed either sufficiently autonomous that his or her own judgments will be accepted or as below the threshold, in which case some surrogate will have to be designated for that purpose. The following case poses problems at the borderline of assessing autonomy in mental health treatment.

CASE 12-2   The Case of the Hostile Bag Lady: Mental Illness and Autonomous
             Behavior

The new city ordinance allowed outreach teams to bring "all incompetent or dangerous or gravely disabled, homeless, mentally ill persons to hospitals, involuntarily if necessary." Since the implementation of the ordinance 2 weeks ago, numerous unwilling, mentally ill, homeless patients had been brought to City Center Hospital's Psychiatric Department, where Olivia Samaria, Pharm.D., worked. One patient in particular, Theresa Farney, a middle-aged woman, had drawn the attention of all of the members on the health care team. Ms. Farney had been forcibly picked up from the streets and brought to City Center Hospital for evaluation on a special ward set aside for the mentally ill homeless. Ms. Farney had been living on the streets in an affluent neighborhood for 2 years, panhandling to get money for food and muttering to herself.

Upon her admission to the emergency room, the physician ordered 5 mg of haloperidol and 2 mg of lorazepam to be administered intramuscularly. Ms. Farney was then transferred to the special ward in the Psychiatric Department. After her transfer to the psychiatric ward, Ms. Farney refused all psychotropic medications. Since all nonemergency decisions about the involuntary administration of antipsychotic drugs had to be made by a judge, a hearing was necessary. Ms. Farney received a lawyer from the American Civil Liberties Union (ACLU).

CASE 12-2 *Continued.*

At the first day of the hearing, Ms. Farney's attorney protested her commitment, argu-ing that she did not have a serious mental illness but was a "professional street person" whose difficulties on the street were a natural consequence of being homeless. The attor-ney pointed out that Ms. Farney was extremely resourceful, considering the circumstances of her life, and that her inadequate hygiene and clothing were the consequence of poverty and homelessness, not mental illness. Although she had often been observed on the street to be angry and verbally abusive, Ms. Farney claimed that her resort to verbal abuse was necessary to fend off unwanted offers of help or potentially harmful actions of strangers.

Dr. Samaria listened to the first day of the hearing with great interest. Dr. Samaria had spent some time observing Ms. Farney on the ward after Ms. Farney had refused the chlorpromazine hydrochloride ordered by her psychiatrist. Ms. Farney had been verbally abusive to Dr. Samaria as she attempted to explain the actions of the psycho-tropic medication that had been ordered for her. Ms. Farney made an obscene gesture toward Dr. Samaria as she angrily left the conference room where they had been talk-ing. Ms. Farney isolated herself from other patients and was often heard to be talking in rhymes or muttering to herself. However, Dr. Samaria was not certain that any of this behavior could necessarily be labeled psychotic.

The second day of the hearing, Dr. Samaria's doubts about Ms. Farney's diagnosis were shared, along with the testimony of several psychiatrists and other members of the mental health team. There was no definitive evidence of the delusions or hallucina-tions characteristic of psychosis. She appeared rational and lucid during the hearings. She denied suicidal or homicidal ideation. Ms. Farney was able to answer questions about the proposed medication. During a past hospitalization, Ms. Farney had received chlor-promazine hydrochloride, which she claimed had made her feel sleepy, light-headed, and "foggy." She did not like the sensation of not being able to think clearly. Also, Ms. Farney prided herself on her independence. She concluded her reasons for refusing the antipsy-chotic medications by stating, "I doubt the medicines will be very effective, I dislike the side effects, and I am wary of all mind-altering drugs."

Dr. Samaria was impressed with Ms. Farney's capacity during the hearings, but she still could not erase the mental picture of Ms. Farney sleeping on an air vent outside of a delicatessen in the middle of winter or of her defecating in the gutter. But even if the judge found in favor of the psychiatrists and approved the involuntary use of antipsychotic drugs, Dr. Samaria was certain that Ms. Farney would likely discontinue the medication once she left the hospital. Involuntary treatment often leads to resentment and even greater reluctance to have any contact with the mental health system in the future. Even after all of the evidence presented at the hearings, Dr. Samaria believed that she would have a hard time determining if Ms. Farney was mentally ill or making an unusual but autonomous lifestyle choice.

Commentary

One of the firm conclusions of the moral debate about health care during the last half of the twentieth century was that competent patients have the moral and legal right to refuse any medical treatment provided that treatment is offered for the patient's own good. As was discussed in Chapter 6, the moral principle of autonomy affirms the right of such patients to make their own choices, even if they turn out to be bad decisions. As will be shown in Chapter 15, the right to refuse treatment is widely believed to hold even in cases in which the result of the refusal is likely to be death.

Were Ms. Farney clearly competent, those who defend the right of competent patients to refuse treatment would permit her to make her own lifestyle choices, however unattractive these choices seem to most other people. However, were she clearly incompetent and unable to understand the nature of her choices, most people would favor having a guardian appointed to make choices in her best interest. Ms. Farney, however, does not completely fit either category.

It makes little sense to talk of people being *completely* competent. Nevertheless, most adults are what can be called *substantially* competent; we treat them as if they were autonomous agents capable of understanding enough about the decisions they make and free enough to be said to be making free choices. However, most people are not totally incompetent either. Even children understand choices to some degree and have some capacity to choose freely, even if that freedom is quite constrained.

Ms. Farney appears to be some place in between. The moral issue that Dr. Samaria must confront is determining what moral offense is committed if she makes a mistake. The healing professions represented here not only by Dr. Samaria, but also by the psychiatrists, traditionally have given highest priority to beneficence and non-maleficence. They are committed to benefiting the patient (even if it sometimes involves violating the patient's autonomy). They should admit that if they presume the patient is incompetent when she really is not, Ms. Farney may suffer discontent. That should count in their calculation of benefits and harms. But if, on balance, they believe that her interests will be served by violating her autonomy, they will conclude that morally they should act paternalistically. Since they give low priority to respecting autonomy, not much wrong is done if they falsely presume she is incompetent.

Conversely, the lawyer from the ACLU is committed to the high priority for respect for liberty or autonomy. Such people believe that it is morally preferable to do what the patient chooses, even if that means risking that the patient will be worse off. For them the error of violating autonomy is worse morally than the error of failing to do what most people would believe is best. Which kind of error should Dr. Samaria risk? She could treat Ms. Farney as incompetent and risk violating her autonomy if she really has the capacity to formulate a life plan and live by it. Or she could treat her as substantially competent and risk hurting her well-being should Ms. Farney make unwise choices. If Dr. Samaria believes that Ms. Farney is autonomous enough that her wishes should be respected, she will have to decide what she should do about the medication that has been prescribed. If administering the medication would be an unethical violation of the patient's right to consent, a case can be made that the prescription should not be filled. On the other hand, failing to cooperate with the treatment plan could end up hurting the interests of someone who is not capable of being responsible for her own welfare. Part of the moral choice is which mistake would be worse. Are there interventions that Dr. Samaria should take in the face of the psychiatrists' commitment to strive to do what they think is beneficial?

Mental Illness and Third-Party Interests

The decisions in the previous section of this chapter posed traditional medical ethical questions of the conflict between benefiting the patient and protecting the patient's autonomy to the extent that it exists. Patients receiving mental health treatment also pose the newer ethical problems of conflict between the interests of the patient and the interests of others within society. These conflicts can arise in the context of confidentiality. (See Chapter 8 for additional cases involving the general problem of breaking a confidence in order to protect the interests of others.) Additional conflicts between the interests of mental health patients and others include situations in which providing good care for the patient will necessarily jeopardize the care that can be given to others. Sometimes these problems arise because of the shortage of resources.

In the following case a potentially violent outpatient threatens the well-being of others. The pharmacist must weigh the freedom of the patient against the interests of others.

CASE 12-3   A Compulsion to Kill: The Mentally Ill and Third-Party Interests

Carl Forbes, Pharm.D., a member of the psychiatric staff at a large community mental health center was familiar with the patient being presented at the facility's weekly care conference. Dr. Whitney Kellogg was describing the progress of Bryant Watson, a 32-year-old man who had been referred by the employee-assistance program at the city's Parks and Recreation Department where he worked as a groundskeeper and landscaper. Mr. Watson was now on a leave of absence because of his erratic behavior, angry verbal outbursts, and one incident of physical assault of a coworker. Because this was a sudden change in Mr. Watson's behavior, his employer viewed him as a valuable employee and wanted him to benefit from intensive, but hopefully short-term, psychiatric care. Dr. Forbes had been dispensing Mr. Watson's atypical antipsychotic medication for the past several weeks and during that time had noted Mr. Watson's gruff dismissal of attempts to counsel him about his medication. Mr. Watson appeared extremely angry and volatile to Dr. Forbes.

Dr. Kellogg intoned, "Mr. Watson is still somewhat hostile and refuses to engage in civil dialogue. He has not been able to clearly articulate the focus of his anger and obsession, but it seems to involve several co-workers and past slights. At times, Mr. Watson has expressed a compulsion to kill. At this point, he is equally vague about how he would carry out this homicidal ideation. I will continue to use risperidone and intensive psychotherapy in his care."

Dr. Kellogg closed the chart, indicating that the team's discussion of Mr. Watson's case was over. Dr. Forbes was highly concerned about what he had heard Dr. Kellogg state. At this point, Mr. Watson was still a day patient, which meant that he arrived at the community mental health center at 8:00 A.M. and left at 5:00 P.M. 6 days a week. Dr. Forbes asked, "Dr. Kellogg, excuse me, but aren't you going to inform the police department of Mr. Watson's violent threats?" Dr. Kellogg responded, "I am not going to do anything of the sort at this stage."

"But, Dr. Kellogg," Dr. Forbes continued, "Mr. Watson is a violent person. Don't we have a duty to report this?" Dr. Kellogg huffed, "We are through discussing this patient, Dr. Forbes."

Dr. Forbes reluctantly accepted that the topic was closed for the present. However, he still felt an obligation to at least warn his coworkers in the Parks and Recreation Department of Mr. Watson's potential for lethal violence.

Commentary

Here Dr. Forbes faces a problem similar to those in Chapters 4 and 8 in which the interests of the patient may not be the same as the interests of third parties. Mr. Watson's interests might best be served by keeping him in the day-patient program, thus allowing him to maintain something closer to his normal life while at the same time receiving substantial clinical care. This may be riskier to others than having him committed to an institution, but arguably it is better for him.

The moral principles suggest two approaches to this problem. First, the social utilitarian form of the principles of beneficence and nonmaleficence would seem to indicate that Dr. Forbes should attempt to estimate the total consequences of both reporting and maintaining the status quo. He would have to try to calculate all of the effects of maintaining Mr. Watson's day-patient status, which is likely to be more pleasant for Mr. Watson and certainly less embarrassing should commitment proceedings result from his threatening behavior. A good utilitarian will also have to consider the disadvantages of maintaining day-patient status: the nervousness of coworkers who must endure his threatening behavior, the horrible effect not only on others, but also on Mr. Watson if he acts out and seriously harms someone, and the possibility that day-patient therapy might not be as effective.

The social utilitarian would then try to envision the effects of reporting: a likely commitment hearing and institutionalization against Mr. Watson's will but also the possibility that harm to others would be prevented.

Traditional health care professionals consider consequences as well, but they limit the consideration to the benefits and harms of each alternative that will accrue to their patient. The impacts on other parties are out of bounds in the calculation. Their moral duty is to remain faithful to their patient.

The morally troublesome case is the one in which the utilitarian, considering consequences to third parties as well as to the patient, concludes that more net good is done by reporting, while the Hippocratic consequentialist, the one who considers only the impacts on the patient, reaches the opposite conclusion.

Dr. Forbes may also feel compelled to take into account the implications of the other moral principles: fidelity, autonomy, justice, and avoidance of killing. For example, if those who limit the morally relevant consequences to those affecting the patient are asked why, they may claim that as health professionals they have promised fidelity to the patient and that this promise requires them to ignore the interests of third parties. However, those who take into account certain consequences to others may point to the principles of justice or avoidance of killing to justify their point of view. Only if there are similar duties of fidelity to those who might be harmed by Mr. Watson's acting out would the principle dictate that Dr. Forbes should also take into account the impacts on others. If his family, for example, were likely to be victims of Mr. Watson's acting out, Dr. Forbes would also have the duty of taking their interests into account. These, of course, would not be duties resulting from his role as pharmaceutical caregiver.

Autonomy may have some implications, depending on whether Dr. Forbes considers Mr. Watson to be a substantially autonomous agent. If he is, then he might be inclined to respect Mr. Watson's freedom. Usually, however, autonomy is limited in cases when it risks harms to third parties. Unlike the previous case, in which it was the welfare of the patient herself that could be served by overriding her autonomy, in this case it is the interests of third parties that are of concern.

The principle of avoidance of killing suggests to those who include it within their ethical theory that when there is a risk that others will be killed there is a separate and independent duty to do what one can to avoid having that killing take place. This might be interpreted as implying that if Dr. Forbes believes that Mr. Watson's behavior runs the risk of resulting in a killing that Dr. Forbes has an independent reason, beyond the harm that could be done, to report the case, if that is what might help prevent the killing.

Finally, the principle of justice as an independent consideration would lead Dr. Forbes to ask who is potentially the worst off and what can be done about it. It might at first appear that Mr. Watson is the worse off. His life seems quite miserable. That could lead to a choice that would serve his interests at the expense of third parties. However, on reflection it might be argued that it is really potential murder victims who would be the worst off. If that is the case, then doing what is necessary to prevent them from ending up worst off would receive independent support from the principle of justice. One who believes in the priority of these principles would still have to balance the competing implications of them, even if collectively they were seen as taking priority over considerations of consequences. If you were Dr. Forbes, what would you do?

Other Behavior-Controlling Therapies

The ethical problems in mental health arise not only in clinical psychology; they must be faced in other behavior-controlling interventions as well. Neurological interventions, including psychosurgery and ECT, require judgments about the concept of mental health.[11] They require judgments about when a patient is autonomous as well as moral tradeoffs between the welfare of the patient and that of other parties.

ECT involves administering electrical charges at voltages high enough to cause convulsions. In some instances the force of the charges has been strong enough, if muscle relaxant medication is not administered, to cause bones to break. The exact effect on the brain is not known, but ECT is considered a highly efficacious treatment in psychiatry.[12]

This imagery of convulsions and brute physical assault raises doubts in some people's minds about the acceptability of ECT. Especially, as in the following case, in which the patient appears to have changed her mind, the pharmacist involved in dispensing medication for ECT faces serious moral issues.

CASE 12-4   A Shocking Ambivalence: ECT Without Consent

When Daniel Purcell, Pharm.D., saw the medication orders for a muscle relaxant and short-acting barbiturate for Georgia Beck, a 60-year-old inpatient, he knew Ms. Beck was scheduled for electroconvulsive therapy (ECT). Dr. Purcell immediately recalled the conversation he had had yesterday with Ms. Beck in the nurses' station of the psychiatric unit where Ms. Beck had been an inpatient for approximately 3 weeks. Ms. Beck had a history of depressive episodes. This was the second hospitalization for severe, nonpsychotic depression. Dr. Purcell knew that the psychiatrist considered Ms. Beck to be medication resistant as far as her depression was concerned.[13]

CASE 12-4 *Continued.*

Ms. Beck had been talking to her husband on the phone, albeit her husband was doing most of the talking. Dr. Purcell heard only an occasional "yes" and "uh huh" from Ms. Beck before she hung up the phone. Ms. Beck sighed and turned to look at Dr. Purcell. "You're on the staff here, right?" Dr. Purcell explained that he was the clinical pharmacist in psychiatry. Ms. Beck continued, "I'm not getting any better even with all the different medications. They want me to have shock therapy, but I can't sign that consent. I am so afraid of it." Dr. Purcell encouraged Ms. Beck to express her fears, thinking they may be based on misunderstanding about the procedure. However, Ms. Beck understood that she was seriously depressed, that the drugs had failed, that ECT would probably cure her depression, and that the risks of ECT were slight compared to the harms of her depression.[14] Yet, even given all this, Ms. Beck could not bring herself to sign the consent.

Now, a day later, Dr. Purcell is faced with an order that clearly means that Ms. Beck is scheduled for ECT. Dr. Purcell called the nurses' station of the unit where Ms. Beck was a patient to see if she had given her consent. The nurse told Dr. Purcell, "No. She's still refusing ECT, but the physician believes she isn't competent to give consent since she's so depressed. We're going ahead with treatment anyway." Dr. Purcell feels that preparing and dispensing the medications is participating in a treatment Ms. Beck doesn't want. Dr. Purcell also has mixed feelings about ECT, believing it is often effective in patients who are unresponsive to standard antidepressants, yet it seems inhumane to force her to undergo a treatment against her will.

Commentary

Dr. Purcell is facing both legal and ethical issues when he considers whether to dispense the medications necessary for Ms. Beck to receive the ECT. Legally, he may be facing the charge that he is dispensing a prescription without a valid consent. Likewise, ethically, his patient's autonomy may be violated if she does not agree to the treatment she receives.

The real issue here is whether Ms. Beck should be treated as a competent patient with sufficient autonomy to be making her own decisions about treatment. She is institutionalized in a mental hospital, but that does not automatically establish her as being mentally incompetent. One important question is whether Ms. Beck signed herself into the institution voluntarily or whether she was committed against her will. In the former case, the hospital staff have already acknowledged that she is competent enough to make choices about her own care. Her right to consent would presumably remain in tact. In the latter case she may have been declared incompetent. Still that does not automatically give the clinician the authority to treat her without consent. A guardian may have been appointed. If so, that guardian will have limited authority to consent to medical treatments in her best interest. That person might be her husband. Dr. Purcell would need to know whether anyone has the authority to consent on her behalf and, if so, whether that consent has been given. In some jurisdictions, however, such as California, legislation has been passed making it difficult for psychiatrists to employ ECT without satisfying many administrative regulations.[15]

Other jurisdictions allow for incompetent patients to refuse ECT. Why would mentally incompetent patients be permitted to refuse specific treatments, such as ECT? In the routine case, minors, the severely retarded, and those who have been adjudicated incompetent can be treated, even over their objections. That is because we presume that such persons lack sufficient autonomy to determine what is in their own best interest. Why would patients who generally lack the capacity to make decisions about their own care be given the authority to refuse in special cases, such as ECT? Surely it is not because ECT is easier to understand. Rather it must be because society recognizes that there are certain situations in which the risks of intervention are believed to be about as weighty as the anticipated benefits. Thus children are sometimes permitted to refuse participation in certain experimental treatments on the grounds that, even though they are not capable of autonomously assessing the alternatives, experimental treatments by their very nature are not known to offer benefits that exceed harms. In such cases, logically, even a less-than-rational choice cannot be known in advance to be contrary to the patient's interest. Some would argue that ECT is so controversial and risks such harms that, like an experimental treatment, it cannot be known by a health professional or by a guardian to be significantly better for the patient than omitting the therapy. If society believes that the proposed treatment is so controversial that the expected benefits cannot be established to exceed the expected harms, then nothing is lost by giving even an incompetent patient a choice.

If Dr. Purcell reaches the conclusion that no valid consent exists for the medications that have been prescribed, he has several options. He could refuse to dispense. He could cooperate with the physician's plan even though he has legal and moral doubts. Or he could ask for further review from the hospital's ethics committee, risk manager, or attorney. Are there other options and which option should he choose?

Future behavior-modifying therapies are likely to involve pharmacological agents that will force pharmacists to face important ethical questions. One area in which pharmacists will play a key role is aversive conditioning. These are therapies in which drugs are used to punish persons or to provide "negative reinforcement" when individuals engage in unacceptable behavior. The following case illustrates this problem.

CASE 12-5   Treating Pedophiles with Aversive Therapy

As the consultant pharmacist to the regional correctional facility, Scott Ennis, Pharm.D., often attended the quarterly meetings of the health care providers associated with the prison. Dr. Ennis was particularly curious about the last item on the agenda, "research project on aversion therapy." John Mugisha, MD, the medical director, explained that a new project would be conducted in cooperation with behavioral psychologists who were interested in studying aversion therapy on pedophiles who were incarcerated for their second offense. The aversion therapy would involve the use of intravenous injections of succinylcholine chloride, a short-acting neuromuscular blocking agent.

Dr. Mugisha went on to explain, "The experiment will attempt to suppress the undesirable behavior of attraction to children by associating photographs of children with the severely frightening experience of the inability to breathe that is the result of injection of

CASE 12-5 *Continued.*

succinylcholine chloride. Of course we will follow standard procedures for obtaining valid consent from all inmates who choose to participate in the study. Additionally, we will take every precaution to protect the physical well-being of the subjects, and the procedure will be done in a setting with complete medical support for resuscitation or ventilatory support in the unlikely event they should become necessary. Furthermore, we will screen out those who are at risk for cardiopulmonary problems, neurological problems, etc."

Dr. Ennis wasn't opposed to all forms of aversion therapy. For example, he had seen good success with disulfiram therapy for alcohol dependence. The severe cramping, diaphoresis, and nausea that accompanied the ingestion of alcohol with disulfiram was certainly noxious enough to keep some patients alcohol-free. The use of succinylcholine chloride seemed different. Dr. Ennis suspected that the inmates who were the targets of the study would be desperate to try anything to get out of prison early. Also, pedophiles often are the victims of violent crimes in prisons, another reason to accept the harms of the study if it meant an earlier parole.

Dr. Ennis knew that the study would involve him insofar as he would have to supply the drug. Should Dr. Ennis cooperate with the study?

Commentary

The first question Dr. Ennis must face is whether the prisoners are sufficiently autonomous to give their consent to this experiment. It might be suggested that they must be mentally ill to have done the things for which they are imprisoned. However, they apparently have not been ruled insane in court. There is no obvious reason why a prisoner, even if he or she suffers a psychopathology that leads him or her to engage in unacceptable social behavior, is necessarily lacking in capacity to give consent for treatment. Many prisoners presumably should be able to understand the nature of the medication, the risks involved, and the treatment alternative. Unlike the patients in Cases 12-2 through 12-4 the prisoners who may receive the aversion therapy are not as obviously mentally impaired.

But they may lack autonomy in another important sense. Autonomous persons are not only in possession of the internal capacity to understand the nature of the choices to be made; they must also be free of external constraints. This raises the question of whether prisoners are free of such constraints. It is the very nature of imprisonment that one gives up claims to freedom. Nevertheless, lack of freedom in certain areas of life does not necessarily rule out the capacity to make choices in other areas. A more difficult question is whether the realization that participation in such research may provide the only realistic chance these people have of getting out of prison. Given the alternative, does the offer to participate in the study constitute an irresistibly attractive offer, and if so, does that mean the prisoners lack adequate autonomy to consent to participate?

The ethics of irresistibly attractive offers deserves more attention. It seems that there is a substantial enticement, but the term *coercion* may not apply in such situations. It is surely not that the prisoners are being forced physically to participate.

When others outside prisons must choose between two jobs or marriage options, one of which is much more attractive, we normally do not conclude that the individual is lacking freedom just because one option seems so much better. Some very attractive offers are said to involve exploitation. This would be the case when the one making the offer could satisfy in some other way the interest of the one receiving the offer. In this case, for example, there are reports that long-acting, gonadotripin-releasing hormone agonist analogues, together with psychotherapy, are highly effective in controlling selected paraphilias, such as pedophila.[16] If Dr. Ennis and Dr. Mugisha had these agents available and were permitted by the legal authorities to use them and offer the possibility of release, then the intentional refusal to offer them in order to recruit prisoners for the aversion experiment would be exploitation. If, however, legal authorities would not condone the possibility of release with the use of the hormone therapy, then the aversion experiment would be the prisoners' only option. Dr. Ennis and Dr. Mugisha would not be exploiting the prisoners.[17]

Dr. Ennis may face other ethical questions, such as whether an adequate consent is the only moral decision he must face. Some might argue that it would be morally wrong to administer aversive therapy even if the person had given a valid consent. Some interventions may be so offensive that pharmacists may feel they have committed a moral offense even if the one upon whom the offense is committed has given an adequately informed and free consent. It is common in the discussion of conditioning to distinguish between positive and negative conditioning. In positive conditioning a reward is given for approved behavior; in negative conditioning a punishment is given for unacceptable behavior. Aversive conditioning is similar to negative conditioning in that the purpose is to associate something very unpleasant with the unacceptable behavior. But what is the significance of the distinction between the morality of positive and negative conditioning? In some cases, the difference between the two may not be as clear as one might believe. When financial rewards and penalties are used, many would claim there is little difference between giving a reward for good behavior and, alternatively, giving someone a basic income and then fining them for instances of bad behavior. It all depends on what is considered the baseline.

In the case of aversive conditioning for sex offenders, it might be claimed that most of us have a natural aversion to the sexual practices that seem to attract this minority. Can we say that the aversive conditioning is merely a method of providing the minority with an aversion that most of us possess naturally? If so, is there anything morally wrong with using the frightening experience of temporary paralysis of the respiratory muscles as a way of providing it?

These last two cases both involve nonstandard or experimental treatments that raise a range of controversial moral issues. It is to the ethics of pharmacist participation in experimentation with human subjects that we now turn.

Notes

1. Roberts, Laura Weiss, and Allen R. Dyer. *Concise Guide to Ethics in Mental Health Care*. Washington, DC: American Psychiatric Press, 2004; American Psychiatric Association Ethics Committee. *Ethics Primer of the American Psychiatric Association*. Washington, DC:

American Psychiatric Association, 2001; American Psychiatric Association. *Opinions of the Ethics Committee on the Principles of Medical Ethics with Annotations Especially Applicable to Psychiatry.* Washington, DC: American Psychiatric Association, 2001; Bloch, Sidney, Paul Chodoff, and Stephen A. Green, Editors. *Psychiatric Ethics.* Third Edition. Oxford: Oxford University Press, 1999.

2. Englebretsen, George. "The Concept of Mental Health." *APA [American Philosophical Association] Newsletter,* Spring 2001, 162–164.

3. Caplan, Arthur L., James J. McCartney, and Dominic A. Sisti, Editors. *Health, Disease, and Illness: Concepts in Medicine.* Washington, DC: Georgetown University Press, 2004.

4. Flew, Antony. "Disease and Mental Illness." In his *Crime or Disease?* London: Macmillan, 1973, pp. 38–48.

5. Conrad, Peter. "The Discovery of Hyperkinesis: Notes on the Medicalization of Deviant Behavior." In Caplan, McCartney, and Sisti, *Health, Disease, and Illness,* pp. 153–162.

6. Veatch, Robert M. "The Medical Model: Its Nature and Problems." *Hastings Center Studies* 1, no. 3 (1973): 59–76. Also see Parsons, Talcott. *The Social System.* New York: Free Press, 1951, chap. 9.

7. Goldstein, Joseph. "Medical Care for the Child at Risk: On State Supervention of Parental Authority." *Yale Law Journal* 86 (1977): 645–670, esp. 669–670.

8. *In re Maida Yetter.* 62 Pa.D. and C. 2d 619 (1973).

9. *New York City Health and Hospitals Corporation v. Stein.* 335 N.Y.S.2d 461 (1972).

10. Faden, Ruth, and Tom L. Beauchamp, in collaboration with Nancy N. P. King. *A History and Theory of Informed Consent.* New York: Oxford University Press, 1986, pp. 235–269.

11. Merskey, Harold. "Ethical Aspects of the Physical Manipulation of the Brain." In *Psychiatric Ethics.* Third Edition. Sidney Bloch, Paul Chodoff, and Stephen A. Green, Editors. New York, NY: Oxford University; 1999, pp. 275–299.

12. Abrams, R. *Electroconvulsive Therapy.* Fourth Edition. New York: Oxford University Press, 2002.

13. Husain, S. S., I. M. Kevan, R. Linnell, and A. I. Scott. "What Do Psychiatrists Mean by Medication Resistance as an Indication for Electroconvulsive Therapy?" *Journal of ECT* 21, no. 4 (2005): 211–213.

14. Holtzheimer, P. E., and C. B. Nemeroff. "Advances in the Treatment of Depression." *NeuroRx* 3, no. 1 (2006): 42–56.

15. California Welfare and Institutions Code. §§5325.1, 5326.7, 5326.8, 5434.2. 1979.

16. Rösler, A., and E. Witztum. "Pharmacotherapy of Paraphilias in the Next Millennium." *Behavioral Sciences and the Law* 18 (2000): 43–56.

17. For further discussion of the differences among coercion, exploitation, and irresistibly attractive offers see Faden and Beauchamp, *A History and Theory of Informed Consent.*

13

Formularies and Drug Distribution Systems

One of the great ethical problems of the twenty-first century is the challenge presented by new drug control and distribution systems. Pharmaceuticals are becoming increasingly expensive. Presently, the percentage of health care expenditures spent on prescription drugs is about 12% and is projected to rise to about 15% by 2014.[1] As the cost of health care rises society will develop ever more sophisticated strategies for containing costs. These will certainly involve efforts to eliminate or control the use of pharmaceuticals that are not cost-effective. Some drugs currently in use can be eliminated if they can be shown to be ineffective for the patient's condition. That should raise few ethical problems. The controversies will arise when health system planners discover that sometimes a very expensive drug is only slightly better than a much cheaper drug. A newly approved agent intended to reduce repeat heart attacks and costing a thousand dollars per patient might, for example, show a success rate that is only a tiny bit better than an older agent costing hundreds of dollars. Even claiming that a new drug is "a tiny bit better" is hard to say with certainty, as there are few head-to-head trials. Most clinical trials of new drugs are versus a placebo. A trade name pharmaceutical preferred by a clinician only because she is more confident in the manufacturer costs, on average, four times the generic equivalent that meets all current standards. A continuous-release hypnotic that is chemically identical to the shorter-acting agent that has been on the market much longer may cost many times more. Systems managers will realize that the savings obtained by limiting clinicians to the cheaper options can do much more good for patients than permitting indiscriminate use of the more costly alternatives. Pharmacists increasingly find themselves on the committees that will set the standards for formularies used by health system pharmacies and insurers responsible for paying for the cost of pharmaceuticals.

In the chapters of Part II, several ethical principles were introduced that are relevant to the decisions setting limits on prescribing and dispensing practices. One of the most obvious principles is the principle of justice. It is explicitly endorsed in the APhA Code's eighth and final principle: "A pharmacist seeks justice in the distribution of health resources." The code explains that the pharmacist is to be "fair and equitable, balancing the needs of patients and society." That could easily justify restraining marginal benefits for a relatively healthy, well-off patient if the savings were used to fund much worse off patients in the health plan. It would be harder to use the principle of justice to constrain benefits for the sickest patients.

Justice is only one ethical principle that is relevant in formulary and drug distribution planning. The principles of beneficence and nonmaleficence also are very relevant. Unfortunately, in many cases, meeting the requirements of these principles can directly conflict with the principle of justice. Slightly limiting the benefit to a well-off patient might make sense from the perspective of justice, for example, using a very good headache remedy rather than the latest, most expensive drug. Even slight compromises of the patient's interest would seem to violate the principle of beneficence, at least in its Hippocratic form, which requires that the health provider do as much good as possible for the patient.

Some of the other ethical principles in Part II may also be relevant in deciding which drugs are included in a health system pharmacy. Although placeboes may be effective in certain settings, they may be seen as violating the principle of veracity or fidelity. Autonomy may require permitting patients to refuse the most-effective agents in favor of less-effective alternative medicines. The principle of avoiding killing will influence how pharmacies stock and dispense potentially lethal abortifacients and drugs with euthanasia potential.

The task of this chapter is to apply all of these principles to the new issues of creating formularies and controlling the distribution of pharmaceuticals through drug distribution systems. Cases involving each are presented here.

Formularies

Formularies are lists of drugs approved for use by a particular hospital, health plan, or government.[2] Most hospitals or health organizations have a multidisciplinary committee called the Pharmacy and Therapeutics (P & T) Committee that is responsible for the development and operation of a formulary in addition to policy development and sometimes medication use processes or guidelines.

The formulary system—because it has attempted to outline the scientific data on a medication, including its toxicities, untoward side effects, safety profile, and beneficial effects—has been a controversial method of appraising medication therapy. While the pharmaceutical industry promotes the virtues of a brand name medication, the formulary system evaluates the virtues and defects of that medication in comparison with other brands with similar therapeutic uses.[3]

A number of issues, problems, and opportunities have resulted from systems such as formularies that attempt to control the distribution of drugs. The following is a partial list: (1) the increasing complexity of new drugs, especially biotechnology drugs, is challenging the capabilities of the P & T Committee staff-support function, (2) regulatory agencies, payers, prescribers, members of managed care organizations, and legislative bodies are questioning and challenging the drug formulary decision making process, and (3) beneficiaries of insurance plans often want everything covered at no additional cost.[4] The following cases deal with the ethical implications of formularies and other types of systems to control drug distribution.

Eliminating Unproven Therapies

One of the most troublesome problems with the creation and administration of drug formularies is the challenge of new therapies. They are often expensive and many have unknown side effects when they emerge and come to the attention of prescribers or patients. It is natural to want to try the newest therapies. Especially when a patient faces a critical illness these therapies are tempting even if they are unproven. Not to mention that they are aggressively promoted by the pharmaceutical industry sales force.

CASE 13-1   Avastin for Breast Cancer: Eliminating Unproven, Expensive
Therapies

When the new, targeted cancer drugs came out, Hilde Reagan, Pharm.D., had hoped they would replace chemotherapy and make cancer treatment easier on her patients in the large oncology unit where she worked. However, that was not the case with most of the drugs. Many of the new drugs, like bevacizumab, worked only when combined with traditional chemotherapy. This was particularly troubling since the cost was so high, about $50,000 per year. As a member of the P & T Committee, she knew that the increase in overall survival in first line-treatment of metastatic colorectal cancer with the addition of bevacizumab was on average about 4.7 months. This made Dr. Reagan even more concerned about the costs. For these reasons, bevacizumab was not an approved drug on the hospital formulary.

Dr. Reagan had heard about preliminary results of a few studies focusing on the addition of bevacizumab to standard chemotherapy with breast cancer and non–small cell lung cancer (NSCLC). It appeared that bevacizumab had acceptable tolerability but extended overall survival by only a little over four months in breast cancer patients and less than two months in NSCLC. The annual cost would be higher since treatment for breast cancer and NSCLC require higher doses. Although bevacizumab had not yet been approved by the FDA for use in breast cancer or NSCLS, Dr. Reagan suspected that one of the oncologists would soon request it for this use.

Sure enough, the next day Dr. Reagan saw orders from Gerald Horchow, MD, for paclitaxel and bevacizumab for Eugenia Packer, a 44-year-old woman with locally recurrent breast cancer. Dr. Reagan spoke to Dr. Horchow, "Are you asking that we consider placing bevacizumab on the formulary? You know that the FDA has requested more data before making a decision about bevacizumab for breast cancer. It is just not clear yet if it has any significant impact let alone issues with the cost. It would cost about $8,000 a month for the bevacizumab." Dr. Horchow replied, "If it gives Ms. Packer a few more months, I think we should consider it. That's why I ordered it."

Commentary

Ethicists have questioned whether the manufacturer of bevacizumab, a monoclonal antibody, is justified in the price it charges for the drug.[5] Dr. Reagan, however, has no control over the charge that the manufacturer has put on the drug. She is limited to the localized question of whether her hospital should include it among the drugs available within their facility. P & T Committees and formularies became a necessity in hospitals following the advent of Diagnosis Related Groups (DRG) and per diem reimbursement. These prospective payment systems created incentives to become more efficient. Formularies allowed hospitals to reduce expensive inventory by stocking fewer products and buying in volume—a smaller list of drugs, which created competitive bidding by drug companies. Looking at the problem from the traditional Hippocratic perspective that has been the ethic of both pharmacists and physicians, neither the pharmacist, Dr. Reagan, nor Dr. Horchow, the physician, have reason to question the use of the bevacizumab. The Hippocratic ethic requires the clinician to do what is best for the patient. That seems to include using a very expensive, if minimally beneficial, agent.

Some might question whether Dr. Reagan or Dr. Horchow can assume that the drug will really benefit Ms. Packer. It is not FDA approved for breast cancer, and the preliminary estimate of an average of four months of extra life from the drug when used for breast cancer may prove false after more studies are completed. This, however, confuses the question of whether there is enough evidence for the FDA to approve claims on the drug label of proven life-extending benefit with the different question of whether Ms. Packer would be reasonable in deciding that the benefits of trying the drug exceed the anticipated harms for her. Even though the estimate of four months of life extension are preliminary (and it is conceivable that the drug's effects could actually shorten her life), she is not irrational if she bases her decision to use the drug on whatever information is available. She may have imperfect information but unlimited hope, as do many patients, family members, and clinicians. As long as she values even a short addition to her life expectancy and there is more reason to believe that the drug will lengthen than shorten her life, she has a reason to agree to Dr. Horchow's recommendation. They would, of course, have to factor in other benefits and harms anticipated—not only the side effects of the bevacizumab, but also the side effects of the chemotherapy, the added discomfort from additional months of living with breast cancer, and so forth, but as long as she sees the estimate of net benefit to exceed the harms, she would not be unreasonable in deciding she wants to try the drug. The fact that her health insurance is going to bear the financial costs eliminates that factor from her direct concern.

Even though Hippocratic pharmacists and physicians would seem to be locked into a moral perspective that would require using any drug, no matter how costly, as long as it was estimated to offer more expected benefit than harm to the patient, other moral perspectives provide a different view. From the point of view of the insurer—whether it is a hospital or a traditional insurance company—adding an expensive drug to the formulary that will offer relatively modest benefit to subscribers may be unwise. If the insurer is a profit-making entity, its profits will suffer. Even taking into account indirect marketing advantages of being able to claim that the insurer provides such expensive benefits, it is hard to claim that including the drug serves the company's interests. Even a nonprofit insurer—private or governmental—has good moral reasons why expensive therapies, especially unproven ones, should be excluded.

If a pharmacist or physician continues to take the traditional Hippocratic perspective, that may be a good reason why he or she should be excluded from institutional resource allocation decisions such as those made by P & T committees. From the perspective of institutional ethics, approving whatever is best for the individual patient regardless of the costs and the impacts on others in the institution is hard to defend. At least the interests of other patients served by the institution must be taken into account.

A standard method used by health planners to take the interests of groups of people, such as patients, into account is to do a cost-benefit or cost-effectiveness analysis. These strategies examine the cost per unit of benefit of alternative uses of the institution's resources or the comparative costs of alternative ways of accomplishing some agreed upon end. In health care the standard unit of benefit is sometimes taken as the quality-adjusted life-year or QALY. This approach looks at the amount of benefit from a resource calculated in the number of years (or days) of benefit per unit of resource. The years of benefit are adjusted to the quality of life produced, so that 10 years of added life with a quality estimated to be 80% of normal would be considered equal to 8 years with normal health (or 20 years at a level of health judged to be 40% of normal). This method enables health planners to compare widely diverse therapies, including some that have an impact on extending life but of a poor quality as well as some that do not extend life at all but improve the quality of life. In order for the approach to be used, standard estimates must be determined not only of what the effects of a therapy will be, but also how people generally evaluate the improvement in the quality of life that results. Put in financial terms, health planners calculate the cost in dollars per QALY.

Although it may sound crass to decide whether drugs are included in formularies based on the cost per quality-adjusted year expected, when the choices are viewed comparatively, many consider them defensible. Since there are never enough resources in a health plan to do everything that any patient would ever desire, it seems wise to invest in the treatments that offer the most QALY's per dollar. It seems foolish to spend a $1 million to add 1 year to a terminally ill patient's life when the same $1 million could add 10 or even 100 years if used for other patients. As a rough rule, Americans are typically willing to spend about $100,000 per quality-adjusted life-year.

These calculations often are too complex and time-consuming for individuals like Dr. Reagan to do, but in many cases information is available that local P & T Committee members can use. In the case of bevacizumab, the cost per quality-adjusted life-year is considerably more than the $100,000 figure. Although the drug in this case may cost about $100,000 to extend the lives of 3 patients by 4 months each, there are other costs involved, including the chemotherapy, hospitalization, and professional services that make the cost much higher.

The moral theory standing behind these cost-benefit calculations is utilitarianism—the idea that one should maximize the net benefit from the use of scarce resources. The approach is grounded in the moral principles of beneficence and nonmaleficence. If Dr. Reagan and Dr. Horchow are committed to beneficence and nonmaleficence without limiting their application to the individual patient, they will almost certainly have to reject the use of bevacizumab and its inclusion in the formulary.

There is a final moral principle that Dr. Reagan must consider. As was discussed in Chapter 5, utilitarian ethics driven by the principles of beneficence and nonmaleficence often conflicts with the implications of the principle of justice, which rejects the notion that it is necessarily morally right to choose the course that will produce the greatest net benefit for the people affected. Justice requires looking at the way the benefits and harms are distributed within the community of those affected. Most contemporary theories of justice call for the adoption of practices that arrange resources so as to benefit the worst-off people. This makes P & T decisions more complex.

The first problem with applying the principle of justice to P & T decisions is in figuring out who is the worst off. It seems at first that Ms. Packer is a candidate for being among the worst off. She is suffering from breast cancer that threatens her life. If she is among the worst off, then even an unproven therapy that offers only a few months of extra life at compromised quality may be justified from the perspective of the principle of justice.

One reason that the Hippocratic perspective of focusing exclusively on the individual patient is inadequate for P & T decisions is that it fails to consider how well off or poorly off other patients are. Many patients in hospitals are very sick. Determining that Ms. Packer is among the worst off is a difficult task. Moreover, a sophisticated justice approach considers not only who is the worst off at the moment, but who might be the worst off at some later time if resources are used for the bevacizumab rather than other purposes. Putting the money into an aggressive immunization program may not only be more cost-effective, it could also spare some patients from suffering from even more burdensome diseases at some future point. Even within the pharmacy budget some other use of the funds could prevent some more burdensome condition. A rigorous justice approach to P & T decisions would require identifying patients who presently are the worst off or may be the worst off at some later time and targeting the limited budget to that use.

The key to Dr. Reagan's decision is not only the complex estimates of who would benefit most from pharmacy resources and who is the worst off, but how the principles of beneficence and justice should be integrated into a final decision. If bevacizumab loses on both beneficence and justice grounds, Dr. Reagan's decision may be relatively easy. If, however, it loses on one principle but wins on the other—loses on beneficence grounds but wins on justice grounds, for example—then she must decide how to resolve the conflict among the principles. She will have to decide whether to balance the competing claims or to give priority to one principle or the other. Utilitarians and justice theorists differ over which principle should get priority.

Eliminating Proven but Marginally Beneficial Therapies

Similar questions may arise in other formulary decisions. A drug may be questioned not because it is unproven or terribly expensive, but because its expected benefits are considered trivial. If the drug were extremely inexpensive, perhaps the modest benefit could be ignored, but some drugs are relatively costly when considering the small benefit they promise. The following case poses this problem.

CASE 13-2   Antibiotic for a Child's Otitis Media

Harvey Silverstone, Pharm.D, noticed the large number of prescriptions the pharmacy was receiving from pediatrician Dr. Linda McAdoo for the antibiotic Omnicef suspension (Cefdinir) at $55.56 per bottle. He encountered Dr. McAdoo in the lunchroom one day and asked her about them.

Dr. McAdoo told him that many of the prescriptions were for children with otitis media with effusion (OME), a common infection for which there is a high rate of spontaneous resolution. Before Dr. Silverstone could press her on why she was using an antibiotic for an infection in which bacteria are involved in less than 50% of the cases, she commented that she knew that antibiotics were not recommended and that, in any case, medical evidence had accumulated showing that long-term ill effects of OME are rare. She went on to say that nevertheless the condition can be unpleasant, even if it is a relatively benign infection. Dr. McAdoo explained that parents bringing their children to her were invariably distraught and desperately wanted her to do something. It is a common problem among physicians that patients want some action. Dr. McAdoo observed that often that means writing a prescription. Since without a culture she could not know for sure that the infection was not bacterial and because there was a small chance that the antibiotic would help, she felt that this, combined with the psychological benefits of prescribing something, justified her prescriptions.

Extensive use of antibiotics when they are not necessary can lead to the development of resistant strains of bacteria. This could eventually mean that some child will develop an infection from the resistant strain and suffer serious consequences because antibiotics had been used too often to attempt to treat minor infections, especially those that the antibiotic is very unlikely to help. Dr. McAdoo was aware of all of this but commented that her job as a clinician was to benefit her patient, not to protect society from some eventual social problem.

Dr. Silverstone had always accepted the common wisdom that antibiotics were being overused and should be avoided except in cases in which they are necessary to avoid serious medical problems. The antibiotics, he believed, should be saved for the truly most needy cases. Still, he acknowledged to himself that the risks of today's antibiotics are very low and that there was some small mathematical chance that Dr. McAdoo's patients had a bacterial infection that would respond to the antibiotic. He realized that, if he focused solely on the individual patient, Dr. McAdoo was making a good case, but he knew that collectively such uses of antibiotics were posing a social risk and were using pharmacy resources for a relatively trivial purpose. The infection would probably not respond to the antibiotic, and the harms from the condition were not permanent in any case. Dr. Silverstone thought a clinical guideline should be developed to encourage physicians to use the wait-and-see prescription (WASP) for OME whereby parents are asked not to fill the prescription unless the child is not better or worse in 48 hours. All patients would receive oral ibuprofen suspension and otic analgesic drops. Research findings indicated that the WASP approach substantially reduced unnecessary use of antibiotics.[6] He knew that present policy permitted the facility's physicians to prescribe for any purpose they deemed worthwhile as long as a drug was included in the formulary, but Dr. Silverstone was convinced that this policy made no sense. The mere fact that omnicef suspension was very beneficial for some uses did not justify letting physicians use it when the drug was almost certainly not going to be effective and would only offer marginal benefits in any case.

Commentary

The moral conflicts in this case are similar to those raised in Case 13-1. From a Hippocratic point of view, Dr. McAdoo makes a case that prescribing the antibiotic will produce some benefit—psychologically and just possibly medically as well. As long as the benefit, however small, exceeds the risk of side effects, she can make a case for her prescriptions.

From the point of view of social utilitarianism, however, the prescribing practice is hard to defend even if it may offer more benefit than harm for individual children that Dr. McAdoo is seeing. The moral problem is whether Dr. Silverstone and Dr. McAdoo should take a moral social perspective or remain loyal to the interests of the individual patient.

There is one significant difference between this case and Case 13-1, where it can be argued that the patient who was prescribed the very expensive and only marginally beneficial drug was among the worst off. She was terminally ill and statistically speaking could survive for only a few more months. As was demonstrated earlier, whether she really was among the worst off is difficult to determine, but such a conclusion could at least be defended. If so, she would have a claim of justice to the use of the pharmacy resources, even if it was inefficient, that is, even if the same dollars invested in other patients would do more good.

In the present case, the children who would receive marginal benefit were suffering from a temporarily painful condition but would almost certainly suffer no permanent harm, although some have argued that delaying treatment could lead to hearing loss or speech alterations in a minority of cases. It is hard to imagine how they would qualify as being among the worst off. Thus, these patients were less likely than the patient in the previous case to qualify as having claims of justice on pharmacy resources. These children appear not to deserve the antibiotic from either a utilitarian or a justice point of view. Dr. Silverstone thus faces the remaining practical question of whether there is some policy that the P & T Committee could pursue to discourage the prescribing practices of Dr. McAdoo and her colleagues, whether that be simply an educational program about the wait-and-see prescription for the treatment of OME or a more radical solution of developing a policy of P & T Committee actions to permit formulary decisions that are diagnosis-specific.

Eliminating Proven but Cost-Ineffective Therapies

Unproven therapies and marginally beneficial ones are not the only kinds of cases facing those responsible for formularies. Perhaps the most common problems are caused by proven therapies that offer cost-ineffective benefits. When compared to alternatives they offer significant benefit but benefit that is only marginal compared with other, much cheaper alternatives. In the era when the platitude was that health professionals were supposed to do what was best for their patients, these medications were prescribed even though the benefit at the margin was often very small in comparison to the costs. In an era of cost-conscious medicine, pharmacists in their role as formulary writers cannot afford the luxury of condoning every such medication. One example involves the use of an additional agent for preventing nausea that accompanies chemotherapy.

CASE 13-3   Marginal Benefit from an Additional Antiemetic Agent

Jennifer Lavadan, Pharm.D., worked in the oncology department of a large county hospital and clinic in a major urban center. Because of the location of the hospital, most of the patients were indigent. Therefore, most of the funding and reimbursement came from county and state welfare programs. The hospital formulary committee, of which Dr. Lavadan was a member, controlled drug expenditures with a tight hand, using a blending of cost-effectiveness analysis, peer review, and continuing medical education to evaluate drug purchases. Recently the American Society of Clinical Oncology (ASCO) had updated its antiemetic guidelines that previously had been approved in 1999. The 1999 guidelines for preventing high emetic risk included 2 drugs: 5-HT3 serotonin receptor antagonists, such as dolasetron, granisetron, ondansetron or palonosetron, and dexamethasone. The 2006 guidelines added aprepitant to the 5-HT3 serotonin receptor and dexamethasone. The 3-drug combination is recommended for patients receiving chemotherapeutic agents of high emetic risk. By adding the aprepitant, the cost of the regimen increased by approximately $329.

At the formulary committee, this change in the ASCO guidelines caused quite a bit of discussion, particularly among the pharmacists and physicians who worked with oncology patients. Dr. Lavadan summarized their main concerns, "The primary benefit of aprepitant, based on data from randomized controlled trials, is that it increases the complete response rate, which is defined as no emetic episode and no use of rescue therapy in patients receiving highly emetogenic chemotherapy. The absolute benefit, that is, no nausea or vomiting, is about 20%, or to put it simply, about 1 in 5 patients will benefit from the addition of aprepitant. However, because 5-HT3 serotonin antagonist plus dexamethasone remains a very effective regimen and because of the high cost of the aprepitant, I recommend that the standard of care here should be to reserve aprepitant for selected patients, those who fail the 5-HT3 serotonin antagonist plus dexamethasone regimen." The unspoken message was that the hospital could not afford to offer the top recommended guideline treatment.

Commentary

As with the first two cases in this chapter, a Hippocratic ethic would seem to support the use of the agent in this case. The benefit is clear—1 patient in 5 will avoid the unpleasant effects of nausea and vomiting. Unless fear of side effects offsets this benefit, the aprepitant is necessary to benefit the patient.

Just as clearly, the problems are apparent from the social utilitarian perspective. The economic costs are significant—increasing the cost of the regimen by $329. The benefits are transient and relatively modest—not occurring in four out of five patients at all and merely avoiding an unpleasant but time-limited problem in the fifth patient. From a utilitarian perspective, the case can be made for the exclusion of the aprepitant.

For decisions such as this, there is an alternative to asking pharmacists and other decision-makers who are professionals associated with the health care institution to make a judgment call. They could determine the yearly costs of the inclusion of the drug in question and ask subscribers or citizens responsible for the health insurance premiums whether they would be willing to pay the marginal costs. When this strategy is used to determine what is ethical (rather than what is in the subscribers self-interest), a condition is often imposed to make those who are asked take a more objective, neutral view. They are asked to imagine that they do not know when making the decision whether they would be the one who needs the drug. They might be the one on the chemotherapy whose nausea would be prevented with the extra expenditure, they might be one who would take the aprepitant and not need it, or they might be one of the great majority of subscribers who will never be in the position where the drug is an option. They could even be asked to imagine that they have no idea what their chances are of benefiting from the drug (imagining that they have no genetic information, family history, or record of their general medical condition). If they were to render an opinion about whether they wanted their health care insurance to fund the drug under these conditions (and to pay the extra costs of the insurance that would result), they would be deciding under what philosophers call the veil of ignorance.[7] While in the real world we are not blind to our particular situations in this way, it helps us imagine what would be appropriate from a more neutral point of view. Since we can easily imagine that, if we needed an additional drug to avoid the nausea of chemotherapy, we would be quite ill, we might think of such persons as among the worst off and therefore appeal to the principle of justice as a reason to support funding of the drug, even though the majority of such patients would not actually benefit and those who would benefit only transiently.

There is an additional moral principle that could come into play in this case. The principle of autonomy holds that actions or policies (such as P & T policies) are morally right insofar as they respect the autonomous choices of individuals who have significant degrees of autonomy. This might lead to a policy of excluding the aprepitant as a drug included in coverage funded by Medicare, Medicaid, and private insurance but stocking the drug in the pharmacy on the condition that those who freely choose to do so could have the additional agent at their own expense. This, of course, poses problems of fairness—people who are equally sick and have an equal chance of benefiting from the drug would not have equal access.

Some who incorporate the principle of autonomy into their ethics believe that such an approach is inappropriate for basic medical care because everyone should be equally entitled to such care, but they might find this acceptable for a second tier of services that are desirable but not essential as part of a basic tier.

Such a defense presents problems for those who believe that health insurance decisions should be based on what is deemed to be medically necessary. The acceptance of a second, optional or luxury tier of services suggests that some treatments, while beneficial, are not an essential entitlement.

Appeals to Override Formularies

If a health care institution is to have a closed formulary that offers no benefit for nonformulary drugs, exceptional cases will eventually produce problems. A patient may have a serious side effect from one agent when a therapeutically equivalent one could be substituted without causing the problem. If the therapeutically equivalent drug is not included in the formulary, then the interests of patients who have idiosyncratic reactions to the approved agents will be left stranded. Logic tells us that there must be a mechanism for an exception in these special cases.

A rare problem can result when a generic version of a drug is manufactured with an element that causes a reaction in some patients who have an unusual sensitivity to it; or, more commonly, it can arise, as in the following case, when pharmacies operate under policies that mandate the substitution of different drugs that are therapeutically equivalent but that may cause different side effects in certain patients.

CASE 13-4   Overriding Formularies: Therapeutic Equivalents That Cause
             Different Side Effects

Marilyn Cross was not surprised when her physician, Frieda Wells, MD, told her that the deep cough and cold she could not seem to get rid of was "walking pneumonia." Ms. Cross knew she was sicker than she had been last year when she had gotten bronchitis. Dr. Wells told Ms. Cross that she would need an antibiotic and was about to write a prescription when Ms. Cross stated, "I don't want that antibiotic you gave me last year when I had bronchitis. It gave me diarrhea. I was running to the bathroom too much. Could I have something else?" Dr. Wells looked in Ms. Cross's medical record and noted that last year she had prescribed cefuroxime axetil (Ceftin). "I'll write an order for something different that is less likely to cause loose stools. It's called Vantin." Dr. Wells then wrote a prescription for cefpodoxime proxetil. When Ms. Cross got her prescription filled she took the time to read the drug line on the prescription label. It said, "Cefuroxime axetil." Ms. Cross asked the pharmacist, "Is this Vantin?" The pharmacist replied, "No, but it's the therapeutic substitution. Vantin is not in the formulary." Ms. Cross replied, "But this isn't the drug that my physician prescribed. She and I talked about this. We agreed on another drug so I wouldn't have the side effects I did the last time. I don't understand how you can disregard what the doctor ordered and what I want!"

Commentary

Pharmacies have good reason for limiting the drugs that are made available to their patients. In addition to questions of inventory, drugs that are therapeutically equivalent may not necessarily be "price equivalent." It is possible that the manufacturer of Ceftin agreed to a lower price to get into the formulary or may have other reasons for charging less. The price relationship may be fluid. There may be other reasons that the manufacturer agreed to a lower price for this drug. Perhaps they would get more drugs into the formulary, called bundling, by making a deal with this drug. Whatever the reason in this case, it makes sense that pharmacy formularies would limit the medications that normally are available to patients.

That being said, therapeutic exceptions exist for all drugs, i.e., if a specific patient has a bad side effect or does not tolerate one drug over another, thus the closed formularies typically have exceptions' policies. It is possible for this patient to get a therapeutic exception approved, but it probably will not be easy. Procedures for exceptions would typically involve the patient's physician making a case for the patient as to why the formulary alternatives are not appropriate treatment options. This request would be reviewed by the exceptions/clinical review area at the health plan. That is probably what should happen here. Additionally, the patient might be a member of a health plan that has a tiered benefit package that allows her to have a particular drug for an additional co-pay.

It is much harder for inpatients in hospitals to get exceptions to the formulary, as they are not as informed as outpatients about what they are receiving, and hospital formularies are almost always more restricted than outpatient drug benefits groups. Also, the hospital as provider of the product would have to special order the drug in question.

Controversy may arise when the reasons given seem trivial in relation to the reasons for originally placing the limits on which drugs are available. A case in which a patient has had an anaphylactic reaction to the listed antibiotic should have no difficulty getting a substitution. If the patient's objection to the listed agent appears trivial, however, some mechanism will be necessary to adjudicate the issue. A patient's complaint that she thought a drug might have previously given her a headache will be harder to handle, for example. Likewise, appeals for nonformulary alternatives will be easier to accept when the cost difference is small rather than large. Ms. Cross's complaint is an interesting intermediate case. Diarrhea is not anaphylaxis, but it is not a vague belief that a drug caused a headache either.

Similar moral controversy might arise if the patient's objection to the formulary drug were nonmedical. Consider the case in which a patient was angry with a manufacturer because she believed that in the past the company had manufactured a drug that had harmed a family member and had not settled a lawsuit appropriately. Patients surely have a right to boycott manufacturers for these or other reasons, but should these count in adjudicating appeals for exceptions to formularies? What about a patient who prefers a manufacturer of a similarly priced nonformulary product because the patient owns stock in the company?

Physician Behavior with Drug Company Influence

Physicians and other health professionals may have other reasons in addition to problems of idiosyncratic patient reactions for influencing formulary decisions. One of the most persistent of these issues is drug company influence. This can come in many forms—drug company representatives in the hospital or pharmacy, goodwill through sponsorship of continuing education programs, and interactions with pharmacists and physicians. In the following case, a manufacturer cultivates the goodwill of a hospital physician who happens to be a member of the P & T Committee, first by inviting him to attend an educational seminar and then by including him as a paid member of the company's speakers' bureau. Eventually the physician buys shares in the company. The issue is when these relationships become unethical.

CASE 13-5   Conflict of Interest on a P & T Committee

James Hadler, MD, a rheumatologist, serves on a community hospital's P & T Committee. The committee is currently reevaluating remittive agents or disease-modifying antirheumatic drugs (DMARDs) in the formulary. Members were concerned that some expensive DMARDs were not being used appropriately. A proposal had been made by one committee member to reduce the number of DMARDs in the formulary to provide a more efficient pharmacy with better control of inventory.

Dr. Hadler had recently been invited to a meeting at a luxury resort in Palm Beach, California. The focus of the meeting was Jointease, one of the DMARDs that the P & T Committee had been reviewing. He received a $2,000 honorarium just to attend the meeting. Dr. Hadler had doubts about Jointease but was impressed by the evidence-based research findings. He gradually became convinved that he could use Jointease for some patients for which other agents had not proved to be effective. On his return home he used Jointease for several of his patients who were pleased with it.

Dr. Hadler urges the P & T Committee to keep Jointease on the formulary and lift the current limits placed on using it. The week after the P & T Committee met, Dr. Hadler received a visit from the manufacturer's detail man, who invited him to join the company's advisory board. Dr. Hadler's responsibility would be to provide any advice about Jointease and his experience with it. He would receive an honorarium of $1,000 a year and might, in addition, be invited to present his experience at seminars for which he would receive additional compensation. Dr. Hadler agreed to serve on the board. After serving for a year, Dr. Hadler informed his financial advisor that he thinks the company has a bright future and asks him to move some of his retirement funds into the company.

Commentary

Members of the P & T Committee face many conflicts of interest. Standard policy requires, at minimum, that they disclose these conflicts. If the committee does not have a routine procedure for disclosing conflicts of interest, Dr. Hadler surely has an obligation to initiate a conversation with the committee chair. The more complex problem is determining when a conflict exists. Another problem is in deciding whether some conflicts are sufficiently grave that more should be done than mere disclosure.

Some conflicts are so apparent that there is little difficulty determining that they call for action. Some financial arrangements are clearly designed to influence the behavior of the health professional. In one case, a company in a medically related business offered stock only to pharmacists and physicians who were in a position to influence the use of the company's product. Moreover, they were offered stock on unrealistically favorable terms—the money to buy the stock would be a low-interest loan to be paid back entirely out of profits from the stock ownership. The arrangement was a no-risk offer of financial reward that was surely designed to get the health professionals to take a favorable view of the company and to behave in ways that would improve the company's business. Some of these sweetheart deals are now illegal, but whatever their legal status, they doubtless pose ethical problems. If Dr. Hadler buys stock in the company making Jointease, it is obvious he must, at a minimum, disclose his special arrangement.

Merely buying stock in the company on terms available to any investor also can pose a conflict of interest. Dr. Hadler will benefit financially from the success of the company. Ownership of a drug company's stock by a P & T Committee member needs to be disclosed. Standard policy permits some exceptions, for example, if the ownership is through a publicly traded mutual fund in which the investment decisions are entirely in the hands of a mutual fund manager. If Dr. Hadler owned the company stock in this indirect way he might not even know it. The moral rule seems clear: ownership in a company in such a way that it could reasonably influence the committee member's decisions needs to be reported.

The other relationships Dr. Hadler has with this company raise more complicated issues. Membership on the advisory board no doubt provides a useful service to the company, and Dr. Hadler's time deserves compensation, but the arrangement can easily lead to abuse. The company is likely to make such offers only to people who are useful to it. The fact that Dr. Hadler had a favorable opinion of the company's product was probably relevant. Dr. Hadler surely realizes that his membership on the board and the compensation that goes along with it are more likely to continue if he makes positive contributions.

The initial offer to attend the meeting for which he was paid is somewhat more subtle but can be seen as a marketing strategy by the company. The company knew that Dr. Hadler was a potential prescriber of its product. In one case, a national drug manufacturer maintained a database containing all physicians in the country and listing their specialties from which it could be determined whether they were likely prescribers of the company's drugs. It also had a record of the specific prescribing practices of the physicians (obtained by review of pharmacy prescription files). Those physicians who were in the top tenth of all prescribers for the classes of drugs manufactured by the company were singled out for special offers, such as the meeting Dr. Hadler attended. This company even had the foresight to exclude those high prescribers who were already writing for the product the company wanted to promote. Whether the purpose of inviting Dr. Hadler to this meeting was to promote Jointease, the invitation certainly has that appearance. Many would hold that such invitations should be reported to the P & T committee as potential conflicts of interest.

Other financial relations with pharmaceutical manufacturers raise similar questions. Phase four (or postapproval) clinical trials often involve recruiting health professionals to participate by reporting their experiences with the new agents. These clinicians are compensated for their involvement. These arrangements have the appearance of paying health professionals to use (and report on) the new drugs the company is trying to promote. Surely not every pharmacist or physician who accepts payment for serving as a clinical investigator or speakers' bureau member is taking the money as payment for using or recommending the drugs being promoted, but the arrangements smack of a conflict of interest. At least they need to be reported to the P & T Committee if a member receives such compensation.

Reporting conflicts of interest is required by the moral principles of fidelity and veracity. Fidelity requires keeping faith in relationships. A P & T Committee member has made a commitment to the institution to make honest and untainted contributions to the committee's work. Reporting even the appearance of a conflict of interest is necessary. The real issue is whether the situation calls for more than mere reporting. A member who is paid by a manufacturer of a drug under consideration by the P & T committee may need to withdraw from any action on that company's agents. The more difficult issue is whether a similar problem exists if the member has a financial relationship with a competitor. Being paid by the competitor of Jointease would reasonably pose about as much of a conflict of interest. The committee itself needs to articulate clear policy on conflict of interest, including what financial and nonfinancial conflicts might exist, what disclosures are needed, and what steps need to be taken beyond disclosure.

Drug Distribution Systems

In addition to the use of formularies, a second emerging trend in pharmacy is posing moral problems for pharmacists, the sociological changes taking place in the way prescription drugs are distributed. In place of the corner pharmacy or even face-to-face encounters between pharmacists and patients at hospital or clinic pharmacies, new distribution systems are changing the ways that patients receive their medications and that pharmacists interact with them. The nature of the pharmacist-patient relationship as well as the responsibilities of the pharmacist are shifting. Sometimes these changes are as modest as changing the person in the clinic pharmacy who has face-to-face contact with patients. In place of the pharmacist, a technician or clerk may be the one who takes in prescriptions and hands medications to patients after the prescriptions are filled. In such cases, the pharmacist is still on the premises and theoretically available to interact with the patient, if the patient takes the initiative and asks for a consultation. In other cases, however, when face-to-face contact is completely eliminated, there seems to be no realistic chance for the patient to ask questions of the pharmacist. The HMO patient now orders refills online and has the prescription mailed to his or her home without ever speaking to another human being, let alone having an in-person conversation. Even more remote are the mail-order pharmacies that remove contact between pharmacist and patient and the international alternatives made use of in order to obtain less expensive medications. This section addresses some of the moral problems inherent in these new drug distribution systems.

Mail-Order Pharmacies

Increasingly, patients are choosing to get their prescriptions filled through the mail. In some cases, prescription benefit plans actually require doing this in order to reduce the costs of prescriptions, although in the end, the cost reduction may not be that great. In mail-order pharmaceuticals there is a bigger discount per unit, but it is doubtful that providing increased days supply of drugs is really cost-effective.

The economic benefits of mail-order pharmacy are attractive. There are efficiencies related to being able to serve much larger groups of patients, thus reducing overhead. Pharmacists can work more efficiently and avoid slow periods. One of the potential sources of efficiency, however, is morally controversial. Pharmacists avoid face-to-face meetings with patients, thus reducing the time spent in patient counseling and the other service-oriented aspects of pharmaceutical care.

CASE 13-6   Counseling Patients Using Mail-Order Pharmacies

Chase Sumerfield, Pharm.D., the owner of several retail pharmacies tried to do everything he could to compete with all of the mail-order pharmacies that had sprung up over the past several years. Most of the mail-order pharmacies were owned and operated by pharmacy benefit managers (PBMs) and were formidable competitors. He knew that if he didn't change certain practices he would not only lose prescription revenue but could also face a loss of revenue from items like shampoo and facial tissues that customers bought on their way to pick up their prescriptions. Dr. Sumerfield started to provide the 90-day fill quantities commonly provided by the mail-order pharmacies. He knew that he also could start his own mail-order operation, but this conflicted with his firmly held belief that patients should have the benefit of face-to-face counseling about their medications. If he started a mail-order option, he would, he felt, be lowering the standards of pharmacy practice. He realized that not every patient wanted or needed counseling, but the option was there if the patient was physically in the pharmacy.

Dr. Sumerfield's dedication to face-to-face counseling was put to the test when Marya Eckels and her 12-year-old daughter, Sonia, presented themselves at the counseling window of the pharmacy where Dr. Sumerfield was working one weekend. Although the Eckels used to purchase all of their prescription medications from Dr. Sumerfield's pharmacy, they had not done so in several months. Dr. Sumerfield noticed the Eckels's absence because Sonia had moderate to severe asthma and took several prescription medications, including a bronchodilator as needed. Dr. Sumerfield hadn't seen the Eckelses in more than 2 months.

Mrs. Eckels placed a new inhaler on the counter, one that had not been dispensed by Dr. Sumerfield's pharmacy and stated, "I know you haven't seen us lately, but Jim's health coverage included a mail-order benefit, so we have been getting our prescriptions that way. But I hope you can see your way clear to help us even though we didn't get this from you. Sonia just started on this inhaler, and we're just not sure how to use it. I knew that you could show her how to use it appropriately. Could you help us?"

Dr. Sumerfield noted that the inhaler was a corticosteroid, which indicated that Sonia had severe asthma. He also knew that using the inhaler appropriately could mean less unscheduled doctors' visits and trips to the emergency room for Sonia. However, he was more than a little irritated that the Eckels were buying their medications from a mail-order company yet were seeking counseling from him. He wondered what his obligations were to the Eckels, since his pharmacy didn't dispense the inhaler.

Commentary

The problem in this case is not only the relative difficulty of patients receiving counseling from mail-order pharmacies, but also the imposition placed on the traditional, brick-and-mortar store-based pharmacist to provide, free of charge, a service amounting to covering for a competitor. The mail-order pharmacy should be offering this information to Mrs. Eckels. It is possible that it has a telephone number that patients can call with questions, but, in fact, few patients take advantage of this option. In other words, Dr. Summerfield is being asked to substitute for the ones who have achieved an economic advantage to the point where they threaten the very existence of his pharmacy.

Regardless of whether the mail-order pharmacy should be providing this service, does Dr. Summerfield have a moral obligation to respond to his patient's questions? For some, that may depend on whether the Eckelses remain under his care. If they have ceased to utilize his pharmacy, he might argue, they no longer are his patients and, therefore, his duty to counsel no longer pertains. While that might satisfy some, the fact remains that there is a patient, a 12-year-old girl whose medical welfare depends on getting her mother's questions answered competently.

Some ethics incorporate a distinction between moral duties and behaviors that are meritorious but not required. Charity is sometimes analyzed in this way. Those activities that are beyond the call of duty are called *supererogatory*, that is, they are manifestations of good character but not strictly morally required. It seems that it would at least be a noble act of kindness for Dr. Summerfield to answer Mrs. Eckels's questions in order to serve Sonia's welfare. Would it be his duty to do so, or would it merely be supererogatory?

Drugs from Canada

A version of the development of mail-order pharmacies is the increasing willingness of patients to attempt to save money on their prescriptions by getting their drugs from Canadian pharmacies. The FDA claims that this activity is illegal, but many patients, especially those living near the border, regularly go to Canada to obtain prescription drugs. Short of inspections at the border to confiscate drugs imported illegally because they are not in compliance with FDA requirements, there is little that can be done to stop these activities.

Critics of the efforts claim that the FDA cannot assure the safety of the manufacturing of drugs obtained internationally; in fact, they cannot even assure that the ingredients are what they are claimed to be. In response, defenders of the action indicate that the Canadian authorities have adequate protections that are the equivalent of the FDA and that there is no evidence that drugs from Canadian pharmacies are any more dangerous than those obtained in the United States. In response to the charge that patients cannot even be assured that their Canadian prescriptions are being filled by reputable pharmacists, defenders point out that the same is true for those who use U.S.-based mail-order pharmacies.

One example of the debate over accessing drugs from Canada has emerged in the effort of Montgomery County, Maryland, to give county employees the option of obtaining their prescriptions from Canada.

CASE 13-7   Drugs from Canada for Montgomery County, Maryland, Employees

---

On November 1, 2005, the County Council of Montgomery County, Maryland, passed a bill requiring officials to give county employees and retirees the right to obtain lower-cost prescription drugs from Canada.[3] The proposal, which passed 6 to 2, would permit 12,500 county employees and retirees to choose to turn to a particular Canadian health benefits company, Canusa, based in Windsor, Ontario, and could potentially save the county between $15–20 million according to estimates. (Other estimates placed the figure much lower). Individuals would thereby help their county, preserve county resources, and possibly save on co-payments. The plan, if it ever overcomes substantial

CASE 13-7 *Continued.*

legal hurdles, could be expanded to other employees of the school system, planning agency, Montgomery College, and the Suburban Sanitary Commission, thus impacting as many as 85,000 people. It could also serve as a pilot for other government agencies to opt for cheaper Canadian drug sources.

The FDA, alarmed by these developments, dispatched a top official to emphasize that it held that the importation of drugs was illegal as well as unsafe. They have held this in spite of the fact that many of the drugs would have their origins in U.S. manufacturing plants, be imported to Canada, and then "reimported" to the U.S.

In the face of persistent opposition from the FDA, the county has suspended the development of its plan, and it sued the FDA in an attempt to obtain a waiver to permit its implementation. In August 2006, a U.S. district court dismissed the suit. A decision about appeal is still forthcoming. Political changes that would modify the FDA position also could reinstate the plan.[8]

Commentary

The Montgomery County proposal is interesting because it comes from a government agency for a county that includes the home of the FDA. It is a large, suburban Washington, DC, county with great resources for public policy advice. Its proposal addresses many of the more obvious problems with efforts to obtain less expensive pharmaceuticals by going outside the United States. A single source would be involved, a health benefits company that can be reviewed and checked for quality. Participants would be free to use the plan or get medications from more traditional sources. While no source of pharmaceuticals can be guaranteed to be completely safe and reliable, the risks to those who take advantage of such a plan would be quite small. Many if not all of the drugs would be manufactured in the United States under FDA supervision and would be scrutinized further by Canadian regulatory agencies.

Libertarians and others who give weight to the ethical principle of autonomy would surely support the county proposal. They have long questioned the foundation of FDA efforts to protect consumers from taking risks no matter how small they may be. A more subtle problem is whether there are long-term American interests in addition to the purported concerns about drug safety. The policy of having drug companies offer the same medications at different prices in different countries rests in part on the awareness that markets vary. People in developing countries, for example, cannot afford medications at prices charged in the United States. Presumably, manufacturers will strive to keep net profits at a high level. If the American market shrinks and more drugs are purchased overseas and in Canada, profits will fall. That should lead to corresponding increases in prices in the other countries. In a perfectly free market, Canadian drug prices would increase so that eventually the savings would disappear. Is there a case to be made for restricting international prescriptions so that poorer countries can maintain a less expensive supply while richer countries pay more? Do their arguments from the perspectives of public benefit and justice offset the libertarian concerns for autonomy that would support the Montgomery County plan?

CASE 13-8   Pharmacy Promotion of a Medicare Part D Plan

As he returned home from the chain community pharmacy where he attended a short presentation by the pharmacist on Medicare Part D, Lawrence Keller decided he was more confused about the new Medicare drug benefit than when he left his house earlier that evening. He threw the brochure the pharmacist distributed on the desk. None of the brochures he had picked up over the past several weeks were clear about the advantages of signing up for the new prescription drug coverage in his particular case. Mr. Keller was a relatively healthy 70-year-old widower. Presently, he only took two medications, an antihypertensive and an anticoagulant, neither of which was very expensive since he took the generic versions. It was clear to him that if he didn't sign up now he would have to pay higher premiums if he enrolled later on. Then there was that "donut hole" or coverage gap that all the brochures mentioned. Mr. Keller thought the whole thing was confusing. He just didn't have enough information to understand how the drug benefit would affect him, making it difficult to pick the best plan if he were to choose one at all. How was he supposed to weigh risks when he didn't know what his future would look like? He felt like he was being pushed to make a decision on the government's clock, not his own, and without a clue as to how to gauge the risk he might be taking. Also, he wasn't sure what the chain pharmacy stood to gain if he signed up for their plan.[8]

Commentary

The emergence of the federal Medicare prescription drug plan poses many ethical and policy problems. It is the nature of insurance to pool risks and shift costs. Subscribers will know better what their costs will be, and they will be protected from the potential risk of needing very expensive pharmaceuticals in the future. The central ethical question is what is a fair allocation of the costs and shifting of the burdens? A hazard of all voluntary insurance is that rational people will desire the insurance if they believe they will have significant expenses that are covered and will avoid the insurance if they believe their expected costs will be low. Thus insurers will want to avoid letting subscribers buy policies after they know what their need for medications will be. On the other hand, since Medicare is a program primarily for the elderly, many people will have some knowledge of their need for drugs when they first become eligible. Assuming the plan is not mandatory (as basic Social Security is), strategies must be imposed to minimize the risk that people will buy Medicare Part D only when they discover they have a need for expensive drugs. That explains the feature of the insurance that increases the premium as one gets older at the time the decision is made to subscribe.

Insurers also want to create incentives to avoid frivolous use of marginally needed drugs. At the same time, the larger society does not want to drive the unfortunate into bankruptcy if they need pharmaceuticals that are extremely expensive. Hence, the "donut-hole." If people know that after a certain amount of drugs are covered more fully, the consumer will have to pay a larger portion of the costs, an incentive is created to use drugs cautiously to make sure one avoids drug use that will be more costly. At the same time, compassion requires resuming more complete coverage of costs beyond the point that people could reasonably afford to pay. The Medicare program is a political compromise designed to protect people from having to pay for a basic first-tier of pharmaceuticals and also protect them from catastrophic costs while simultaneously making them cost-conscious, responsible users of the insurance.

Another political decision involved maintaining a role for the private sector in issuing insurance. Rather than a single-payer, government-managed insurance plan, the commitment was made to keep the private sector insurance industry involved. Some have suggested this would provide competition that would increase the efficiency of the system.

The result was that there are many different drug insurance plans from which people can choose, and private, for-profit firms have devised competing plans that, while meeting certain requirements, offer a bewildering variety of options from which consumers can choose.

Only a relatively small set of problems with Medicare Part D present ethical problems that directly concern pharmacists. They will necessarily have to contend with patients who have made bad choices and do not have adequate coverage for medications that they eventually need to have. Pharmacists will have to determine whether they have any responsibility to provide charity services for those who have chosen the wrong insurance plan or avoided drug coverage altogether. They will have to respond to patients who reach the "donut-hole" and can no longer afford to pay for pharmaceuticals that they had been receiving during the period when they had coverage for more of the costs.

A new issue that pharmacists will confront is what role they should play in promoting plans and how they should respond to potential conflicts of interest. In Case 13-8 Mr. Keller is receiving his Medicare Part D education from a retail chain pharmacy. No doubt pharmacies have a strong interest in these plans. They provide a source of payment for drugs that can increase the market for drug sales and relieve pharmacists of the embarrassing problem of patients who cannot afford to pay for needed pharmaceuticals. At the same time, the pharmacy has an interest in which drug plan its customers choose. No doubt the education offered by the pharmacy organizing the presentation of Medicare Part D attempted to provide a fair survey of the options, but it is also true that the pharmacy stands to benefit more from some plans than others. In fact, some of the plans may actually have financial arrangements with the chain sponsoring the presentation. At least the pharmacy may understand that it will have better, more complete, or more efficient payment from some plans than others. Thus the presentation poses the problem of conflict of interest if the pharmacy ends up having to compare plans that are more and less attractive to the pharmacy. Certainly it would be ethically unacceptable for the presentation to favor an insurance plan that is favorable to the pharmacy at the expense of providing fair and accurate information for Mr. Keller. Should retail pharmacies stay out of the Part D education, or is there any way they can participate fairly?

Notes

1. From Table 118, "National Health Expenditures Survey—Summary, 1960–2003, and Projections, 2004–2014." *Statistical Abstract of the United States: 2006.* Washington, DC: U.S. Department of the Treasury, Bureau of Statistics, 2006.

2. Bowman, L. A., M. S. Adams, and A. Christopher. "Information Resources in Pharmacy and the Pharmaceutical Sciences." In *Remington: The Science and Practice of Pharmacy.* Twenty-first Edition. Joseph P. Gennaro, Editor. Philadelphia: Lippincott, Williams, & Wilkins, 2006, p. 68.

3. Scott, B. E., B. L. Senst, and M. Thomas. "Hospital Pharmacy Practice." In *Remington: The Science and Practice of Pharmacy,* p. 2259.

4. Penna, P. M., and D. Giaquinta. "Impact of Pharmaceutical Care on Managed Care." In *Pharmaceutical Care.* C. H. Knowlton and R. P. Penna, Editors. Bethesda, MD: American Society of Health Systems Pharmacists, 2003, pp. 274–275.

5. See Dan Brock. "How Much Is Life Worth?" *Hastings Center Report* 36, no. 3 (2006): 17–19; and Lyseng-Williamson, K. A., and D. M. Robinson. "Spotlight on Bevacizumab in Advanced Colorectal Cancer, Breast Cancer, and Non–Small Cell Lung Cancer." *Biodrugs* 20, no. 3 (2006): 193–195.

6. Spiro, D. M., K. Y. Tay, D. H. Arnold, J. D. Dziura, M. D. Baker, and E. D. Shapiro. "Wait-and-See Prescription for the Treatment of Acute Otitis Media: A Randomized Control Trial." *Journal of the American Medical Association* 296 (September 13, 2006): 1235–1241.

7. The term appears in the classic work on justice by John Rawls, *A Theory of Justice.* Cambridge, MA: Harvard University Press, 1971, pp. 136–142, although he uses the concept in a somewhat different way.

8. The case is based on Craig, Tom. "Council Approves Canadian Drug Bill: Montgomery Effort to Cut Costs Raises Risk of Legal Action." *Washington Post,* November 2, 2005, p. B1; "Maryland's Montgomery County Sues FDA to Allow Pilot Prescription Drug Reimportation Program." *Kaiser Daily Health Report.* Available at http://www.kaiser network.org/daily_reports/rep_index.cfm?hint=3&DR_ID=35615 (accessed January 24, 2007); and "U.S. District Judge Dismisses Montgomery County, Md., Lawsuit Seeking to Overturn FDA Decision against Prescription Drug Reimportation Waiver." *Kaiser Daily Health Report.* Available at http://www.kaisernetwork.org/daily_reports/rep_index. cfm?hint=3&DR_ID=39424 (accessed January 24, 2007).

14

Experimentation on Human Subjects

Many of the great controversies in health care ethics have focused on problems in research involving human subjects. The research done by the Nazis gave rise to the Nuremberg trials that exposed to all humankind the outrageous things that could be done in the name of medical science. Those trials gave rise to the Nuremberg Code,[1] the first international document from public sources setting out an ethic for research on human subjects.

It may come as a surprise to some that, taken literally, the Hippocratic ethic does not permit research on human subjects, at least if research is defined as activity designed to gain knowledge rather than to help a specific patient. The Hippocratic code says that everything a health care worker does should be to benefit the patient according to the clinician's ability and judgment. It is the very nature of medical research, however, that the purpose is not to benefit the individual subject, but to produce generalizable knowledge for future use by people as a whole. (Some people distinguish between therapeutic and nontherapeutic research, the former referring to research on treatments that can potentially benefit a patient, but even in these cases, all of the research procedures—the randomization and data gathering—are undertaken to produce knowledge, not to benefit the patient.)

The various codes of ethics of the health professions differ considerably on these matters. Some follow the Hippocratic Oath in pledging commitment to the welfare of the individual patient. Others follow more traditional religious and secular ethics from outside medicine focusing on the rights of subjects as well as their benefit and opening the door to consideration of the common good and the welfare of others beyond the individual. The 1994 revision of the APhA Code of Ethics for Pharmacists contains some of each perspective. On the one hand, much like the Hippocratic Oath, it commits member pharmacists to promote the good of every patient. On the other hand, it incorporates commitments to other principles, such as autonomy, honesty, and justice, notions not included in the Hippocratic ethic. The interesting cases are those in which respecting patient autonomy or being honest with patients or promoting justice in the distribution of health resources may not be what is best for the patient. Also, by having the pharmacist commit to promoting the good of "every patient," the APhA Code may imply that pharmacists who embrace the APhA Code are not focusing on the welfare of the individual patient in the same way as under the Hippocratic Oath. This could mean that pharmacists who subscribe to the APhA Code are more open than the Hippocratic Oath to activities that help patients as a group rather than the individual patient, such as conducting research for the benefit of society. That could provide a basis for pharmacist participation in medical research that is lacking in the Hippocratic tradition.

Health professionals have, of course, faced difficult situations in which known therapies were not successful. In some of these cases, they might, in desperation, try something new, hoping it will help. Sometimes such attempts might be called "experimenting," but they do not constitute medical research as generally understood. Trying something new on a patient can be called *innovative therapy*. It is used in the same way as any other therapy because, everything considered, it is believed to be the best thing to do for the patient. Even a Hippocratic health professional could accept such innovation.

Medical research in a more formal sense is quite different. It often involves randomization between two or more therapies. The therapies are chosen precisely because it is not known which is better. The process of randomization and many of the tests performed on the subjects are not done to benefit the patient; they are done to produce knowledge for the welfare of society. Some of these experiments on human subjects may even involve normal subjects or patients who are not suffering from the condition being studied. They surely are not involved for their personal medical benefit. None of these research interventions could be justified in advance as being best for the individuals; none could be justified under the traditional Hippocratic ethic or any health profession code that requires its members to work solely for the welfare of the individual patient.

During the Nuremberg trials, a critical choice had to be made. Either the medical community could return to the Hippocratic notion that every intervention had to be for the benefit of the patient (thus eliminating randomized trials, systematic data gathering, and the use of normal subjects) or it could modify the Hippocratic tradition, providing exceptions in the case of medical research that would justify some actions by health professionals not based on the good of the immediate patient but, rather, the welfare of the community or of other individuals.

The health care community, and the public at large, took the latter course and developed an ethic that permitted the use of human beings under certain carefully defined conditions. The Nuremberg Code spells out one version of these conditions. For one, the good being sought must be important and not obtainable by other means.[2] This requirement necessitates calculating the risks and benefits of the research proposal, a set of issues that are taken up in the first section of this chapter. These calculations would provide some protection but not nearly enough. Theoretically, the Nazi experiments could have been designed to produce really important information not obtainable by other means. In fact, some have claimed that at least some of the Nazi research was pursuing some important research questions.[3]

In order to provide further protection, the writers of the Nuremberg Code placed as the first, and perhaps most important, new requirement the provision that the consent of the subject be obtained. The code called voluntary consent "absolutely essential."[4] This provision, as was noted in Chapter 6, is grounded in the ethical principle of autonomy. Informed consent in research will be taken up in the last section of this chapter in preparation for additional cases raising consent issues that will be covered in Chapter 15.

Other provisions in the Nuremberg Code include protection of privacy and confidentiality (to be explored in the second section of this chapter) and equity in subject selection (to be taken up in the third section).

In examining the ethics of research on human subjects, other professional and public codes that have emerged since the events of Nuremberg will be important to consider. The World Medical Association developed its Helsinki Declaration in 1964. That Declaration was revised and extended by the Twenty-ninth World Health Assembly in Tokyo in 1975 and again in Venice in 1983, in Hong Kong in 1989, in South Africa in 1996, and in Edinburgh, Scotland, in 2000.[5] While covering many of the same requirements of Nuremberg, it is a professionally generated code written by the world association of medical societies. In some ways it differs from Nuremberg not only in its origins, but also in its content. For example, while Nuremberg insists on the autonomous informed consent of all subjects, the Declaration of Helsinki recognizes that in some cases it is necessary to do research on infants, children, the severely retarded, or critically ill, who are not mentally capable of consenting. The notion of surrogate or guardian consent, and the moral limits of such consent, are introduced in the Helsinki Declaration.[6] The APhA Code requires member pharmacists to respect the autonomy and dignity of each patient, but it is silent on what should happen, in either research or therapy, when the patient lacks autonomy.

In the United States, the American Medical Association adopted a specific code for research on human subjects in 1966.[7] The 1994 APhA Code does not directly address pharmacist participation in research. Its seventh principle recognizes that the pharmacist should serve community and societal needs. This might be taken as a basis for legitimating pharmacist participation in pharmacological research. But the earlier principles affirm that the pharmacist should avoid actions that compromise dedication to the best interests of patients. Since many research procedures ask patients or normal subjects to take some modest risks with their well-being in ways that are not in the patient's interest, this provision could be interpreted as excluding participation in such research. The cases in the fourth and fifth sections of this chapter explore pharmacist conflicts of interest and introduce issues involving informed consent.

In the public arena, the U.S. federal government has long been concerned about protection of human subjects but increased its level of attention in the 1960s. By 1970, the first federal guidelines designed to protect human subjects were issued by the Department of Health, Education, and Welfare (HEW, now called the Department of Health and Human Services [DHHS]).[8] In response to several dramatic cases in the 1970s and 1980s involving alleged abuses of human subjects, formal regulations were established. These included requirements that all research funded by DHHS be reviewed by local institutional review boards (IRBs) made up of health professionals and laypeople capable of assuring that the welfare and rights of human subjects are adequately protected.[9] These were revised and extended to cover virtually all federal government research in 1991.[10] Several minor revisions have occurred since then, most recently in June 2005. Other countries have similar codes governing research with human subjects.[11] The following cases reveal some of the major problems raised in assessing the ethics of such research.

Calculating Risks and Benefits

The earliest efforts to protect human subjects focused on the assessment of risks and benefits. As was fitting the earlier, more Hippocratic ethic focusing on benefiting patients and protecting them from harm, the primary attention of those reviewing research was directed toward research that posed significant risks. They were not as concerned about protecting the rights of subjects who were involved in research posing little or no risk. For example, the reviewers were not focused on the possible inequity of a research project conducted exclusively on low-income patients as long as those patients were not at substantial risk. They also were not concerned about whether potential subjects gave their informed consent to be studied as long as they were not going to be placed at much risk of injury. In contrast, more recent codes, including the federal government's,[12] pay attention to at least some of these issues of the rights of subjects as well as simply making sure that the subjects are not injured. While the APhA Code does not refer specifically to human-subject research, it does stress respecting patient autonomy and dignity as well as promoting the patient's good.[13] This includes matters of honesty as well as confidentiality, plagiarism, and fraud.

Assessing the benefits and harms and determining how the risks to the subjects should be related to the benefits envisioned for the society was the central task in the early years of human subject research. The following case reveals some of the problems in making such assessments.

CASE 14-1   An Experiment of Last Resort: Calculating Risks and Benefits

---

"There are two basic reasons that advances in antipsychotic drugs are so few and far between," Kenneth Higgins, M.D., Ph.D., intoned. "One is the stigma that is still associated with mental illness. The other is the fact that the people these drugs will help are incapable of petitioning for the development of new agents. They must rely on the efforts of the few advocacy groups interested in mental health and researchers like us at Ethitech Pharmaceuticals." Dr. Higgins, a representative of Ethitech Pharmaceuticals, was addressing a group of psychiatrists and clinical pharmacists on staff at Meadowlake Mental Health Center, a private institution. Meadowlake was known in the mental health community as an excellent facility of last resort. The medical and pharmacy staff were being approached to participate in Phase II of a clinical study of an atypical antipsychotic agent, AP-1. Alberta Billings, Pharm.D., one of the clinical pharmacists at Meadowlake, listened intently to Dr. Higgins's description of the risks and preliminary benefits of the drug.

AP-1 was atypical not only in its action, but also in its side effects. Although the drug showed great promise in patients labeled "treatment resistant," there was a potentially lethal

CASE 14-1 *Continued.*

side effect: aplastic anemia. In addition, several subjects developed tics or minor tremors around the eyes and corners of the mouth that were not eradicated by the drugs traditionally used to treat other neurological reactions. Furthermore, these neuromuscular side effects did not completely disappear when AP-1 was discontinued, although they did diminish.

"However," Dr. Higgins continued, "one must weigh these harms against the good AP-1 appears to provide. The core group of patients who do not respond to traditional pharmacological interventions and all of the psychological and social therapies your fine institution can provide need more help. The quality of their life and their ability to function are marginal at best. One could easily consider chronic mental illness to be life-threatening since the risk of suicide is a major factor in the morbidity and mortality of schizophrenia, accounting for approximately 10% of deaths in patients with this condition.[14] I don't need to remind you of the sense of frustration and disappointment your patients experience because there seems to be nothing you can do to make them better, that is, a functioning member of society. AP-1 appears to be able to reduce the risk of suicide attempts by approximately 75–80%. Also, AP-1 puts the patient in a position to benefit from the variety of therapies you offer to help them return to a life outside of an institution."

Dr. Billings agreed that it would be a great benefit indeed if any of her chronic, mentally ill patients could begin to meaningfully participate in life. However, she was deeply concerned about the risks to the subjects. How meaningful would life be if a subject developed aplastic anemia? How would subjects cope with permanent tics and tremors? She knew that Meadowlake would never undertake a clinical drug trial without completely complying with federal regulations to protect human subjects, including justifying the benefits in comparison to the risks. It seemed to Dr. Billings that weighing the risks and benefits in the case of AP-1 was more complicated because all traditional therapies had been tried and found clearly wanting in this core group of patients. Perhaps AP-1 was the only hope for patients who have the most severe symptoms and are resistant to standard treatments.

Commentary

The issues faced by Dr. Billings, the clinical pharmacist at Meadowlake Mental Health Center, are in many ways typical of clinical trials. It may, at first, appear that there are no great ethical or value issues. However, at least three are worth considering: whether patients in a mental health facility can give their consent to participating in these trials, whether adequate consent is the only moral issue raised, and how one assesses the potential benefits and harms of such experimental therapies. The first question—whether these patients can give an adequate consent—will be addressed in the final section of this chapter as well as in Chapter 15.

The second issue is whether obtaining a valid consent from either the patients or their surrogates settles the matter. Federal regulations require that IRBs address no fewer than 7 different criteria for reviewing research protocols, only 2 of which concern matters of consent.[15] The regulations insist on assessment of whether consent will be sought and whether it will be documented properly, but they also impose several other tasks, including assessment of protection of confidentiality (which will be treated in the next section of this chapter) and equity in subject selection (which will be taken up in the following section). Three of the criteria listed deal with the risks and benefits of the research. The IRB must determine (1) that the risks to subjects are minimized and (2) that they are reasonable in relation to anticipated benefits to the subjects and the importance of the knowledge that may reasonably be expected to result from the research. It must also determine (3) that adequate provisions are made to monitor the data collected to assure the safety of the subjects. The implication is that a research proposal could have impeccable consent and still fail to pass muster if these other provisions are not satisfied.

Determining risks and benefits is a deceptively complex task. Of course, it is the very nature of research that no one knows precisely what the effects will be. If that were known, it would no longer be research. All that Dr. Billings and others responsible for the decision about conducting this study can do is render their best estimates based on available information. In this case, the hoped-for benefits are substantial. This will serve, at least at first, as an antipsychotic agent of last resort for a group of people who are destined to long-term hospitalization if an adequate treatment cannot be found. Additionally, the drug supposedly reduces the risk of suicide attempts. These are potentially substantial benefits. But the side effects also are potentially substantial. Aplastic anemia is a serious problem, as are neuromuscular side effects. That they might not be controllable even after the AP-1 is discontinued is particularly alarming.

Determining the frequency of these problems is one issue, but determining their seriousness is another. The seriousness of the harms as well as the extent of the benefits is difficult to quantify. For instance, in order to assess this protocol one must determine how bad it is to experience tics or tremors. One must also quantify how bad death would be for these patients. We assume that death would be a terrible outcome, but some people are beginning to suggest that some conditions are worse than death. For them, a risk of death as a side effect for a treatment-resistant patient who is desperate might not be seen as the ultimate bad outcome.

In order to make a valid assessment, Dr. Billings will also have to have some sense of how good the benefits are if they occur. In this case the benefits presumably are the overcoming of a psychosis, the creation of opportunities for ancillary therapies, and potential deinstitutionalization. Most of us would consider these important benefits, but how can Dr. Billings know just how important they are for her patients? For some of these assessments the patient may be one of the independent variables. He or she may have values and preferences that must be known in order to decide how good a benefit is and how bad a harm is. It seems likely that different patients will make the trade-off among these risks and benefits differently. For some, the risks would not be worth it. They should be the ones who refuse to participate if asked to do so. Others may find the risks of harm and the benefits of the AP-1 about equal, making the investigational agent appear to have about the same value as not trying it. These are patients at what can be called the indifference point[16] or equipoise.[17] Based on what they now know, they are indifferent about both the experimental agent and the standard treatments (which in this case might be continued hospitalization and treatment with less-effective antipsychotics). It is under these circumstances that most analysts say that a randomized clinical trial would be acceptable. It makes no difference to the patient whether he or she gets the standard treatment or the experimental one.

It should be clear that, in order to be at the indifference point, one must envision some potential disadvantages of the experimental compound as well as some advantages. That appears to be the case with AP-I. We are left, however, with a question of whether the judgment of the patient (or surrogate for the patient) should always prevail. Are there ever cases in which the investigators, IRB members, and others at the institution should find the experimental agent so risky that the trial should be prohibited, even if the patient or surrogate is willing to try it after getting a fair explanation of the risks? That may be one of the issues for Dr. Billings here. Does the potential for deaths and for serious neurological side effects make this the kind of study that the staff of the facility should prohibit, even if some patients are willing to try it? If not, are there ever such proposals? In cases in which the IRB or institutional authorities prohibit a trial in the face of willing, consenting patients, would the prohibition be blatant paternalism, and if so, would this kind of paternalism be all right?

There may be situations in which some patients are willing to try an experimental compound even though the IRB members, investigators, or institution managers consider the risks to be too great. There may be cases in which Dr. Billings or an IRB member would conclude that they would not be willing to volunteer themselves but that patients should be given the chance to do so, provided they are adequately informed and their consent is freely given. Sometimes the indifference point for institutional officials differs from that of potential subjects.

Privacy and Confidentiality

A second major issue in the ethics of research involving human subjects is protection of privacy and confidentiality. The general issues of confidentiality were examined in Chapter 8. One moral basis for the requirement that medical professionals maintain confidentiality is an implied promise to do so. If that is the basis, then the underlying moral principle is fidelity or promise-keeping. The key then is what is promised.

Traditional Hippocratic ethics would permit breaking of confidences when the clinician believes that doing so would benefit the patient. Sometimes, of course, the patient might not agree with that judgment. Newer codes, those reflecting a more patients' rights approach, include a stronger confidentiality requirement. According to those codes, if the clinician believes that the patient would benefit from disclosure of confidential medical information, he or she must ask the patient. If the patient agrees, there is no problem, but if the patient insists that the confidence be kept, then it must be.

The second basis for breaking confidence involves situations in which the clinician believes that disclosure would benefit not the patient, but others in society, for example, disclosing information to other specific individuals who may be at risk or law enforcement officials. Many codes now accept the need to break confidence if there is a serious threat of bodily harm to others. While the APhA Code does not, that of the AMA does.[18]

Confidentiality becomes a critical issue in research involving human subjects when medical information in a patient's chart could be useful in the research enterprise. Sometimes the risk is that others will be able to identify the patient as a subject of a study. In other cases, the problem is that the investigators themselves will obtain information that the patient does not want disclosed to strangers, even if the ones getting the information happen to be legitimate researchers.

Some researchers assume that it is acceptable to search a patient's medical records for research purposes provided that the patient is not identifiable in the published study. Others hold that even if the patient is not identifiable, the fact that investigators are entering the medical record itself constitutes a breach of confidentiality, unless the patient has given permission. The following case reveals how the issue of confidentiality can arise in the research setting.

CASE 14-2   Data Mining a Pharmacy Benefit Plan's Prescription Records

Aristide Breton, Pharm.D., is the director of a pharmacy benefit management (PBM) subsidiary of a health insurance company. Dr. Breton previously worked as a community pharmacist. During his work in community pharmacy, he recalled being asked once or twice by pharmaceutical representatives if they could look through his prescription records to see how their particular product was faring against the competition. Dr. Breton was quite clear that this was inappropriate and always flatly turned down their requests. He believed that the information on the prescription was confidential.

Now in his role as director of a PBM, Dr. Breton was again approached for information but this time on a much larger scale. Because of advances in computer technology, the kind and amount of information available on the drug claim forms processed on a daily basis by the PBM were considerably greater than that available in a single pharmacy's prescription records. Not only could one track the amount and kind of prescriptions a particular drug card beneficiary was receiving, one could also view the prescribing patterns of any physician or group of physicians. It was the latter information that was requested by investigators sponsored by a pharmaceutical manufacturer. Dr. Breton received a research proposal requesting information on physician-prescribing patterns for serotonin antagonists in a 3-state region. It was possible for the PBM to screen out any information about particular patients, so their confidentiality would be protected. It was also possible to screen out specific information about individual physicians. However, it would still be possible to determine from the data the penetration of a particular product within a particular market. Although the stated purposes of the study were worthwhile research goals, Dr. Breton suspected that the real purpose of the study was to give the manufacturer information about where their product was being used in order to target marketing efforts. Dr. Breton wondered if the same duty to protect the privacy of individual patients and prescribers applied in this broader sense to the information in the drug claims.

Commentary

Current federal regulations permit certain exemptions to the general requirement that research involving human subjects must be reviewed and approved by a local IRB. These exemptions include studies in which there is no possibility of harm to the subject, provided the data are collected in such a way that there are no identifiers.[19] These exceptions include record searches and the use of pathological and diagnostic specimens. Likewise, the Health Insurance Portability and Accountability Act (HIPAA) does not require permission of patients to review data that are provided in a way that subjects cannot be identified. In this case, neither patients nor physicians, either of which might be considered research subjects, can be identified, so this research could be construed to be legal.

Some IRBs, however, have realized that there are cases in which subjects may object to the research even though they are not at risk. For example, some subjects may object to the purpose of some studies. Even though they cannot be hurt physically by their records being used, they may nevertheless be offended (and have their autonomy violated) if they unwittingly are made to contribute to a project of which they disapprove. The search of the database proposed by a pharmaceutical manufacturer might be such a study. Some beneficiaries of the insurance company might object to providing data for this purpose. They might have developed some reason for not wanting the drug to succeed in the market, or they may simply not want to contribute to the company's marketing efforts. They might assume that a commitment has been made to them that their data will not be used for this purpose. In this case, the physicians might object as well. Does it matter whether a commitment has been made to keep the data private, or do the data belong to the insurer so that it has the right to use the data for its purposes, including cooperating with the manufacturer?

One way in which some subjects may be offended (and have their autonomy violated) if they are used in research without their knowledge or consent is if the study reveals confidential information about them to people they do not want to have it. This problem can arise even if the patients and physicians in the study have data about them collected without any identifiers. For example, such a study could reveal that 100% of the physicians in a given community are high prescribers of a controlled substance, such as oxycodone, or that an unusually large number of patients in this same community are users of antipsychotic medications.

The second way that confidence can sometimes be broken even though identifiers are not collected occurs when the one collecting the data sees a patient's chart. In this particular case, however, no one would physically look at a patient's chart or record. The data would be generated by computer with patient identifiers deleted. Does this protection of the data from the eyes of the investigator make a difference?

As was discussed in Chapter 8, the right to confidentiality is sometimes grounded in the principle of fidelity and the duty to keep promises—implicit or explicit. Is such a promise made with regard to insurance records? It is a standard practice for insurance companies to ask subscribers to sign a waiver of confidentiality that permits the insurer to share data with third parties. Would the waiver apply to this situation? Would it make a difference if the party seeking the data was a drug manufacturer or a nonprofit group or government body? Or is the right of the patient to confidentiality more fundamental such that an explicit clarification that the insurer is not promising such broad confidentiality would be unethical?

Another way of arguing that the patient has a right to confidentiality in this case is to appeal to the principle of autonomy. Does autonomy give the patient the right to control the use of his or her medical information and exclude research uses without explicit consent?

One approach to this problem used by IRBs in some hospitals involves, first, a statement in the admission consent form that specifies that records (as well as body wastes, remaindered blood, and other products without value to the patient) may be used for research without the patient's consent. Signing the admission consent simultaneously grants approval of the research without further consent. It can be called an "uninformed" or "blank-check" consent. Arguably, an insurer could rely on a similar method.

As long as its use is limited to records, wastes, and the like, this might avoid the violation of autonomy by relying on the beneficiary's explicit consent. However, there is a problem. Even patients who generally have no objection to their records being searched for research purposes or their body wastes being studied may occasionally find some element of some specific study objectionable. Furthering the economic interests of one manufacturer might be such a feature that triggers objections from people who usually would be willing to cooperate in research. To overcome this problem, some IRBs have adopted the policy of treating all research of this sort, which is legally exempt from IRB review, as expedited review research whereby certain protocol reviews, such as minor changes in the methods, can be reviewed by a single committee member or subcommittee. Only if the reviewer sees a significant problem will the protocol be taken to the entire committee. Would that approach be sufficient to protect beneficiaries in cases such as Dr. Breton's, or does either the fact that the data are controlled by an insurer or that the study would be funded by a manufacturer change the situation?

In opposition to concerns about protecting the patient's right of confidentiality is the concern for the good of the society or groups, a good that presumably will be served if research is conducted in an efficient manner. It is possible that Dr. Breton's cooperation with the party requesting the data will indirectly serve patient's interests by generating income for the insurer and thereby lowering premiums.

The ethical principle that would support such efforts is normally beneficence, the principle examined in the cases of Chapter 4. Utilitarians would argue that, in principle, if significant good can be accomplished by the research, then the rights of subjects can be overridden. In this case possibly most subscribers would not object, although a minority probably would. Is the subject's right to confidentiality such a right that if the good were great enough the investigator could have access even if the subject objected?

Equity in Research

In the previous case we saw that the ethical principles of fidelity and autonomy might be relevant in assessing research protocols. Another ethical principle that can sometimes place limits on pursuit of social benefits of research is the principle of justice. The importance of the principle of justice in assessing medical research involving human subjects has been discovered quite recently. A federal government commission report called the Belmont Report was the first to mention justice with regard to research.[20]

There are two areas in which questions of justice can arise in research involving human subjects. The one that has received the most attention is subject selection. We have begun to realize that certain groups of people have tended to be particularly vulnerable to being asked to be research subjects. Often these are persons who generally are viewed as oppressed: the lower-income, ward patients who have very limited options in getting care or prisoners who have even fewer options.

More recently, questions of justice or equity have been raised in the design and conduct of the research. If poorly off people are recruited as subjects (perhaps because they are the only ones who have the condition being studied), some people are claiming that they also have claims of justice to make sure that the research is designed in ways that are as beneficial as possible to them. For example, instead of making seriously ill patients come to the hospital for tests needed in a protocol, justice may require sending a nurse to their home, making it as easy as possible on them to participate. Some studies have even had their designs modified—reducing the number of tests or the length of the study—to help protect particularly ill research subjects. The case in this section poses the question of the ethics of equity in subject selection.

CASE 14-3   Recruiting Subjects from the Clinic for Indigents

---

This was the first time that Adam Hislop, Pharm.D., had presented a proposal to the IRB of the Cedar Groves Medical Center. Naturally, he was somewhat nervous. Dr. Hislop was a coinvestigator on a drug study of beta-blocking agents. He had been chosen to present the proposal to the IRB because his research colleagues thought it would be a good learning experience.

As soon as the Chair introduced Dr. Hislop and opened the floor for questions, Nancy Goldman, MD, a family practitioner and long-standing member of the IRB, spoke. "Before we discuss any other aspect of your study, I want to focus on how you propose to recruit subjects for your comparative study of beta-blockers. It appears that you plan on recruiting all of your subjects from the Hamilton Street Clinic. In case you didn't know, the Hamilton Street Clinic was established to serve the needs of the poor. Also, the majority of the patients are black or other racial minorities. By limiting recruiting to the clinic, you are taking advantage of a particularly vulnerable population."

Dr. Hislop attempted to reply, "We chose the Hamilton Street Clinic because that is where we have set up a hypertension clinic, so the subjects would be easy to recruit."

"Just because the patients are available doesn't necessarily make them the ideal targets for a research study. I propose that you and your colleagues revise the section of your proposal that describes how subjects will be selected for inclusion or exclusion and then resubmit the proposal. I will not approve it as it stands," Dr. Goldman firmly stated.

The rest of the IRB concurred with Dr. Goldman. Dr. Hislop met with his coinvestigators and revised the subject-selection portion of the proposal. In the revised proposal, the subjects would be recruited from the West and North Street Clinics instead of the Hamilton Street Clinic.

Once again, Dr. Hislop was present at the IRB meeting to answer questions about the revised proposal. Dr. Goldman was not pleased with the revisions in subject recruitment and said so.

"You and your colleagues just can't seem to get this right," Dr. Goldman began. "The first proposal was limited to poor minorities. Now, you have limited it to a sample that will largely consist of suburban-dwelling, white males if you only draw from the West and North Street Clinics. Elimination of the exploitation of vulnerable groups does not mean that you should uniformly exclude vulnerable subjects from your research study. I suggest that your goal should be to fairly represent the groups affected by the research in question."

Commentary

The regulatory requirement that subjects must be selected equitably is rather new. It poses what may often be a direct conflict between the principle of justice, which requires distributing the benefits and burdens of the research enterprise fairly, and the principle of beneficence, which requires that the investigator maximize the benefit he or she can be expected to produce.

Researchers have long gravitated to vulnerable, low-income populations for their research subjects. These populations have been easier to recruit, perhaps because they believe that if they do not cooperate they will not get needed medical care. It is thought that they ask fewer questions and comply more readily with the investigator's requests.

If this is true, then recruiting such subjects is an efficient way to conduct research. It is not only permitted, but mandated by the principle of beneficence (unless, of course, such a policy would produce a backlash jeopardizing the research enterprise). The principle of beneficence holds that, other things being equal, one should do as much good as possible with resources that are available. It mandates choosing the efficient research design unless there is some moral reason to the contrary. Justice is one such principle. Thus, Dr. Hislop, at least in Dr. Goldman's eyes, has encountered what may well be a direct conflict between the principles of justice and beneficence. The issue here is how the two competing claims can be reconciled.

As we saw in the previous case, federal regulations require that a series of criteria be satisfied in order for a study to be approved by the IRB. These include the requirement that the study produce benefits to society that justify the risks but also that equity in subject selection be satisfied. It also requires adequately informed consent (often believed to be grounded in the principle of autonomy) as well as confidentiality (seen by some as grounded in the principle of fidelity).

The ethical question is whether each of these must be satisfied before a research project is considered ethically acceptable. Must consent, confidentiality, and selection equity all be fully assured before Dr. Hislop can turn to his claim that significant benefits can be expected from completing his study? Or does morality support compromising these earlier requirements (grounded in autonomy, fidelity, and justice) for the sake of the principle of beneficence so that if the expected results are believed to be valuable enough certain liberties can be taken with consent, confidentiality, or equity? Should Dr. Goldman insist that subjects be recruited equitably from other more affluent hospitals as well as the Hamilton Street Clinic?

The revised protocol of Dr. Hislop presses us to further clarify the implications of the principle of justice or equity. Recruiting from the West and North Clinics apparently skews the selection of subjects in another direction. Does it violate the principles of justice to select only relatively well-off suburban-dwelling, white males, and, if so, why? One might argue that it is worse science to select a sample biased by being limited to one sociological group, but would doing so be unethical? Also, if hypertension is more common in minority males, can a case be made that these subjects must be included in adequate numbers so that they would stand to benefit more from such a study?

In recent debates over the ethics of subject selection, minority groups and women have claimed that it is unfair *to them* if they are left out of medical research.[21] In cases in which benefits accrue, medical or financial, they are left out. Also, if data are gathered only from middle-class white males, we will have less reason to believe that we know what the effect of the drug is on minority, low-income, and female patients. In extreme cases, groups who may be excluded as a matter of protocol have complained that their rights have been violated. This has occurred with women of childbearing age who traditionally were excluded from drug studies due to the fear that the drugs could affect any offspring if the woman should happen to be pregnant. Increasingly women have demanded the right to participate as vociferously as low-income and minority subjects have articulated their right to avoid being the only subjects recruited. Would it satisfy Dr. Goldman if Dr. Hislop revised his protocol to recruit from the three clinics in such a way that the subjects mirrored the socioeconomic distribution of the community or distribution of disease? Would he also have to stratify for gender, age, religion, psychological state? If so, how should he respond if the biostatistician tells him that with so many subgroups, he must radically increase his sample size? How should Drs. Hislop and Goldman resolve these conflicts?

Conflicts of Interest in Research

While much traditional discussion of the ethics of research involving human subjects has focused on the conduct of the investigator vis-à-vis the subject, increasing attention is being given to the moral status of the investigator and his or her relationship to the funder of the research. This moral relation is, in a way, independent of the problems addressed thus far: assessment of benefits and harms, confidentiality, and equity. It is also independent of the consent issues to which we turn in the final section of this chapter.

The essence of being an investigator conducting scholarly research is what used to be called objectivity or neutrality. Today, we are beginning to recognize that pure objectivity or neutrality is an impossibility. We will always be influenced by our cultural, religious, familial, and economic interests. Nevertheless, we still maintain the goal of minimizing the distortion that can come from letting outside agendas and loyalties shape research. It has been a serious enough problem for the investigator to resolve the conflicts between his or her research goals and loyalty to the subject as patient. When strong influences from funding agents or others claiming loyalty penetrate the research enterprise, the problem of the investigator becoming a "double agent" can become overwhelming. Still, a source of support is inevitable, and that funding agent will have an agenda that will come into play. Investigators may try to hold these outside influences at bay, but as we see in the following case, that can be a difficult task.

CASE 14-4   Profiting from Enrolling Subjects in Research

Heloise Gato, Pharm.D., was the first clinical pharmacist on the Oncology Service at the City Medical Center to receive funding directly from a pharmaceutical manufacturer to conduct a formal, premarket evaluation of the safety and efficacy of a new antiemetic. Dr. Gato had submitted the proposal for the study to the IRB and received their approval. Felix Cannon, Pharm.D., a new pharmacy resident working with Dr. Gato on the study, had been reviewing the study protocol and budget as part of his orientation.

"Wow," Dr. Cannon said, "I didn't realize we would be getting a $3,000 capitation payment for each patient we entered in the study. Where does the money go?"

Dr. Gato responded, "The capitation money goes to pay for our data management costs, our time, and additional medical expenses incurred by the study, such as blood work."

"Are we going to pay the subjects?" Dr. Cannon asked.

"Yes," Dr. Gato replied, "Each subject will be paid $100 for completing the 10-page questionnaire we've developed regarding their dietary intake and symptoms."

"Let's see. So we're going to enroll 50 subjects at $3,000 each. That's $150,000 minus the $5,000 we're giving to the subjects, minus the data manager's salary that's listed here at $27,000. So we'll have about $118,000 over our costs barring any unforeseen medical costs. What are we allowed to do with the excess money?" Dr. Cannon queried.

"We're allowed to use the excess funds for travel to professional meetings, equipment and supplies, and to support other studies that are not funded," Dr. Gato answered.

"It seems to me that it would be very tempting to enroll a patient in a study with this kind of financial incentive for the investigator when another treatment might be as effective as the one being tested in the study," Dr. Cannon reflected. "You might start seeing patients in light of the new equipment you could purchase because of their involvement in the study. Do we tell potential subjects about this direct financial benefit? Do we tell them about the source of the funds?"

The informed consent form that had been approved for the study did not include information about the source, amount, and mechanism of funding for the study. Dr. Gato had not really given this aspect of the study that much thought until Dr. Cannon raised these questions. Dr. Gato wondered if she would be unduly influenced by the extra funds she would gain from the study. She also wondered if full disclosure required that she inform subjects about the source of funding.

Commentary

It seems obvious that Dr. Gato should not recruit subjects into the study solely for the money if they would be better off taking some other antiemetic. Let us assume that Dr. Gato, when she thinks about it, insists she will not be influenced by the financial incentive to include inappropriate patients. Several problems still remain.

First, which patients are considered appropriate? Is there anything wrong if patients who probably would do acceptably well on standard antiemetics are diverted to this agent in order to complete the marketing development? Assuming they are told that they have the right to choose the standard treatment, would it be wrong to ask them to try the new agent using the $100 incentive? The risks to the patient are not great, but they do exist. The risks include the possibility that the new agent will not be effective and that it may have some side effect not previously identified. The payment is, at least in part, for the inconvenience of filling out the questionnaire. One might also assume that part of the payment is compensation for taking the risk that the antiemetic will not be effective.

It is commonly held that some incentives to subjects can be so powerful that they exert undue pressure. Some people would claim such incentives are coercive, but others prefer to limit that term to more direct physical force that limits the options people have. What is offered here is not force that limits options, but an additional option that was not previously available. The issue is whether this offer distorts the patient's choices so severely that it constitutes undue pressure. Begin the moral assessment of this case by reflecting on whether the patients are subject to undue pressure.

A second problem Dr. Gato must face is whether she is really capable of avoiding undue pressure herself. No one would criticize a manufacturer who paid real costs for medications and personnel needed. If the study is justified at all, reasonable payment for the costs also must be justified. Costs must surely include payment for the time of all personnel involved. This would include Dr. Gato and her staff as well as the data manager. If City Medical Center were a profit-making institution, it seems it would have a right to a reasonable profit as well. If it is not for profit, it still can be expected to accumulate a reserve for the kinds of functions Dr. Gato says will be funded by the extra income. But just as some incentives may offer undue inducement to potential subjects, some incentives to investigators might also be excessive. How should Dr. Gato determine when the incentive is excessive?

One of the keys in assessing incentives is sometimes called the criterion of *publicity*. This criterion holds that, for a policy to be moral, one should be willing to publicize it. In this case, Dr. Gato should be willing to disclose to others, i.e., to colleagues, potential subjects, and the general public what the incentives are that shape the program. This implies that Dr. Gato should include an account of the funding in the consent process.

Some funding relationships seem important to the decision of the potential subject to consent to be in a study. Most believe that morally controversial sponsors should be disclosed. There is less agreement on whether the amount of funding should be. As we shall see in the final case in this chapter and in those of the Chapter 15, a key question is whether the potential subject would find the information relevant in deciding whether to consent to participate. The moral objective is to promote the autonomy of the potential subject.

Informed Consent in Research

In earlier cases in this chapter, the requirements of confidentiality and equity in subject selection, grounded in the principles of fidelity to promises and justice, provided reasons why some would place limits on research, even if it is believed to be well designed and is likely to produce significant benefits for society. These two ethical principles, which do not focus on maximizing good consequences, could potentially hold social beneficence in check, thereby protecting the rights of patients regardless of whether societal benefits are lost in the process.

Another way in which societal interests come into conflict with the moral requirements of other principles of ethics is when they jeopardize individual autonomy. That may be the most critical moral conflict in Case 14-4, as the autonomous choices of both investigator and subject may be constrained by conflicts of interest. A final way in which societal interests may conflict with other moral requirements arises in the area of informed consent. As was shown in Chapter 6, the consent requirement is often grounded in autonomy rather than utility. Consent is required according to the principle of autonomy, even if the health professional believes that more benefit to the patient or society might result if the consent requirements were ignored.

This conflict between autonomy and social benefit arises frequently in cases in which investigators believe that consent should be waived or modified in order to assure greater societal benefit from the research. The next case illustrates this problem.

CASE 14-5   Consent for Randomized Assignment of ACE Inhibitors

It seemed to Sherman Sharp, Pharm.D., Director of Ambulatory Pharmacy Services for Mountain Region Medical Center, that there was another new angiotensin-converting enzyme (ACE) inhibitor introduced every month. Dr. Sharp suspected that a significant number of these new ACE inhibitors were "me too" drugs or merely additional compounds that appear after an initial drug has established the therapeutic niche. There did not appear to be noticeable differences in the effectiveness of these compounds, but there was a major difference in price. With this information in mind, Dr. Sharp presented the following research proposal for a clinical study to the Medical Advisory Board at their monthly meeting.

"I propose," Dr. Sharp began, "that we compare and contrast the clinical effects and reports of side effects of the various ACE inhibitors by conducting a study that will control for bias in reporting on the part of physicians. The study design would only involve ACE inhibitors already approved by the FDA. We routinely use 5 of the newest ACE inhibitors. With your support and approval, I would like to randomly assign your patients to these 5 drugs. Of course, we would set up standard dosing schedules for each drug prior to the study, but after the study began, you would only have to order a generic ACE inhibitor, and I would randomly assign one to your patient. There would be no need to inform the patients that they are part of this comparative study since the drugs are already approved and the patients would likely have received one of these drugs anyway."

The Medical Advisory Board unanimously approved Dr. Sharp's proposal and noted that studies like this were needed since physicians didn't have time to seriously examine the clinical differences in drugs in the same therapeutic category. However, the proposal was not uniformly accepted by the pharmacy staff. When Dr. Sharp presented the proposal to his staff, Angus McConnell, Pharm.D., a long-time employee queried, "Even though these drugs are already approved, don't we still have to get patient consent?"

Commentary

Dr. Sharp seems to assume that as long as he is conducting a randomized trial of several apparently similar ACE inhibitors, all of which are standard treatments in clinical use, he is under no obligation to obtain the patient's informed consent. That assumption is not warranted. As the pharmaceutical care literature makes clear, some form of consent is needed even for standard medications. Patients at least need to be told appropriate information about side effects. In some cases they may want to be told the name of the drug they are taking. It is a mistake to assume that consent is only required for experimental drugs or research protocols.

What Dr. Sharp is proposing, however, is a research protocol, and it may be that additional information needs to be disclosed in such cases. Assuming that Dr. Sharp is conducting a piece of research designed to produce generalizable knowledge, he is involved in some interventions that have purposes unrelated to the normal therapy. For example, the randomization itself is not part of standard treatment; it is a research intervention. Moreover, he will record data, perhaps asking his patients questions about how well the treatment is doing, maybe using a standardized questionnaire. None of these is part of standard therapy. As long as there are research interventions designed to produce generalizable knowledge (whether it will be published or not) most commentators would hold that a research consent is required.

There is also a question of the cost to be faced. Is Dr. Sharp planning to charge each patient the usual charge for his or her medication, or will the charge be the equivalent of the least expensive (with the additional costs being borne by the institution as part of its research costs)? If patients are being asked to bear the extra costs solely for research purposes, surely that is something they would like to know. If the 5 ACE inhibitors are apparently so similar that clinicians cannot tell the difference, it seems reasonable that clinicians would want to prescribe the cheapest for their patients or at least give them the chance to choose it.

Getting that consent may be inconvenient for Dr. Sharp. Sometimes investigators defend ignoring the consent on the grounds that patients would not object as long as all the treatments are standard. Does such an argument or the worry about the inconvenience of having to get consent justify waiving the consent in this case? Current federal guidelines specify that under special circumstances consent can be waived provided the risks are minimal. Presumably they are here. (The risk that is relevant is the marginal difference between getting the drug chosen by the physician and being randomized among the 5 medications.)

However, 3 other conditions also must be met before consent can justifiably be waived. First, there must be no other way that the study could be conducted. Second, the subjects must be debriefed afterward (telling them the nature of the research and why they were not asked to consent in the first place). Can Dr. Sharp meet either of these conditions?

Finally, the regulations say that if consent is to be omitted, the rights of the subject must not be adversely affected."[22] This poses a paradox. It is often held that one of the rights of the subject is to consent to participate in research. If that is one of the rights of subjects, the only cases in which consent could be waived are those in which the right to consent has been respected.

Before turning to the next chapter, consider Dr. Sharp's situation. He apparently has 5 treatments to choose from and is legitimately perplexed about which is better. Presumably any one of them would be an accepted treatment. Additionally, there are few postapproval, head-to-head comparison studies conducted by pharmaceutical manufacturers, so the findings would be a real contribution to answer the question about which ACE inhibitor is better. Yet it is precisely in situations where drugs appear to be equally efficacious that, under the principle of autonomy, patients should be informed of their options and permitted to choose among the plausible options, basing their decision on whatever criteria they might choose, including cost, preference for one of the manufacturers, dosage form, convenience in administration, etc. It may be that whether Dr. Sharp considers his intervention research or therapy, he has a consent problem. It is to the role of consent in therapy that we now turn.

Notes

1. "Nuremberg Code, 1947." In *Encyclopedia of Bioethics,* Revised Edition. Vol. 5. Warren T. Reich, Editor. New York: Free Press, 1995, pp. 2763–2764.

2. "Nuremberg Code, 1947," pp. 2763–2764, point 2 of code.

3. Caplan, Arthur L., Editor. *When Medicine Went Mad: Bioethics and the Holocaust.* Totowa, NJ: Humana Press, 1992; Annas, George J., and Michael A. Grodin, Editors. *The Nazi Doctors and the Nuremberg Code: Human Rights in Human Experimentation.* New York: Oxford University Press, 1992.

4. "Nuremberg Code, 1947," pp. 2763–2764, point 1 of code.

5. The current version of the Declaration of Helsinki as well as some of the history are now available on the Website of the World Medical Association, http://www.wma. net/e/policy/b3.htm (accessed June 2, 2006).

6. Declaraiton of Helsinki, points 24–26.

7. American Medical Association. "Ethical Guidelines for Clinical Investigation." In *Encyclopedia of Bioethics.* Vol. 4. Warren T. Reich, Editor. New York: Free Press, 1978, pp. 1773–1774.

8. U.S. Department of Health, Education, and Welfare. *The Institutional Guide to DHEW Policy on Protection of Human Subjects.* Washington, DC: U.S. Government Printing Office, 1971.

9. U.S. Department of Health and Human Services. "Final Regulations Amending Basic HHS Policy for the Protection of Human Research Subjects: Final Rule: 45 CFR 46." *Federal Register: Rules and Regulations* 46, no. 16 (January 26, 1981): 8366–8392.

10. U.S. Department of Health and Human Services. "Federal Policy for the Protection of Human Subjects; Notices and Rules." *Federal Register* 46, no. 117 (June 18, 1991): 28001–28032.

11. U.S. Department of Health and Human Services. Office for Human Research Protections. *International Compilation of Human Subject Research Protections.* 2007 Edition. Washington, DC: Office for Human Research Protections. Available at www.hhs. gov/ohrp/international/HSPCompilation.pdf, accessed Oct. 13, 2007.

12. U.S. Department of Health and Human Services. "Federal Policy for the Protection of Human Subjects." *Code of Federal Regulations* 45 Part 46. Revised June 18, 1991. Reprinted March 15, 1994. Revised June 23, 2005.

13. American Pharmaceutical Association. "Code of Ethics for Pharmacists." Washington, DC: American Pharmaceutical Association, 1995.

14. Meltzer, H. Y., R. Anand, and L. Alphs. "Reducing Suicide Risk in Schizophrenia: Focus on the Role of Clozapine." *CNS Drugs* 14, no. 5 (2000): 355–356.

15. U.S. Department of Health and Human Services, "Federal Policy for the Protection of Human Subjects; Notices and Rules," pp. 28001–28032, especially, esp. pp. 28015–28016.

16. Veatch, Robert M. *The Patient as Partner—A Theory of Human-Experimentation Ethics.* Bloomington: Indiana University Press, 1987, pp. 210–211.

17. Freedman, Benjamin. "Equipoise and the Ethics of Clinical Research." *New England Journal of Medicine* 317 (1987): 141–145.

18. American Pharmaceutical Association. "Code of Ethics for Pharmacists." Washington, DC: American Pharmaceutical Association, 1995 [Principle II]; American Medical Association. Council on Ethical and Judicial Affairs. *Code of Medical Ethics: Current Opinions with Annotations; 2004–2005 Edition.* Chicago: American Medical Association, 2004.

19. U.S. Department of Health and Human Services, "Federal Policy for the Protection of Human Subjects; Notices and Rules," p. 28012.

20. National Commission for the Protection of Human Subjects of Biomedical and Behavioral Research. *The Belmont Report: Ethical Principles and Guidelines for the Protection of Human Subjects of Research.* Washington, DC: U.S. Government Printing Office, 1978.

21. Garber, M., and R. M. Arnold. "Promoting the Participation of Minorities in Research." *American Journal of Bioethics,* May–June 6, no. 3 (2006): W14–20.

22. U.S. Department of Health and Human Services, "Federal Policy for the Protection of Human Subjects; Notices and Rules," p. 28017.

15

Consent and the Right to Refuse Treatment

Issues of informed consent that arise in medical research were discussed in the final case of the previous chapter. Informed consent has also emerged as a central issue in therapeutic medicine, at least in the last half of the twentieth century.[1] Recent informed consent literature reveals its increasing importance.[2]

It is striking that the Hippocratic ethical tradition has no provision for consent of the patient for any treatment. Its central ethical approach was to assume that the health professional could figure out what was in the interest of the patient and act accordingly. The Hippocratic Oath actually prohibits the health care professional from sharing any medical knowledge with patients.[3]

It was not until the twentieth century that consent of the patient became morally important. Its moral foundation is generally not in the moral principles of doing good and protecting from harm but rather in the key principle of Western political philosophy: self-determination or autonomy. As was shown in Chapter 6, autonomy as a moral principle requires that people be allowed to make life choices according to self-generated life plans. In health care this means choosing alternatives that fit with one's own goals and purposes. One of the important ways in which the current APhA code differs from the Hippocratic Oath is in its explicit commitment that a pharmacist "respects the autonomy and dignity of each patient."[4] Technically, the code never refers to patient consent, but it does interpret the commitment to autonomy to convey obligations that are the moral equivalent of consent:

A pharmacist promotes the right of self-determination and recognizes individual self-worth by encouraging patients to participate in decisions about their health. A pharmacist communicates with patients in terms

255

that are understandable. In all cases, a pharmacist respects personal and cultural differences among patients.[5]

The realization that different health care choices will be appropriate for different life plans is one of the most revolutionary in the health care ethics of the twentieth century. At first, the only requirement was that the patient actually agree to the treatment. A key legal case in 1914 summarized the emerging notion by ruling, "Every human being of adult years and sound mind has a right to determine what shall be done with his own body; and a surgeon who performs an operation without his patient's consent commits an assault, for which he is liable in damages."[6]

We gradually began to realize that it was possible for a patient to consent to treatment and still not be informed about the choices being made. It was not until the 1950s that concern began to emerge that consent be informed and voluntary.[7] That introduced several important questions into the discussion of consent. The first section of this chapter focuses on what can be called the *elements of consent*, that is, the types of information that need to be transmitted for consent to be adequately informed. The second section looks at cases involving questions of the *standards of consent*, referring to the question of what standard of reference should be used in determining whether a sufficient amount of a particular type of information has been transmitted. The third section examines questions of whether the information transmitted is comprehended and whether the consent is adequately voluntary. Finally, the fourth section addresses whether incompetent patients can be expected to consent and what role parents, guardians, and other surrogates can play in giving approval for medical treatments for those who are legally incompetent to do so themselves.

The Elements of a Consent

An adequate consent to treatment must be informed. For it to be informed it must contain several types of information (sometimes called elements),[8] not only information about the benefits and harms, but also their probabilities of occurring as well as information about treatment alternatives. There may be other kinds of information that patients would desire as well, including information about the costs of the treatment, inconvenience, the time consumed, risks relating to confidentiality breeches, any changes in lifestyle that will or could result from treatment, and the competence of the provider. As was revealed in Case 14-4, some patients might want to know about the funding source or if the researchers are receiving a large fee for each subject recruited. The following

---

CASE 15-1 Therapeutic Privilege: The Case of the Placebo Narcotic

Over the past 6 months, Daniel Bast, Pharm.D., had become well acquainted with Sandy Lego. The first time Ms. Lego entered the University Clinic pharmacy where Dr. Bast worked, he noted the dark circles under Ms. Lego's eyes, her hollow cheeks, and guarded movements. At that time, Ms. Lego presented a prescription for methadone 15 mg BID. The drug was unusual for a patient who wasn't suffering pain from a terminal illness, so Dr. Bast called the prescribing physician, Boyd Schrader, MD, for information about Ms. Lego's medical

[handwritten margin note: Schloendorff Case (Benjamin Cardozo) — common law — result of surgery performed without pt. consent]

CASE 15-1 *Continued.*

condition. Dr. Bast wanted some assurance that Ms. Lego had a medical problem severe enough to warrant long-acting opiate therapy for chronic, nonterminal pain.

Dr. Schrader explained, "Ms. Lego has incapacitating headaches of unknown etiology. She has had numerous tests, seen a variety of specialists, and we have no explanation. The headaches started when she was 16 years old and have increased in intensity and duration over the last 7 years. She has tried many different kinds of pain management and combinations short of narcotics. She has a history of depression and has expressed some suicidal ideation when the pain was particularly severe. At this point, I am willing to try a long-acting opiate for her chronic pain."

Dr. Bast filled the prescription and instructed Ms. Lego on the proper use of the medication. As Ms. Lego left, Dr. Bast stated, "Please let me know if you have any further questions or problems with the medication. Also, let me know how it works."

Ms. Lego called back later that week to say that the pain was finally under control. She said, "I don't have to spend my day in bed in a dark room." Later in the month, Ms. Lego called to say that she was able to return to classes at a local community college and a part-time job. It appeared that the methadone was effective. Dr. Bast became accustomed to filling the refills for Ms. Lego.

Now, after 6 months of drug therapy, Ms. Lego stopped by the pharmacy and said, "Dr. Schrader changed my medication. He said this would be better for me." Dr. Bast was surprised to see that Dr. Schrader had changed the prescription to a decreased dose of methadone. Dr. Bast called Dr. Schrader to ask for clarification. Dr Schrader said, "I have grown increasingly uncomfortable with the unknown risks of the chronic use of methadone therapy. I want you to prepare decreasing doses of methadone so that we can get her off the narcotic over the next several weeks. I know that if she knew of this, she would not agree and might become depressed or worse. For her own long-term welfare, we must not let her know what we are doing."

From his office, Dr. Bast could see Ms. Lego in the pharmacy waiting area as he spoke to Dr. Schrader. He remembered how she looked that first day compared to how she looked now, clear-eyed, alert, and pain free. He wasn't certain that this change in drug therapy was truly in Ms. Lego's best interest.

cases show how pharmacists may face problems in deciding whether patients have been given enough information for their consent to be adequately informed.

Commentary

The traditional ethic of medicine commits the health professional to doing what will benefit the patient according to the professional's ability and judgment. That is what is required by the Hippocratic Oath. In the culture of that period, however, patients were never told what medication they were receiving. The use of benevolent deception for the patient's good was a rather common practice. That surely is what the physician, Dr. Schrader, had in mind when he changed Ms. Lego's prescription without telling her. This approach, in which deception is used therapeutically, has been referred to as *therapeutic privilege*. It is supported by an ethic in which the only moral goal is the welfare of the patient.

In recent years, that ethic has been challenged. Part of the challenge has come in the form of a commitment to the moral principle of autonomy in which the patient is given the right to be informed of the medication he or she is receiving and to decide whether to agree to the proposed treatment course. We now believe that in many cases it is in the patient's interest to be informed. In a mobile society, it is often for the good of the patient that he or she knows the name of the medication being taken. That means that even those committed to the traditional paternalistic ethic of patient benefit would usually now support disclosing the name of the medication to the patient. They might even insist that the patient understand the therapeutic rationale so that the patient can cooperate fully in the therapy.

In rare cases, though, physicians and pharmacists remain convinced that providing reasonable information about the name of the medication, the dose, and the therapeutic strategy may not be in the patient's interest. That seems to be Dr. Schrader's attitude in this case. The pharmacist, Dr. Bast, is not completely convinced that decreasing the dose and discontinuing the methadone is in the patient's interest. Thus, he might even object to Dr. Schrader's strategy on more traditional Hippocratic grounds. He might have another concern, however. He might acknowledge that the clandestine weaning is good for the patient but still doubt that it is showing adequate respect for her. He could believe that she has a right to be treated as an autonomous agent with the right to be informed about the essential features of the treatment plan, and this belief could force him to the conclusion that there is no way to follow this treatment plan without telling the patient that the medication change really involves weaning her off the opiate.

Just what kinds of information must be disclosed in order for a consent to be adequately informed? Usually we are concerned about the risks and the benefits of the medication. Here, of course, the most serious risk would be the withdrawal symptoms, which are not life-threatening, from coming off the narcotic. She might also need to be told that one possible side effect of decreasing the methadone in this case would be the return of her debilitating headaches. Since disclosures may produce self-fulfilling prophesies, a good Hippocratic pharmacist would be strongly opposed to disclosing this, while one committed to the principle of autonomy would surely insist that this risk be disclosed.

The kinds of information that must be disclosed are sometimes called the *elements* of consent. In what kinds of information might Ms. Lego be interested beyond the risks and the benefits of this medication? One kind of information that often is included is the alternative therapies available. Continuing the narcotic would be one alternative. If alternative therapies include continuing the methadone, that would have to be disclosed. What other alternatives could be presented as part of an adequately informed consent?

Among the other elements of a consent that might need to be transmitted are the costs of the alternatives, other providers who might be involved, which treatments are covered by insurance and which are not, and the extent of disagreement, if any, among health professionals about the feasibility of the treatment. Further studies are necessary to establish safety with long-term use of methadone for chronic, nonterminal pain. Should she be told about this uncertainty regarding the risks of long-term therapy? In some special cases there may be additional information as well. In Case 14-4, it was a fact that the pharmacist would receive a large incentive from a pharmaceutical manufacturer to get patients into a clinical trial. Information about special funding, the name of the manufacturer, and so forth, may sometimes be information that is relevant to the patient in deciding whether to consent to the therapy being proposed.

In the doctrine of informed consent, the key criterion for deciding which kinds of information are to be included in the disclosure is what would reasonably be meaningful or useful information to the patient in deciding whether to agree to the proposed therapy and deciding that the consent was adequately informed. No rational person would want to be "fully informed." It is not even clear what that would mean since there is an infinite amount of information that one theoretically could provide about any medication: its chemical formula, the details of the manufacturing process, the complete details of all clinical trials, etc. It is conceptually impossible for anyone to be fully informed, and we would cease to find the information relevant or interesting long before we ran out of things that could be said. The goal is "adequate" information for the patient to make a choice.

Once the categories or elements of information are understood, there still remains the question of just how much of each kind of information must be provided. This requires assessment of the alternative standards for consent.

The Standards for Consent

In the previous section we saw that there are several elements of information that could be part of a consent (such as the competence of the provider) that normally are not told to patients but that nevertheless are potentially very important. Probably if pharmacists asked their colleagues (fellow professionals and members of other health professions), they would find that, in similar situations, their colleagues usually would not disclose this potentially important information. This practice of nondisclosure raises an important question: should the consensus of one's colleagues be the standard for deciding what must be disclosed?

Deciding what to disclose based on what one's colleagues would disclose is what is called the *professional standard*. Traditional legal and moral practice relied on the professional standard for determining what must be disclosed.

Beginning about 1970 the standard began to change. There emerged what is now called the *reasonable person standard*.[9] It replaces the idea that one is required to disclose what one's colleagues similarly situated would have to disclose with the idea that one is required to disclose what the reasonable person would want or need to know in order to make an informed choice for or against the proposed treatment. The argument is that if the goal is to give information needed in order to make autonomous choices, then it really is not decisive what professional colleagues similarly situated would disclose. They may also have developed a practice that does not provide the patient with everything he or she wants or needs to know. Only telling what one needs to know will do the job.

The reasonable person standard makes a controversial presumption: that what the reasonable person would need is what a particular patient would need. But what about the patient who is unique, who would like some information that the typical reasonable person would not want? Or what about the patient who is unique in not wanting some information that the typical reasonable person would need? Some are now proposing a *subjective standard*.[10] It would require disclosing what the actual patient would want or need to know rather then either what professional colleagues would disclose or what the reasonable person would need to know. The following case requires the pharmacist to choose which of these three standards is appropriate.

CASE 15-2   Explaining Phenytoin Side Effects: The Problem of Adequate
               Disclosure

The Neurology Clinic, where Warren Kindelin, Pharm.D., worked, was part of a large, ambulatory care center for veterans and their dependents. Dr. Kindelin helped establish a number of pharmacist-run clinics for antihypertension drugs, antilipemic agents, and anticoagulant therapies, with good results. Dr. Kindelin was working with Anne Stone, MD, Medical Director of the Neurology Clinic, to determine the feasibility of an anticonvulsant pharmacotherapy clinic for patients who had been under treatment for seizures for at least 1 year.

Dr. Kindelin accompanied Dr. Stone and several other neurologists as they saw patients in the Neurology Clinic. He listened as they discussed the risks and benefits of various types of anticonvulsant medications and any alternative therapies with each patient. After a week of observing the procedures in the Neurology Clinic, Dr. Kindelin and Dr. Stone met to formalize plans for the pharmacy clinic. Dr. Kindelin stated, "Before we begin discussing details about how the pharmacy clinic will operate, I have a few questions to ask you regarding the type and amount of information you and the other neurologists disclose to patients about the drugs you use to treat their seizures. For example, let's use the drug phenytoin, since it is so commonly prescribed. I notice that you and your colleagues routinely disclose all of the plausible benefits to patients. However, of the many risks associated with the drug, you disclose only 5 or less. Why is that?"

Dr. Stone responded, "Well, I think my colleagues would agree that it is critical to disclose information about risks. Of course you can't tell each patient about every risk. There are just too many. I try and share information about risks that I believe are most likely to occur."

"I'm not so sure about that," Dr. Kindelin said. "There are numerous risks that you and your colleagues didn't disclose that I think would be important for patients to know about before deciding what drug treatment is best for them. For example, I only occasionally heard a neurologist disclose the risks of lymphadenopathy, gastrointestinal disturbances, or hirsutism when discussing phenytoin. Granted, some of these risks are not life-threatening. However, a risk like hirsutism occurs in approximately 5 out of every 100 patients taking the drug, and the extra hair does not go away after the patient stops taking the medication. Don't you think patients should routinely be told about all of these risks?"

Dr. Stone answered, "No, I don't. Frankly, I believe that detailed disclosures would make patients less likely to correctly adhere to their prescribed regimens. I think patients would have less confidence in their drugs as a result of the kind of detailed disclosure that you are recommending. I am certain that all of the neurologists in our clinic meet the standard of practice regarding the amount and kinds of information to be disclosed to patients."

Dr. Kindelin said, "The fact is that neither one of us is a patient. What patients want to know may be very different from our perspectives as health professionals. It would be helpful to empirically explore this issue as we set up protocols for the anticonvulsant pharmacy clinic."

Commentary

In fact, the views of seizure clinic patients have been studied empirically.[11] Ruth Faden and several of her colleagues at Johns Hopkins University School of Hygiene and Public Health asked patients in a seizure clinic how many of 16 named benefits they would like to be told about. In the case of pediatric patients they asked the parents. They also asked the neurologists in the clinic how many of these risks they routinely disclosed to their adult and pediatric patients. They learned that the patterns of physician disclosure ranged, in the case of adult patients, from 86% who would disclose gingival hypertrophy and 83% who would disclose dose-related ataxia all the way down to small percentages who would routinely disclose rare but reported events, such as hyperglycemia (3.2%), lupus (3.9%), and clinical neuropathy (4.7%). Adult patients said that they wanted much more information: from dose-related ataxia (98%) and dose-related sedation (96%) down to hyperglycemia (77%) and drug-related mortality (71%). In general, patients preferred detailed and extensive information regarding risks and alternatives.

Assuming that one has an estimate (or in this case hard data) on what clinicians tend to disclose and what patients say they would want to be told, the intriguing question is what standard should be used in determining what counts as a morally or legally adequate disclosure. Dr. Stone seems to be appealing to what is often called the *professional standard*, under which the clinician is obligated to disclose what his or her colleagues similarly situated would disclose. If a legal charge of failing to get an adequately informed consent is brought against the clinician, the defense would be to bring in colleagues similarly situated to testify about what they would have done.

Assuming the professional standard was used, there remains a question of just what percentage of one's colleagues would have to favor disclosure before it became a standard. Would it be 50%, 95%, or what?

Assuming that there is a duty to get an informed consent in such cases, Dr. Stone and Dr. Kindelin must realize that they cannot tell patients literally everything about any drug. There are virtually infinite effects that could occur, many of which patients clearly would not be interested in learning about. There is no way they can tell *everything*. Knowing what to disclose depends on which standard is appropriate. According to the traditional professional standard, clinicians need tell only what their colleagues similarly situated would claim. Dr. Stone maintains, probably correctly, that other physicians would not have disclosed all the details about even the 16 named side effects of the medication. If Dr. Stone can show that her colleagues would not have said more than she did, is that not a sufficient defense of her actions?

The *reasonable person standard* holds that she must tell what the reasonable person would want to know before consenting. The patients at the clinic studied by Dr. Faden apparently had a strong desire for substantial information. A majority expressed a desire to know about each of the side effects mentioned. That, of course, does not imply they want to know "everything." If there are countless things that could be said about any pharmaceutical, some of them are surely so trivial or irrelevant that learning about them would not be worth the time and energy required.

The moral principle behind this reasonable person standard is autonomy: the patient must be told what he or she needs to know to make an informed choice, even if the information is upsetting. Dr. Stone's concern about patient adherence to regimen or fear of side effects dissuading the patient from taking needed medication may not be definitive according to the principle of respect for autonomy, as seen in the cases of Chapter 6.

Some patients may have unusual desires when it comes to what they are told. Some may want to know less than the typical patient. If the patient says he or she has been told enough, is that sufficient to satisfy the ethical principle of autonomy? What about the patient who wants to know more than the typical patient? Some people are now advocating what is called the *subjective standard* whereby a patient should be told information that fits his or her needs. This would seem to conform to the principle of autonomy even better than the reasonable person standard.

There is a problem with this subjective standard, however. How can the clinician know what the individual patient's need for information is? In some cases, clinicians may know or have reason to know that the patient's needs are atypical. The patient may be in a profession where predictably she would have special concerns about injury to hands or legs or certain mental functions. Some are now arguing that if the clinician knows or has reason to know that the patient's needs are atypical, because of what is known about the patient or what the patient discloses, then information must be disclosed according to the subjective standard but that, otherwise, the reasonable person standard should be used.

The reasonable-person standard poses some problems of its own, however. Just as with the professional standard, one problem is just what percentage of patients desiring information would count as evidence that the "reasonable patient" would want to know? Would it be justifiable to disclose only those items for which more than 50% wanted to know? If so, that suggests that up to 50% of the patients would not be given information that they desired. That could mean that 50% of the time a patient's autonomy would be violated, what many would take to be a high rate of moral error.

We might try to remedy this problem by telling any information that only a small percentage of patient's would want to know, say, 5% or 10%. That policy, however, would still leave some patients not getting certain pieces of information they would want in order to make an informed choice. There will always be some information-hungry patient who wants to know more. There would be no way of guaranteeing that a patient got every last piece of information relevant to making his or her decision without disclosing everything—a task we have already suggested is impossible. The logic of the principle of autonomy implies that a clinician should withhold information only if he or she has strong reason to believe that the patient would not want it. This can be expressed in terms of what percent chance one would be willing to take of withholding a piece of information necessary for the patient to decide autonomously about consenting to the drug. Defenders of autonomy claim that they would not be willing to take a 50% risk or even a 20% or 10% risk. Would a 5% error in assuming the patient would not want the information be tolerable, or should it be more or less than this chance?

These concerns about figuring out what patients would want to know have led to suggestions of a combined standard. Under it, patients would have to be told information according to the reasonable person standard adjusted according to what the clinician knows or has reason to know is unique about the patient's interests.

Comprehension and Voluntariness

It is not enough that the patient be adequately informed if the consent is to satisfy the requirements of the principle of autonomy. The information must also be understood, and the consent must be voluntary. Consent may be constrained either because the information, though communicated, was not understood or because the individual's choice was somehow not voluntary.

Understanding is jeopardized when the words cannot be comprehended because they are unfamiliar, either because the patient is not a native speaker or, even if he or she is a native speaker, the terms are simply too complex. Psychological factors, such as stress from an illness, also may make the information incomprehensible.

Even if the patient understands, the consent may not be voluntary. The patient can be constrained externally by undue physical or psychological pressures or internally by mental illness or compulsion.[12] The following cases raise the problem of whether a consent is based on adequate comprehension and voluntariness.

CASE 15-3   Consenting to the Risks of an Antipsychotic: Capacity to Consent

Patrick Merron, MD, a psychiatrist, and Lisa Riha, Pharm.D., both work in a county mental health hospital and clinic. The two health professionals routinely review the progress of patients Dr. Merron has admitted to the facility, particularly in the area of psychopharmacology. Dr. Merron specializes in the care of the chronic mentally ill. Thus the majority of his patients are clinically challenging. Many of them have gone through the depressing cycle of being admitted in a psychotic state, receiving treatment, reaching a functional level, and being discharged to outpatient care only to repeat the process.

Dr. Merron and Dr. Riha were reviewing the medical record of Wendy Sterling, a 30-year-old woman with a history of chronic schizophrenia and numerous admissions to psychiatric facilities. Ms. Sterling's mental illness began when she was 14 years old. Her parents, Morton and Rita Sterling, have remained involved in her care despite the toll it has taken over the years on both their emotional and financial resources. Ms. Sterling was most recently admitted for a psychotic episode that ended with her wandering around her parents' neighborhood in a nightgown in subzero weather. Ms. Sterling has been treated with two different atypical antipsychotic medications with poor results. Dr. Merron and other members of the health care team are scheduled for a patient care conference with Ms. Sterling this afternoon to discuss treatment options.

Dr. Merron opened Ms. Sterling's medical record and sighed. "I think that we are going to have to turn to an injectable formulation of either haloperidol or fluphenazine. Treatment with 2 different atypical antipsychotics has failed. I have been reluctant to chronically treat her with a typical antipsychotic due to the unfortunate adverse effects that accompany their use, but she has a history of noncompliance, so an injectable drug is the way to go."

CASE 15-3 *Continued.*

"I assume you are talking about tardive dyskinesia and tardive dystonia (TD) as the adverse effects you are worried about," Dr. Riha responded. "Even though patients are not always aware of the manifestations of TD, it can be distressing and sometimes disabling. I am also troubled by the fact that there is no successful treatment for the disorder and that it can continue after the medication is discontinued," Dr. Riha added.

"I feel caught between balancing the benefits of treatment with these medications and the risks of developing persistent TD," Dr. Merron said.

"Since we're talking about this, I would like to bring up another area of concern—informed consent. Are you going to bring this adverse effect to the attention of Ms. Sterling?" Dr. Riha asked.

"No," Dr. Merron quickly replied. "You seem to forget that only a week ago Ms. Sterling was restrained from walking into the center of a semifrozen pond in her nightgown. I do not think she is cognitively organized enough to appreciate the information."

Dr. Riha said, "I spoke with her today, and she meets what I would consider to be the elements of competence, that is, she understands information about her care and the risks and benefits it entails. She also appreciates that the information applies to her particular case. I think she should be told."

"I disagree," Dr. Merron stated. "In my experience, patients like Ms. Sterling may appear to be competent. You find, however, that after you make a good faith effort to educate them and involve them in the decision-making process they fail to recall what you told them and often forget the fact that you talked to them about the side effects of their medication. If she gets TD, we'll discontinue the drug and hope that the effect isn't permanent."

Dr. Riha decided to let the matter drop though she still believed that Dr. Merron had an obligation to disclose this devastating and potentially irreversible risk to Ms. Sterling and that Ms. Sterling was capable of making her own decision about the medication.

Commentary

Ms. Sterling is a resident in a mental health facility and has been diagnosed as having chronic schizophrenia. It might be assumed that she is not mentally competent to be informed about the side effects of the antipsychotic drugs she is receiving and to give consent. This is not necessarily the case, however. Just because she is in a mental institution does not necessarily mean that she cannot give a legally effective consent to treatment. In fact, many people sign themselves into such institutions. They realize they need such help. Clinicians routinely take such signing in as effective consent to treatment. The law does not automatically assume a lack of competence just because one is in a mental institution.

Even if she were deemed incompetent, that would not settle the issue of whether she has a right to be informed. There are good reasons to inform people of certain side effects, even if one assumes that the patient is not competent to give or to withhold consent to treatment. Small children, for example, are routinely told about the negative effects of an injection. ("This may sting a bit.") It might be advisable to alert an incompetent adult to report certain side effects if they are experienced. Doing so, of course, increases the risk that the patient will report the effects, perhaps even if they are not actually experienced, but in various cases there are good reasons to inform a patient even if she is not competent to consent.

In this case there seems to be disagreement over Ms. Sterling's mental state and whether she is competent to consent to treatment. Health professionals have a duty to assess the capacity of a patient to render judgments in such situations, but they do not have the legal authority to declare incompetence. Only a court can do that. This leaves clinicians, such as Drs. Merron and Riha, in an awkward position. They cannot legally treat without an effective consent, and consents from incompetent patients are not effective consents, yet they do not have the authority to declare the patient legally incompetent, even if she is institutionalized because of her mental condition.

Adults are presumed to be substantially autonomous agents with the capacity to consent until proven otherwise. Yet it would be terribly dangerous for health professionals to presume all adults in fact have such capacity. The duty of providers is to make an initial assessment, seeking outside consultation if that seems necessary. Some patients are so clearly lacking in capacity that little formal assessment is needed. Others, such as Ms. Sterling, may be sufficiently near the threshold of adequate capacity that drawing the line can be extremely difficult.

One strategy is to make the assessment and then, if the provider believes that the patient lacks capacity, ask if the patient would be willing to let a surrogate act on her behalf. The surrogate might be the next of kin or someone else appropriate for the surrogate role. In a number of states, the next of kin is now designated by law to have the authority to act on behalf of an incompetent adult. In the case of children, the child is presumed incompetent, and the parents have the authority to act on the child's behalf. If the patient concurs in transferring the decision-making authority, most would accept this as adequate. There may be no explicit legal authority for such transfer, but it is routinely done and, absent ill-will on the part of the people involved, has apparently never caused any legal trouble. Likewise, if the patient is so incoherent that she cannot object, it is generally presumed that the transfer of authority to the surrogate is appropriate. If Ms. Sterling is believed by Drs. Merron and Riha to be incompetent, this is one approach they could use.

If the clinicians believe the patient lacks capacity but the patient herself insists that she should be her own decision-maker, then a more serious problem arises. The clinicians lack the capacity to declare her incompetent. In such a case, there may even be dispute among the caregiving professionals about whether she is competent. The only safe course legally is to seek judicial review if the patient and the caregivers cannot reach agreement.

The other possibility is that the clinicians believe that she possesses the capacity to give an adequately effective consent. Since the patient is an adult, that would be the initial presumption. Of course, even the competent patient possesses the right to ask significant others for assistance in reaching a decision. Assuming Ms. Sterling approved, there would be no barrier to transferring decision-making authority to her parents, even if the clinicians believed her to be competent to consent.

There is one last possibility suggested by Dr. Merron's actions. He seems to believe that she lacks the capacity to consent and that he therefore has the right to treat her without any consent at all. Is that an option available to him? If not, what should Dr. Riha do if she believes Dr. Merron is proceeding without adequate consent?

In the previous case, the mental capacity of the patient made the consent problematic. In other cases, such as the one that follows, constraints on the choices available to the patient are what call the quality of the consent into question. Some people may have the mental capacity to assess the choice they are making but still raise questions about whether they are making a substantially voluntary choice to agree to a therapeutic intervention. They may be lacking adequate information or, as in the following case, they may have been given a reasonable amount of information. If their choice is constrained by external circumstances of confinement or other limits on their options, some are inclined to say that the choice is coerced and therefore not free or voluntary. Is it possible for the prisoner in this next case to make a voluntary choice to agree to the proposed medication?

CASE 15-4   Chemical Castration or Prison: Is There Really a Choice?

"So I'm damned if I do and damned if I don't. That about sums it up doesn't it, Doc?" James Ginter flatly stated to Hal Mason, Pharm.D., Director of Pharmacy in the Regional Correctional Facility. Dr. Mason watched as Mr. Ginter paced in the small counseling area of the prison infirmary. Mr. Ginter had been convicted of first-degree criminal sexual assault. His charges arose from acts of sexual intercourse with his 12-year-old stepdaughter. Mr. Ginter had already been convicted once before for child molestation and placed on probation. He received behavior modification after the first incident. For this second offense, Mr. Ginter was sentenced to 15 years in prison to be served in the Regional Correctional Facility plus a $25,000 fine, reduced to 1 year with 4 years probation if the prisoner agrees to castration by chemical means and psychotherapy. Dr. Mason was asked to explain the action, side effects, and adverse reactions of the most commonly used hormone for this purpose—medroxyprogesterone acetate (MPA)—to Mr. Ginter. Dr. Mason explained, "MPA has been shown to be effective in the treatment of sex offenders. We aren't really sure how it lowers libido, but it does. There also seems to be a sort of tranquilizing effect on the brain. The drug is given either by weekly injections or a depot form of injection that can be given every 3 months. The side effects include weight gain, mild lethargy, cold sweats, hot flashes, nightmares, hypertension, elevated blood sugar, shortness of breath, and lessened testes size."[13]

Mr. Ginter asked, "Will these side effects go away if I quit taking the drug?"

Dr. Mason replied, "As far as we know, yes. If you take the drug with some form of psychotherapy, the success rate is good."

"I hate shots," Mr. Ginter shuddered. "It seems to me that this is too harsh of a punishment. I mean they're going to be putting something in my body that will work all sorts of ways. From what you've said, I probably won't be able to have any kind of sex, even the legal kind with an adult. If I don't agree to these shots, then I'm locked up for 14 more years. Some choice."

Dr. Mason knew that there were several programs in other jurisdictions in which imprisoned paraphilias, or sexual deviants, were voluntarily participating in the study of MPA, talk therapies, and control groups. It appeared that those in the MPA groups were significantly less likely to reoffend. However, Mr. Ginter was not being asked to participate in a study. He was being asked to choose between two unappealing alternatives: chemical castration or prison.

Commentary

It appears that Dr. Mason, the pharmacist in this case, has given Mr. Ginter substantial and fair information about the medication being proposed and that Mr. Ginter has the mental capacity to understand the choice. In fact, he may understand all to well that he either takes the medication and has a chance of being released from prison or refuses and remains incarcerated for 14 more years. But is Mr. Ginter free to consent or refuse the medication? Is he being coerced by the forced choice between two unattractive options, and if so, does that negate the voluntariness of his consent?

Mr. Ginter is not being physically coerced in the sense of being held down while the medication is injected against his will. He seems to have a real opportunity to accept or decline the offer. But one is tempted to say that the alternative (14 years in jail) is so awful that he is de facto forced to agree to the drug. The issue seems to be one of whether one can be said to be coerced when the only available alternative is very unattractive. By comparison, some might say that the MPA is "coercively attractive" even if it presents potential side effects that Mr. Ginter finds very unpleasant.

Sometimes people are forced into choices through circumstances beyond their control. When one of the options seems traumatic but nevertheless much better than the alternative, we might say the choice is forced. If a parent is asked to consent to a liver lobe donation after being told by a transplant surgeon that a live donation is the only way that his or her child's life can be saved, for many the choice presents no real option. The donation is so attractive compared with the death of the child that there is no doubt in the mind of the parent that the donation must be made.

But the overwhelming power of the option should not be taken to imply that the parent's autonomy is being violated. The surgeon in this case seems to have no other alternatives to present. We tend to exonerate the surgeon if there is no other alternative available to him as a solution to the problem. The choice of the parent can be said to be autonomous if it fits with the parent's consistent life plan. Assuming this is a loving parent who has previously made sacrifices for his or her child, it is perfectly understandable that the donation of a liver lobe fits the parent's life plan. It can be a forced choice and an autonomous one at the same time.

Dr. Mason presents Mr. Ginter with what may be a forced choice that is very attractive compared with the alternative. His case differs from the surgeon who offers the parent the chance to donate in that there may be other options open. The society could choose other punishments; it could simply forgive Mr. Ginter, but those do not seem terribly plausible or morally defensible. Moreover, these are options that are probably not within Dr. Mason's control. He seems to be giving Mr. Ginter a choice between the only two options available to him. We certainly would not see Mr. Ginter as more free if chemical castration is removed as an option. In the context of a legitimate incarceration, it is not even clear whether maximizing Mr. Ginter's freedom is relevant. If additional plausible options were available to Dr. Mason and he chose to withhold them, say because he wanted to conduct a clinical trial of the medroxyprogesterone and needed more subjects, then Dr. Mason might be said to be guilty of unethical manipulation of the consent process by withholding legitimate options, but in this case that does not seem to have happened. Does it make sense to say someone is free to choose and can act autonomously in these circumstances?

There is still another kind of case raising problems about comprehension and voluntariness of consent. In the two previous cases, the patients were adults and were, at least initially, presumed to be competent to consent or withhold consent to treatment. The issues were the mental capacity of the patient (Case 15-3) and the constraints on choice created by a prison environment (Case 15-4). There is another kind of problem with comprehension and voluntariness. Minors are presumed to be incompetent. Their parents are their presumed to be proper surrogates for making decisions in medicine and many other important aspects of daily living. Unless they are found to be negligent or malicious, they usually are assumed to be allowed to speak for their children. In the following case, however, a child's wishes challenge the legitimacy of the parents' role.

CASE 15-5 Consent for Incompetents

Ten-year-old Kendra Orr and her mother Shirley were listening to Ralph Anselmo, Pharm.D., as he carefully explained the protocol for the experimental study that Kendra would be a part of for acute lymphoblastic leukemia (ALL). At 10 years of age, when she was diagnosed, Kendra was older than the usual age of onset of ALL, but all of the tests indicated that she had a good chance of survival. The control and treatment groups would both undergo intensive therapy to induce remission, followed by consolidation therapy, meaning shorter courses of chemotherapy over 4 to 8 weeks and rehospitalization. The study would then randomly assign subjects to a 2-year or 3-year group for the final phase, maintenance chemotherapy. The present study was based on previous work that demonstrated excellent survival rates after a 5-year maintenance protocol. The investigators then compared a 3-year protocol to the 5-year protocol and discovered that there was no significant difference in survival rates between the two groups. Now the hypothesis was that there would be no difference between the survival rates of those subjects in the 2-year group as compared to the 3-year group.

The study was approved by the IRB. The investigators were hopeful that the 2-year protocol would be as effective as the 3-year so that there would be one less year of therapy with all its attendant side effects.

Kendra was randomly assigned to the 3-year group. After 2 years, Kendra and her mother met with Dr. Anselmo for a routine review of progress and problems. When Dr. Anselmo walked into the conference room, he knew there was a problem between Kendra and her mother. It did not take long for Mrs. Orr to explain. "Kendra has got it into her head that she is through with the treatment and wants to quit now that she's made it to the 2-year point. I disagree, I think she should stay in the 3-year group and finish the therapy," Mrs. Orr stated.

Kendra, now 12, reacted to her mother's statement. "I understand that there are two groups in this study and that I just happened to get in the 3-year group. I could have ended up in the 2-year group, and we wouldn't have to argue about this. I'm tired of looking all swollen and puffy. I look like a freak. There are lots of kids in the 2-year group anyway. I've just decided that I'm going to be one of them."

Mrs. Orr turned to Dr. Anselmo, "Will you talk some sense into her? I think she should continue with the 3-year protocol."

CASE 15-5 *Continued.*

> Dr. Anselmo stated, "The investigators suspect that the shorter time would be adequate or they would not have allowed subjects to be placed in the 2-year group."
> Mrs. Orr crossed her arms and said, "I am her mother, and I think I should have the final say."
> Kendra began to cry and said, "Don't I have a say in this? I'm the one who has to go through all of the IVs and getting sick."
> Dr. Anselmo knows this is the first group of subjects to reach the 2-year mark, so the data are not in yet to determine if the 2-year protocol is as effective. He also knows that Mrs. Orr is the legal decision-maker, but he is moved by Kendra's arguments. He wonders about several issues. Does Kendra understand the potential risks of her decision to withdraw at the 2-year mark? Whose wishes should take precedence? Is she competent to withdraw from the study?

Commentary

Minor children are assumed to be subject to significant limits in their capacity to make autonomous choices. They may lack the capacity to understand the nature of the alternatives, or they may lack the capacity to be sufficiently oriented to their long-term interests to make a free choice. Parents are presumed to be the legitimate and authorized agents to act on their children's behalf, with a duty to act in their best interest. This presumption extends to choices in health care, including the right to consent or withhold consent for medications prescribed for the minor.

This case adds complexities that challenge these presumptions. First, Kendra, though only 12 years old, seems to have a fairly decent understanding of the choice before her. She is repulsed by the side effects of the medication—an understandable feeling on her part. We recognize that the initial presupposition that minors are incompetent and that adults are competent is, at best, a crude rule of thumb. There is no magic transition point when a youngster reaches the age of majority (18 in most jurisdictions). For this reason, adults, while initially presumed competent, can be declared incompetent by a court. That was a possibility in Case 15-3. It is also true that for some decisions, those below the age of majority can be deemed competent.

The law recognizes 4 instances in which minors will be treated as having the authority to consent on their own behalf. First, according to the *emancipated minor* rule, minors who are married or living substantially on their own may be deemed to have the authority to consent to medical treatment without parental involvement. Kendra, however, is not emancipated.

Second, according to the *mature minor* rule, some minors may be found competent to make substantially autonomous choices. This option is normally reserved for older adolescents who can demonstrate that they have a substantial understanding of the nature of the choices to be made and sufficient autonomy to make a choice consistent with a developed life plan. A mature minor might, as a substantially autonomous person, have the same authority to consent to treatments as an adult. There is controversy over whether clinicians such as Dr. Anselmo have the authority to declare minors mature for the purposes of consenting to treatments. Some clinicians believe they have such authority, but since courts are the only agents with the authority to declare adults incompetent, it seems to follow that they should be the only ones with authority to declare minors competent. Clinicians wanting to play it safe will seek judicial approval before acting on the basis of the consent of a mature minor. That is especially true when a parent, such as Mrs. Orr, is actively objecting to the proposed choice of her daughter and would retain the capacity to press charges against Dr. Anselmo. In any case, even if Kendra seems to understand much of the choice in front of her, she is quite young to be deemed mature for purposes of making a momentous choice about a potentially life-saving chemotherapeutic agent.

There is a third set of circumstances in which minors are deemed capable of authorizing treatment without parental permission. In many jurisdictions state laws authorize minors to obtain certain treatments without parental consent. These often include treatments for venereal diseases, birth control, and, in some jurisdictions, abortion. The reasoning behind these laws is somewhat obscure. There is no reason to believe that a minor is any more capable of making substantially autonomous choices about these treatments than about any others. Moreover, there is no reason to assume that all minors are mature in such matters. One explanation might be that parents have come to believe that for certain treatments it is best for their children if they give blanket approval for treatment without explicit parental consent or even knowledge. Parents might reason that, if the minor had to get parental consent for treatment of venereal disease, that requirement might dissuade the minor from seeking treatment. Parents may believe that it is better in the long run for their minor to be treated than to insist on waiting for parental permission. If so, this is a special case in which the law permits treatment of minors who are not deemed necessarily mature or emancipated without parental permission because it is seen as what is best for the minor.

While that provides a limited basis for a pharmacist to dispense to a minor without parental approval, that does not apply in Kendra's case. If she is not emancipated, not necessarily mature, and not a candidate for these special treatments where parental permission is waived, is there any other reason why Dr. Anselmo might be governed by Kendra's refusal rather than her mother's insistence on the third year of chemotherapy?

Consent for research is the fourth area in which minors are given limited authority to make decisions about participation. We might assume that Kendra is motivated by the short-sighted view that she does not want to put up with the third year of nausea, edema, and other side effects of the therapy and that her mother has a more appropriate long-term view. Mrs. Orr might recognize that a year of discomfort is a small price to pay for the added advantage of a better chance of survival.

But there is a problem with that formulation. Dr. Anselmo and his colleagues have already established that 3 years is no worse than 5 years of the therapy, and they now find the idea that 2 years of therapy may be just as good as 3 years sufficiently plausible that they are willing to randomize youngsters to the two lengths of time. For such a study to be ethical, the null hypothesis must be plausible, that is, there must be real doubt whether the 2-year or the 3-year treatment is better. Since the third year has well-known unattractive side effects, nausea and edema, etc., they must believe that the third year might have offsetting advantages that just about equal the unattractive side effects. They must believe that they are not taking undue risks by placing children in either the 2- or 3-year arms of the study.

If that is true (and it should be if the IRB has approved the study), can Mrs. Orr justifiably believe that the 3-year arm would be in her daughter's best interest? Some might say that if the best oncologists in the world cannot determine whether 2 or 3 years is better, there are no grounds at all for Mrs. Orr to know. If so, why shouldn't Kendra be able to choose, even if her choice is not terribly rational or autonomous? For this reason, in the case of minors who are capable, federal regulations require that, in addition to asking parental permission to enter a minor into a randomized clinical trial, researchers also seek the minor's approval or assent.[14] The reasoning is that, if the null hypothesis is plausible, there can be no preexisting rational preference for one treatment arm or the other and that even less than autonomous preferences on the part of the minor can be honored. That seems to give the minor the authority to veto the parent's permission to include the minor as a subject. Since subjects who have the right to consent (or grant assent in the case of the minor) also have the right to withdraw from a study at any time, Kendra might be said to have the right to end the study at 2 years even against her mother's wishes.

There is one final consideration that could restore her mother's right to keep her in the trial against her wishes. Parents have the right to grant permission for (non-experimental) medical treatment, even against a minor's wishes, because we believe that parents have the ability to choose what is in the minor's best interest. The argument given above suggests that in a random clinical trial no one can have a rational preference for one treatment arm or the other and that therefore there is no basis for the parent to have a strong preference. That assumes, however, that it is irrational for patents or their surrogates to have a strong preference when knowledgeable medical scientists have none. That assumption is worth exploring.

This is a situation in which the medical scientists appear to think that there is some modest reason to believe that 3 years of therapy may be slightly more attractive in terms of survival than 2 years. (If they believed 3 years was much better, they could not morally randomize some patients to only 2 years; if they believed 3 years had no chance of being better, they would not be justified in inflicted the extra year of side effects of the therapy.) Believing the null hypothesis is plausible requires a belief that, when one takes into account survival as well as side effects, the two treatment lengths seem about equally attractive to the investigators. But comparing a slightly better survival chance with the risk of nausea and edema or other side effects is a remarkably subjective judgment call. Different people will make the comparison differently. There is no reason to assume that being an expert in medical science gives one special skills in making such a comparison. In fact, the investigators may be members of special social, age, or gender groups that lead them to give special weight to the pattern of envisioned benefits and risks for one of the arms rather than the other. In this case, male researchers who are oncologists may place great weight on doing whatever it takes to increase chances of survival and may downplay the importance of physical and psychological side effects of the chemotherapy. Oncologists, after all, are known to have a unique commitment to fighting death. Kendra and her mother may have differing subjective evaluations of the benefits and risks involved. Her mother may want to fight her daughter's death with even more zeal than the investigators. If so, it would not be irrational for her to insist that the 3-year treatment was better for her daughter even while the investigators are uncertain which is better. In that case, she would rationally have refused to enter her daughter in the study, knowing that the alternative would be standard 3-year therapy. Kendra, however, may hold values that differ from both her mother and the investigators. She might place higher value on avoiding the side effects. Many adults probably would share such a view.

If that is the case, is there any reason why either the 12-year-old Kendra or her mother should have the authority to pick one option or the other? In the present circumstance of a randomized clinical trial, both parental permission and the minor's assent are needed. That means that the mother could refuse her permission to enter the trial and that Kendra would be forced to receive the standard 3-year therapy. But, since Kendra's assent also is needed, she could block continuation in the trial because she has a preference for the 2-year arm. In that case, however, her mother would have the authority to enter her into standard therapy, which would be a third year of chemotherapy. Who really should have the authority to give consent or withhold it?

Many of the most controversial informed consent cases involve consent or refusal of consent for treatment of a critical or terminal illness. Patients may refuse consent knowing that they may be at risk for dying. In fact, they may actually be wanting to die when they refuse the consent. These issues arise in the cases in Chapter 16.

Notes

1. President's Commission for the Study of Ethical Problems in Medicine and Biomedical and Behavioral Research. *Making Health Care Decisions: A Report on the Ethical and Legal Implications of Informed Consent in the Patient-Practitioner Relationship.* Vol. 1. Washington, DC: U.S. Government Printing Office, 1982; Faden, Ruth, and Tom L. Beauchamp, in collaboration with Nancy N. P. King. A *History and Theory of Informed Consent.* New York: Oxford University Press, 1986; Katz, Jay. *The Silent World of Doctor and Patient.* New York: Free Press, 1984; Beauchamp, Tom L.; and Ruth R. Faden. "Informed Consent: I. History of Informed Consent." In *Encyclopedia of Bioethics.* Third Edition. Stephen G. Post, Editor. New York: Macmillan, 2004, pp. 1271–1277.

2. Katz, Jay, and Angela Roddey Holder. "Informed Consent: V. Legal and Ethical Issues of Consent in Healthcare." In Post, *Encyclopedia of Bioethics,* pp. 1296–1306; Evans, Martyn. "The Autonomy of the Patient: Informed Consent." In *Bioethics in a European Perspective.* Henk ten Have and Bert Gordijn, Editors. Boston: Kluwer, 2001 pp. 83–91.

3. Edelstein, Ludwig. "The Hippocratic Oath: Text, Translation and Interpretation." In *Ancient Medicine: Selected Papers of Ludwig Edelstein.* Owsei Temkin and C. Lilian Temkin, Editors. Baltimore, MD: Johns Hopkins University Press, 1967, pp. 3–64, esp. 6.

4. American Pharmaceutical Association. "Code of Ethics for Pharmacists." Washington, DC: American Pharmaceutical Association, 1995 [Principle III].

5. Ibid.

6. *Schloendorff v. New York Hospital* (1914). In Katz, Jay. *Experimentation with Human Beings: The Authority of the Investigator, Subject, Professions, and State in the Human Experimentation Process.* New York: Russell Sage Foundation, 1972, p. 526.

7. *Salgo v. Leland Stanford, Jr. University Board of Trustees.* 317 P.2d 170 (1957).

8. Beauchamp, Tom L., and Ruth R. Faden. "Informed Consent: II. Meaning and Elements." In Post, *Encyclopedia of Bioethics,* pp. 1277–1280.

9. *Berkey v. Anderson.* 1 Cal. App.3d 790, 82 Cal. Rptr. 67 (1969); *Cobbs v. Grant* 502 P.2d 1 (Cal. 1972); *Canterbury v. Spence,* U.S. Court of Appeals. District of Columbia. 464 F.2d 772, 150 U.S.App.D.C. 263 (1972).

10. President's Commission for the Study of Ethical Problems in Medicine, *A Report on the Ethical and Legal Implications of Informed Consent in the Patient-Practitioner Relationship,* p. 43.

11. Faden, R. R., C. Becker, C. Lewis, J. Freeman, and A. I. Faden. "Disclosure of Information to Patients in Medical Care." *Medical Care* 19, no. 7 (1981): 718–733.

12. Brown, Alan P.; Troyen A. Brennan, Lisa S. Parker, and Kamran Samakar. "Informed Consent: VI. Issues of Consent in Mental Healthcare." In Post, *Encyclopedia of Bioethics,* pp. 1307–1313; Schwartz, Harold I., and David M. Mack. "Informed Consent and Competency." In *Principles and Practice of Forensic Psychiatry.* Second Edition. Richard Rosner, Editor. London/New York: Arnold/Oxford University Press, 2003, pp. 97–106.

13. Drugdex Editorial Staff. "Medroxyprogesterone" (monograph). In *Drugdex(R) Information System.* C. R. Gelman and B. H. Rumack, Editors. Englewood, CO: Micromedex, Inc., 1996.

14. U.S. Department of Health and Human Services. "Additional Protections for Children Involved as Subjects in Research." *Federal Register* 48, no. 46 (March 8, 1983): 9814–9820.

16

Death and Dying

The informed consent issues raised in the previous chapter often arise in the care of terminally and critically ill patients. In the consent process patients must be told of the treatment alternatives. With terminally ill patients, sometimes doing nothing to attempt a cure is among the plausible alternatives. The terminally ill patient (or his or her surrogate) may decline the treatment offered in favor of letting nature take its course. While this is sometimes referred to as doing nothing at all, in fact it normally involves continuing to *care* for the patient while forgoing efforts to *cure*. The pioneering medical ethicist, Paul Ramsey, was one who stressed the distinction between curing and caring and the appropriateness of continuing to care when cure becomes impossible.[1] Others have summarized the moral issues related to terminal care decisions.[2] Often the pharmacist will have responsibilities for continuing to care for the dying patient in order to make him or her comfortable by providing pain-relieving medication.

In the cases of Chapter 9 the problems surrounding the ethics of killing and letting die were examined. Some traditional medical ethics, such as Orthodox Judaism, include the belief that medical professionals always have a duty to preserve life.[3] As was shown in Chapter 9, however, many medical ethical traditions, including those in the health care professions[4] as well as in the U.S. justice system,[5] often distinguish between active killing, which is prohibited, and forgoing treatment, which can legitimately be chosen by the patient or surrogate under certain circumstances. We also saw that deciding what was ethical to forgo is often based on assessment of benefits and harms expected. The doctrine of proportionality holds that treatments are ethically expendable when the benefits expected do not exceed the expected harms to the patient. While some people consider withholding life-sustaining treatments more morally acceptable than withdrawing treatments that have begun, the dominant view today is that there is no morally significant difference between withholding and withdrawing. Thus, those who consider all actions that will result in death immoral will condemn both withholding and withdrawing (as well as active killing), and those who find withholding treatments on the grounds that no proportional benefit is expected likely consider withdrawing treatments acceptable on the same grounds. A treatment may be started because it is believed that expected benefits justify any necessary risks of harm. If, however, the treatment turns out not to offer the benefit originally expected, a patient or surrogate may revoke the consent to treatment, leading to a justifiable withdrawal. Issues of deciding to accept or to refuse treatment are explored in the cases of Chapter 9.

Many of the critical moral decisions related to the care of the terminally and critically ill actually involve the ethical issues of informed consent or the refusal and withdrawal of consent. Both legal as well as most ethical theories consider the moral principle of autonomy to take priority over paternalism. If this is true, then it is acceptable for the substantially autonomous patient, even if treatment is life-sustaining, to decline or to withdraw consent.

There are some other problems related to care of the terminally ill patient that are taken up in this chapter. These are problems that cannot be resolved solely by figuring out the relationship among the duties to benefit the patient, respect autonomy, and avoid killing. The first section focuses on the problems of the definition of death. Then, in succeeding sections, the cases deal with decisions by surrogates for terminally or critically ill patients who are not competent to make their own choices about care, looking first at formerly competent patients and then at those who have never been competent. In the final section, the issue is new controversies over limiting care to the terminally ill patients in order to conserve scarce medical resources.

The Definition of Death

Until the late 1960s, there had been a millennia-old general understanding of what it meant to be dead. With the development of cardiopulmonary resuscitation (CPR), ventilators, and better understanding of pulmonary and cardiac physiology, we have gained greater capacity to intervene in the dying process. We were able to uncouple a series of events that, until then, had always been connected. For the first time moment that cardiac and respiratory function ceases can be separated from the moment that brain function is lost.

During this same period the first human heart transplant took place, and society developed a profound interest in the viable organs that might be taken from dead patients. At the time, bioethicists were asking whether people can be considered dead if their heart and lung functions are continuing but their capacity for bodily integration through brain activity has been irreversibly lost.[6] If such patients can be considered dead, then organs with life-saving potential can be procured. These developments gave rise to what is now thought of as the brain-oriented definition of death. According to it:

> An individual who has sustained either (1) irreversible cessation of circulatory and respiratory functions, or (2) irreversible cessation of all functions of the entire brain, including the brain stem, is dead. A determination of death must be made in accordance with accepted medical standards.[7]

Sometimes health professionals must confront cases that force them to determine exactly what it means for a patient to be dead. In this case we see that the now-fashionable definition based on irreversible loss of *all* brain function (the so-called "whole-brain-oriented" definition) poses problems for clinicians who must struggle with whether to bend the legal requirements for pronouncing death in order to meet the needs of family or financial requirements.

CASE 16-1   His Brain Is Gone, but Is He Dead?

Eileen Caruso, Pharm.D., stood outside Room 6 in the Neurology Intensive Care Unit reviewing the chart of its occupant, Harvey Price. Mr. Price had been involved in a motor vehicle accident in which he had suffered multiple fractures, internal damage, and a serious head injury. Dr. Caruso noted the numerous vasopressor drugs as well as antibiotics and steroids Mr. Price was receiving. Dr. Caruso watched the slow, rhythmic rise and fall of Mr. Price's chest as the ventilator worked to support his shallow breathing. While Dr. Caruso was lost in quiet thought, Daniel Murray, MD, the attending neurologist entered the room and began a thorough neurological assessment. When Dr. Murray finished the exam, he joined Dr. Caruso at the charting table outside the room.

"Well, that confirms it," Dr. Murray stated. "All of the tests indicate that Mr. Price meets the criteria for brain death. His head injury was quite profound, but I went ahead and ordered a few more confirmatory tests, and there's no denying the clinical presentation."

Dr. Murray wrote a short note in the chart and handed it back to Dr. Caruso. Dr. Caruso expected to see an entry pronouncing Mr. Price dead, but instead there were changes in two of the intravenous drug dosages. Dr. Caruso expressed her confusion to Dr. Murray.

"Why haven't you pronounced Mr. Price dead? You just said he meets all of the criteria for brain death," Dr. Caruso said.

"His family won't be able to get here until tomorrow, so I'm going to continue supporting vital functions for at least another day, perhaps more," Dr. Murray responded.

Dr. Caruso partially understood Dr. Murray's intentions. Mr. Price's family would have the opportunity of seeing him while his heart beat and he continued to breathe. Perhaps this would make it easier for family members to part with their loved one. However, these bodily functions were illusory, Dr. Caruso thought, since Mr. Price was dead. Dr. Caruso was also troubled by the costs that would be incurred over the next several days for the medications, treatments, and nursing care Mr. Price would require. It just didn't seem right to bill Mr. Price's insurance company for the critical care he would receive.

Commentary

A brain-based definition of death is now the law in all jurisdictions in the United States and in almost every other country of the world. The only exceptions are China and a few other Asian countries in which there is continuing resistance based, at least in part, on the belief that the presence of life should not be reduced to neurological activity alone. A decade or so ago, Japan passed a law that generally continues to base death on the irreversible loss of cardiac function but that permits death to be pronounced based on loss of brain function if organs are to be procured for transplantation, provided the individual and the next of kin have both accepted the use of brain criteria.[8] The law in most U.S. states specifies that when the death of the brain is confirmed, "Death shall be pronounced." The law leaves it up to experts in the medical community to specify the precise tests to be used to determine brain death.

Once the death of the brain is confirmed, most states appear not to give physicians discretion in deciding whether to pronounce death. There are some exceptions. A few state laws say "Death may be pronounced." It is hard to tell whether the "may" should be taken as granting the physician permission to pronounce death, leaving the decision up to his or her discretion. There are two states that make some provision for patients who hold religious views that oppose death pronouncement based on brain criteria. New Jersey's law gives the patient the right to execute a document stating religious objection.[9] If such a document exists, then death pronouncement must be based on traditional heart and lung criteria. In New York, administrative regulations permit clinicians to take the religious views of the patient into account in deciding whether to pronounce death based on brain criteria. There is no evidence in Harvey Price's case, however, that he had any religious objection to being pronounced dead based on brain criteria.

In spite of the law that states that death "shall be pronounced," some clinicians believe that they have the authority to exercise discretion in deciding when death should be pronounced. Some physicians will insist on waiting until the heart stops beating, apparently still believing, in spite of the law, that the patient is not really dead until the heart stops. Others will exercise discretion for other purposes, including responding to family needs or wishes.

One problem with physician discretion is that it is hard to know how much variation should be permitted. Increasingly, physicians, pharmacists, philosophers, and others are accepting a newer formulation of what it means to be dead. Sometimes called the "higher-brain" definition of death, it differs from the "whole-brain" definition in that it would permit death to be pronounced when all "higher" functions cease irreversibly. While it is not precisely clear what is meant by higher functions, it approximates the view that a person dies when there is irreversible loss of capacity for consciousness. These functions seem to require activity in the cerebrum. This means that someone who has irreversibly lost cerebral function while maintaining some minimal brain stem activity, such as a cough or gag reflex, would be considered dead by the higher-brain formulation but not by the whole-brain formulation. No jurisdiction in the world permits death to be pronounced based on loss of higher-brain activity, yet increasingly people are beginning to support this view.

Dr. Caruso seems concerned that if Dr. Murray exercises some discretion bad consequences will follow. Does the concern about the extra costs involved justify efforts on her part to force Dr. Murray to declare the death immediately? It is important to realize that there is no technical neurological disagreement here. All involved agree that the brain will never again regain any of its normal bodily integrating functions.

Mr. Price's brain is "dead." He is in a condition often referred to as "brain dead." That is a confusing term, however, because it could mean either that the brain is dead in a still living person or that the person as a whole should be considered dead because the brain is dead. If this patient is considered dead for legal and social purposes, then many important events can take place: his wife would become a widow, his possessions could be dispersed according to the provisions of his will, his health insurance would stop funding his medical care, and his life insurance would pay his beneficiary. If he is dead, then the organ procurement team can, with proper permission, take his organs, something that cannot be done while he is alive, even if his brain is dead.

The dispute is not one that can be resolved by any skill in diagnosis or other technical way. The issue is whether society should treat patients like Mr. Price as dead or alive, knowing that some organ systems continue to function even though the brain is gone. If society wants to consider persons alive who retain the capacity to respire and maintain circulation, Mr. Price is alive. If it wants to focus on the bodily integration capacities localized in the brain, he is dead.

If Dr. Caruso and Dr. Murray continue to disagree over whether Mr. Price should be pronounced dead, Dr. Caruso faces another problem. It seems controversial that a pharmacist should be expected to continue providing pharmaceutical care for a dead person. It also seems questionable that Dr. Caruso should knowingly continue to generate costs charged to the insurance company if Mr. Price really is dead according to the law. Should Dr. Caruso have the right to refuse to cooperate in further treatment of Mr. Price if she is convinced that ethically and legally he is now dead?

While the issues in dispute in Mr. Price's case center on whether he should be treated as dead or alive, most disputes in the care of the terminally ill involve patients who by anyone's view clearly are alive. The issue in the cases to which we now turn is whether it is ever acceptable to forgo life support and let the patient die.

Competent and Formerly Competent Patients

The cases in Chapters 6 and 15 address the ethical principle of autonomy and informed consent, the latter usually seen as protecting autonomy. The cases in Chapter 9 address the ethics of killing and letting patients die by examining whether refusals of life-sustaining treatments are ethical and, if so, under what circumstances. Most commentators now generally agree that if a mentally competent patient wants to refuse medical treatment, he or she has the legal—and perhaps also the moral—right to do so.

In order to attempt to avoid certain unwanted treatments, some people are now writing advance directives specifying which treatments they want and which ones they want to refuse.[10] Federal law requires that all patients, upon admission to a hospital or any health facility or care delivery program, such as a long-term care facility or home care, be offered an opportunity to discuss advance directives.[11]

If the patient remains conscious and competent to confirm the advance directive at the time of crisis, normally the patient's wishes will be followed, but most critically ill patients are so ill that they lapse into incompetence. Health providers worry that the patient's wishes may not be adequately clear or that the patient may have changed his or her mind. The following case illustrates the problem.

CASE 16-2   Who Decides What Counts as "Comfort Care"?

Before he lapsed into semiconsciousness, John Garruzo told almost every health care professional who came into his room that he had a living will and durable power of attorney for health care decisions. Mr. Garruzo had been an estate attorney for most of his career. Thus he was familiar with advance directive documents and their role in helping his patients express their wishes about end-of-life treatment decisions. "What kind of role model would I have been if I didn't have a bonafide advance directive?" he asked the nurse on admission. Mr. Garruzo had battled cancer of the prostate for several years before arriving at the hospital this time for a last attempt at experimental chemotherapy. When the laboratory tests revealed that the chemotherapy was doing more harm than good, Mr. Garruzo made it clear that he only wanted "comfort" measures.

Mr. Garruzo and his wife, Patrice, spent his last coherent days together. Mr. Garruzo told Jack Foley, Pharm.D., the clinical pharmacist for the oncology unit, "Remember, you're the one with the drugs, so it's your job to keep me comfortable, right?" Dr. Foley reassured Mr. Garruzo that he would make certain he fulfilled Mr. Garruzo's wishes.

After 3 days of shifting in and out of consciousness and moaning in pain, Mr. Garruzo appeared to be close to death. Dr. Foley stopped by Mr. Garruzo's room and was surprised to find the usually timid Mrs. Garruzo pacing the room in anger. Dr. Foley asked her what was the matter. She replied, "I thought that what I said counted for something. I'm trying to do what John wanted, what he wrote in that living will, but Dr. Keefe has a mind of her own. She just told me that she's going to try another, different kind of chemotherapy. I don't think it's what John meant by comfort care, do you?"

Beverly Keefe, MD, was Mr. Garruzo's oncologist. Dr. Foley checked the medical record, and what he read affirmed Mrs. Garruzo's concerns. Dr. Keefe had written orders for packed cells, followed by chemotherapy and several other medications.

Dr. Foley saw Dr. Keefe at the nurse's station and asked about the present drug orders in light of Mr. Garruzo's clear statements about "comfort" only care at this stage of his disease.

Dr. Keefe responded, "I guess it depends on how you interpret the word 'comfort.' I'm doing what I think is best for Mr. Garruzo, and I think I'm in keeping with his expressed wishes."

"What about his wife's interpretation? After all, she is his official proxy as indicated in his durable power of attorney document. Shouldn't her opinions count now that Mr. Garruzo can't speak for himself?" Dr. Foley countered.

"So what do you think should be done? Or better, what shouldn't be done, Dr. Foley? Should I discontinue the total parental nutrition, the drugs, and just let him die?" Dr. Keefe asked.

Stated this starkly, Dr. Foley paused and wondered what Mr. Garruzo would say at this point in his argument with Dr. Keefe.

Commentary

This appears to be a case in which a patient has executed a valid advance directive indicating his desire not to have prolonged life-sustaining treatment. What possible reasons could the medical staff give to defend a judgment to override the directive?

One problem is that apparently his advance directive was rather vague. It asked for "comfort care," which is open to many interpretations. There is room for controversy in particular if a clinician believes that aggressive, cure-oriented intervention will help make the patient comfortable.

Dr. Keefe indicated two reasons for ordering the chemotherapy and related interventions. She said, "I'm doing what I think is best for Mr. Garruzo, and I think I'm in keeping with his expressed wishes." Each of those reasons for acting needs to be assessed. The moral principle underlying an advance directive from a formerly competent patient is the principle of autonomy. The directive can be analyzed in the context of the patient's continuing right to consent or refuse consent to treatment. Mr. Garruzo's advance directive can be read as constituting a refusal of the treatments Dr. Keefe wants to provide. If so, the physician's belief that the treatments would be what is best for her patient does not provide a justification for treating him against his will.

Dr. Keefe also said that she believed she was acting according to her patient's expressed wishes. That does not seem to be what Mrs. Garruzo thinks, however. If Dr. Keefe appeals to her patient's wishes, she is, in theory, appealing to her patient's autonomy rather than what she thinks is best for the patient. The real issue then becomes whether she has discerned correctly what her patient would want.

When the spouse disagrees with the clinician's interpretation of what the patient would want, who should be authoritative? The empirical evidence suggests that neither family members nor clinicians are very good at figuring out what patients would want but that spouses are better than clinicians.[12] Some argue, however, that it is not so much a matter of who would guess right about the patient's wishes but, rather, who the patient would like to make the judgment. If the patient names his spouse as the one he wants making decisions, he may be willing to accept the risk that she would interpret his wishes incorrectly yet become very distressed if someone else attempted to make an interpretation, even if that person guessed correctly.

Another problem is that clinicians often fear that the patient might have changed his mind after writing the directive. If the patient remains conscious and competent, the judgment can be reaffirmed but not in a case like this. Does the possibility that Mr. Garruzo may have changed his mind justify overriding his wishes?

Some scholars have recently argued that while autonomy requires honoring a patient's expressed refusal as long as he remains aware of his past views, some patients, including permanently unconscious patients, have so lost contact with their former views that they are, in effect, different persons.[13] As such it makes no sense to respect the autonomy of the former person, when a "new person" now exists who may have different interests. If the new Mr. Garruzo's interests are served by the treatment, why should Dr. Keefe be bound by the wishes of the former individual?

The underlying moral issue is whether the principle of autonomy should continue to be relevant when the patient is no longer autonomous. One approach is to apply what can be called the principle of *autonomy-extended,* which holds that an autonomous person's wishes should take precedence unless there is evidence that the patient changed his mind while still autonomous. Is that the appropriate approach here?

Never-Competent Patients

The previous case involved a patient who while still mentally competent had formulated a view about his terminal care and written his wishes into an advance directive. The issue was whether physicians, family, or others had the right to override his directive and who should have the authority to interpret wording in the directive that was unclear. Many patients have never been sufficiently autonomous to formulate a plan about their terminal care. These patients include children or significantly mentally retarded or otherwise incapacitated adults. Other patients who once were competent and could have formulated their plans are no longer competent and left no available evidence of having done so. In such cases, patient autonomy is an impossibility. Some other appeal is necessary. This is often expressed as the standard of patient *best interest*. Someone has to be designated as the surrogate for the patient, perhaps by court designation of a guardian.

Often, however, formal court proceedings are inappropriate either because there is not enough time or because an obvious surrogate is available. For example parents, are the presumed decision-makers for their children's health care, including terminal care. There is increasing agreement that even if the next of kin is not legally designated as a surrogate, he or she is normally the appropriate surrogate.[14] Sometimes problems arise when surrogates make unexpected decisions. The following case illustrates the problems that can arise.

CASE 16-3   May a Residential Facility Director Refuse Life Support for a Resident?

The Greenleaf Home, a state-run facility for the profoundly mentally handicapped, often sent their residents to Midtown Medical Center for treatment. During the winter months it was not uncommon for there to be several admissions a week of patients suffering with pneumonia often complicated by other chronic problems, such as diabetes and congestive heart failure. Floyd Norris was just such an admission to the postcritical care unit. Mr. Norris was 68 years old but had the mental capacity of a toddler. He had been institutionalized since his tenth birthday. He had no known family. The Director of the Greenleaf Home served as the nominal guardian for all residents who had no next of kin or whose family lived so far away that they were essentially uninvolved in the resident's life. On admission, Mr. Norris presented as an unresponsive bundle on a gurney due to long-standing contractures.

Mr. Norris was treated for pneumonia that responded well to antibiotics. Stella Frost, Pharm.D., a clinical pharmacy instructor from a local pharmacy school took a special interest in Mr. Norris. She assigned one of her students to his case. When the student reported at the noon conference that Mr. Norris had audible rales, increased difficulty breathing, and frothy, blood-tinged sputum, Dr. Frost recognized the signs and symptoms of pulmonary edema. She discussed routine medical management of congestive heart failure with the student then suggested that she and the student check the medical record to see what drug orders had been written to correct this potentially life-threatening problem.

There were no drug orders on the chart. Dr. Frost saw Luke Petrie, MD, Mr. Norris's attending physician in the hallway and told him about Mr. Norris's status.

CASE 16-3   *Continued.*

"I know. We're not going to be aggressive with this," Dr. Petrie replied.

"Why not?" Dr. Frost asked. "This is completely treatable with simple, effective pharmacotherapy."

"We've just decided to let nature take its course this time," Dr. Petrie said.

"Who's decided?" Dr. Frost persisted. "I thought Mr. Norris had no family."

"If you must know, the Director of the Greenleaf Home has given his consent to withhold treatment," Dr. Petrie stated and left. Dr. Frost knew that Mr. Norris was incapable of giving his consent. She doubted whether the Director of Greenleaf was a valid surrogate for Mr. Norris. She believed Mr. Norris had the right to this basic kind of treatment. She also knew she would have to act quickly for Mr. Norris's sake.

CASE 16-4   Parents Who Refuse Life Support for Their Baby

Infant Claire McCarthy was delivered at a rural hospital at 34 weeks gestation. The neonatologist immediately recognized serious anomalies: trisomy 21 with partial duodenal atresia, monosomy 18, liver pathology that was possibly transient and reversible, and a cardiac septal defect that with surgery was potentially correctable. The surgeon considered surgery on the duodenal atresia too risky with an infant so tiny. He recommended IV and nasogastric feeding for at least 4 weeks along with an immediate consult with the pediatric cardiac surgeon. Wallace Leaf, Pharm.D., would be preparing several of the special formulas for Claire's nasogastric feedings and cardiac drugs. He was also a member of the ethics committee that would be asked to review the case.

The geneticist had never seen simultaneous trisomy 21 and monosomy 18 in an infant before and could find none in the literature. If anatomical problems are corrected, patients with Trisomy 21 can live many years. It also usually leads to some degree of mental retardation. Monosomy 18 is much more rare. Isolated cases of years of survival are reported in the literature, but most infants die soon. Severe retardation and institutionalization are the norm. The care team believed Claire's medical problems would be synergistic so that even if no **one** would be fatal, combined they were ominous. The clinicians all believed that the infant would not live. They proposed a do-not-resuscitate (DNR) order combined with surgery for the intestinal problems but were concerned about the parents' response. The concern led to a meeting of the hospital's ethics committee.

Claire's parents attended the ethics committee meeting. The mother was distraught but understood the situation. She remained quiet, turning to her husband when the chairman asked what they wanted to do. The father was dressed in a business suit. He was a teacher in a local high school. He expressed himself using fundamentalist religious language. He said, "There is a message from God here. Claire has been a blessing to us, and God will provide." He had consulted with experts at the National Institutes of Health (NIH), lawyers, and their parish priest. (They were members of a group of conservative Catholics who insist on a literal interpretation of the Bible).

CASE 16-4 *Continued.*

He continued, "God's place for Claire is in heaven. I want all treatment, including nasogastric feeding, stopped. Any suffering in the short term will be more than offset by being spared the pain and suffering of many operations and hospitalizations." He claimed that the parish priest said the treatment was morally expendable when it involved grave burden, a position confirmed by the priest who served on the ethics committee.

Dr. Leaf began reflecting on whether he could support the parents' decision or whether he would urge the committee to take action to block the parents' plan.

Commentary

Cases Case 16-3 and Case 16-4 both involve patients who are obviously not competent to make their own decisions about treatment. In Case 16-3, a physician, based on a "consent" from the Director of the Greenleaf Home, is intending to withhold life-supporting therapy for a patient who, for all practical purposes, has no family available to participate in his decision-making. In Case 16-4, the parents are available to step into the role of surrogate decision-makers, but they make a choice that seems controversial.

Mr. Norris, the elderly patient with the pneumonia, has an acute problem that, according to the pharmacist, Dr. Frost, is completely treatable with simple and effective therapy. Of course, the underlying mental condition would not be changed, nor would the other chronic problems, diabetes and congestive heart failure.

For patients who while competent never expressed any views about whether they would like to receive life-supporting therapy, there is general agreement in both law and ethics that the goal is to do what is best for the patient. The *best interest* standard is used when *substituted judgment* (judgment based on the patient's own wishes) is not possible. But what is best for this patient, and who has the authority to decide?

Neither the attending physician nor the administrator of a health facility automatically has the authority to step into the decision-making role. Physicians often assume they are authorized to become the patient's de facto surrogate, but that is not the case. They have the authority to provide emergency treatment on the presumption that the patient would consent, but the doctrine of presumed consent does not extend to withholding life-supporting interventions. If there is time, as there probably is in this case, he needs to turn to some other authority.

One strategy is to seek to have a guardian appointed with such authority. Depending on the circumstances, the courts may have time to act. The proposition being made by the physician and the administrator is a very bold one: that it is in the best interest of Mr. Norris to die, that is, that he would be better off dead. Before such a radical and irreversible decision can be reached, someone with decision-making authority needs to be involved.

Two other authorities are readily available. Dr. Petrie could rely on the view that the Director of the Greenleaf Home is the de facto guardian of its incompetent residents and has the authority to consent or refuse to consent to treatment. Normally there is no basis for that assumption, however. The director may, in some cases, have been so designated, but Dr. Frost doesn't know this (or at least he doesn't say so).

The other possibility is to turn to an ethics committee, if one exists, at the local institution where Mr. Norris is a resident. The ethics committee has the advantage of involving many moral perspectives, people who have had opportunities to reflect about the moral basis for such decisions. But no law gives an ethics committee the authority to speak for incompetent patients, either. Since the ethics committee would be appointed by the authorities of the institution, it would probably reflect the overall moral bias of the sponsor. If the Greenleaf Home has an ethics committee that has strong pro-life tendencies, its committee might almost never agree that stopping life-supporting therapy was best for a patient. If it reflected moral views at the other end of the spectrum (or if the patient was not paying his own way), the committee might be more inclined to see ending life support as what is best. Turning to the committee may merely be an indirect way of asking what the sponsor's moral inclination is—hardly a basis for determining what is really best for Mr. Norris. Does this mean that if Dr. Frost wants to have the decision reassessed, she will have to call immediately for outside intervention?

In Case 16-4, Dr. Leaf is about the make a decision in which the life of an infant may hang in the balance. If there is any autonomy at stake here, it surely is not that of the child. Parents are frequently assumed to have the authority to function as the surrogate decision-makers for their minor children. In this case, however, choosing to withhold feeding of their child would result in certain death. We need to explore the question of when, if ever, parents are permitted to make such a decision.

As in the case of Mr. Norris, the moral and legal standard that is usually put forward for situations like this is the *best interest standard:* choosing the course that will be expected to be best for the incompetent patient. Normally that would be the choice that gave the infant the best chance to survive, but, as was shown in Chapter 9, occasionally that is not be the case.

If the clinician is dealing with a patient whose wishes cannot be known and who has no relatives available, the traditional rule is to do what is possible to prolong life, at least until there has been a careful and deliberate decision, preferably with the help of some formal due process, such as a court review, to forgo further treatment on the grounds it is doing no good. In cases in which patients have family members or other surrogates standing by, however, the decision-making structure may be much more complex.

It is well established that even if autonomous patients have the right to make strange treatment refusal choices in medicine they do not have an unlimited right to do so for their children.[15] Jehovah's Witness parents, for example, do not have the right to refuse life-saving blood transfusions for their children, even if they are sincere in their belief that it is best for them and even if they have the right to refuse blood themselves.[16] Health professionals on their own cannot force treatment against the parents' wishes, but by using legal due process they might be able to obtain a court order temporarily taking custody of the child from the parents for the purposes of authorizing life-saving medical treatment.

Since 1985, such decisions have been structured on federal regulations referred to as the "Baby Doe" rules, which require states to have mechanisms in place to prevent child abuse in the form of refusal of life-prolonging medical treatment.[17] The rules provide 3 exceptions to the requirement that life-supporting interventions must be provided: if the infant is permanently comatose, terminally ill, or suffering from a condition for which treatment would be "virtually futile" as well as inhumane.

At first the committee might conclude that the infant would have to be treated. She was definitely not comatose. She did not seem to be terminally ill either. It is plausible that treatments could be deemed both virtually futile and inhumane, but not everyone would agree. It is debatable also whether the infant could be deemed terminally ill. No single condition could be considered definitely terminal, but the clinicians seemed to be of the opinion that the infant, having to suffer them all together, would not survive for long. Thus, omitting life-prolonging treatments would require a judgment that the treatment would be virtually futile and inhumane or, considering all of the baby's problems, that she is terminally ill.

Moreover, the rules specify that even if one of the exception clauses is met, "appropriate" nutrition and hydration must nonetheless be provided. The clinician's recommendation was for nasogastric feeding and IV fluids. But is nasogastric feeding "appropriate" simply because a clinician recommends it? It seems clear that the feeding and fluids will prolong the child's suffering and that the infant is likely to die anyway. Could it be said that such feeding is inappropriate and therefore not required by the regulations? These are all matters of controversy. No case has tested these positions in the courts. Should Dr. Leaf support the parents' decision, urge them to change their minds, or urge the committee to ask the hospital administrators to take the matter to court to get a court order to treat against the parents' wishes? Most would strive to have the parents do what is best for their child, however that is interpreted, but increasingly committees and others are recognizing that some surrogate decisions may be tolerated even if it is acknowledged that the decision is not the best.

Society may not want to insist on surrogates doing what is deemed absolutely the best for their ward. Determining exactly what is best would be a difficult task, and enforcement of such a requirement would demand constant vigilance and state intrusion on family life. Generally, in matters of family life, such as education choices and discipline, parents are given discretion.

Still there is a limit beyond which surrogates cannot go when acting for their wards. They cannot choose corporal punishment beyond limits. They cannot choose unapproved schools by uncertified teachers. We can call the standard the *limits of reasonableness*. Surrogates, such as parents, according to this standard, would be obliged to try to do what they think is best. If they were within reason, health professionals would try to cooperate in the parents' treatment plan even if they were not convinced it was the best.

Limits Based on Interests of Others

All of the cases presented in this chapter thus far are situated in what can be called a *patient-centered framework*. They focus on patient benefit or patient autonomy.

Either way the goal is to center on the patient. As was shown in Chapters 4 and 5, however, some of the most important ethical conflicts today involve tensions between the patient and others in the society. The principle of social beneficence that underlies utilitarian reasoning holds that actions tend toward being right when they produce the most good overall considering both the good for the patient *and others.*

That is a controversial notion, often rejected in health care ethics in favor of a more exclusive focus on the welfare of the patient. As demonstrated in Chapter 5, however, there is another way that the interests of others can enter the picture, and that is through the principle of justice, which holds that actions tend toward being right if they distribute goods to those who have special claims. Egalitarian justice, which dominates modern nonutilitarian thinking about justice, usually interprets this to mean distributing health care on the basis of need. Since terminally ill patients would normally be thought of as being in great need, they might, according to egalitarian interpretations of justice, have claims to resources that cannot be sustained solely on the more utilitarian notion of maximizing total benefit to the society.

Terminally ill patients often require extremely expensive treatments, and those treatments often do not have much chance of producing substantial benefits. If we calculate expected benefit by multiplying the possible benefit times the probability of that benefit, the expected benefit can be very small. Hence, increasingly there are controversies over the ethics of allocating expensive treatments to the terminally ill. The last case in this volume introduces what may be one of the most critical issues of health care ethics in the future. The health professionals here have both patient-centered and social reasons for stopping treatment, even though the result may be the death of the patient.

CASE 16-5   Futile Treatment: Diagnostic Surgery on a Man Who Appears to Be Dying

---

Dennis Stading, Pharm.D., recognized Clyde Rushton's name as soon as he read the medication orders. Seventy-year-old Mr. Rushton had been admitted 3 times in the past year to the hospital for a variety of acute and chronic problems. Mr. Rushton had a series of debilitating strokes, the last leaving him aphasic but able to communicate with a letter board and nonverbal gestures. In addition, he was a labile diabetic and, despite good skin care, had developed several decubiti on his heel and coccyx. Somewhere along the line, he developed a methicillin-resistant *Staphylococcus aureus* (MRSA) infection, Dr. Stading recalled.

During his lengthy illness, Mr. Rushton was always accompanied by his sister, Bertha. Dr. Stading decided to drop in on the Rushtons and see what had brought him to the hospital this time. Dr. Stading found that Mr. Rushton had a gastrointestinal bleed of unknown etiology, pneumonia, and blood sugars in the 600+ range. Dr. Stading joined the attending physician and students as they entered the room for morning rounds. Ms. Rushton was at her brother's bedside. Mr. Rushton looked very pale and cachectic to Dr. Stading. In fact, Dr. Stading thought, "He looks like he is really dying this time." Dr. Eric Lufty, the head of internal medicine, spoke first, "Well Mr. Rushton it seems that in addition to all of your other health problems, there is some bleeding going on somewhere. In

CASE 16-5 *Continued.*

order to specifically find out what the problem is, you would have to undergo a battery of diagnostic tests. We're not certain you would tolerate these procedures well. Besides, there is a palpable mass in your abdomen, and we assume that this is the source of the problem. There is a good chance this could be a malignancy. So even if we diagnose the problem, there is little chance you would survive the surgical procedures to correct it. I'm afraid we've reached the end of the road."

"Whose road?" Ms. Rushton asked. "You mean to tell me you're not going to fix this?" Ms. Rushton turned to her brother, "Clyde, do you want to get this bleeding stopped and find out what the trouble is?" Mr. Rushton nodded an emphatic "yes." Ms. Rushton turned back to Dr. Lufty, "Just because my brother's old and has a lot of health problems doesn't mean you should just brush him off," she said. Dr. Lufty muttered, "We'll talk later," as he and the students left the room.

As the team made its way down the hall, Dr. Lufty said to Dr. Stading, "Did you see that poor man? He wouldn't survive a lower GI let alone exploratory surgery. Besides all that, the MRSA causes additional problems putting him at high risk for infection and delayed wound healing. Throw in diabetes and you have just about an impossible picture."

Dr. Stading also thought about the cost of such a picture. He wondered what the Medicare-approved HMO to which Mr. Rushton belonged would think of the efficacy of all these diagnostic tests when the prognosis was so grim.

Commentary

Dr. Lufty seems convinced that it is not really in Mr. Rushton's interest to have the exploratory surgery. Since Mr. Rushton will probably die without it, he needs to have a very strong case before concluding it is not in his patient's interest, but his case seems quite persuasive. Mr. Rushton may well die from the procedure itself. In his condition the increased risk of infection and the expected delay in wound healing, together with the diabetes, make it very likely that the surgery would not do Mr. Rushton any good. Surely treatment that cannot benefit the patient is not morally appropriate.

Ms. Rushton seems to read the situation differently, and maybe Mr. Rushton does as well. Mr. Rushton responded to his sister's questions and seemed to convey that he wanted the intervention. The first question is whether he is competent to consent (or refuse consent) to the surgery. If so, then his sister's role is that of an advisor, friend, and family member. She might influence his thinking, but she does not have the power to act on his behalf. However, if Mr. Rushton is not competent, then Ms. Rushton, as next of kin, is the most obvious person to speak for her brother. In most hospitals she would be the presumed guardian. In many jurisdictions, the law makes this clear. In others, usually no one calls into question the presumption that the next of kin is the legitimate surrogate. In a few states (such as New York and Missouri) familial surrogates may not have the authority to refuse life-supporting therapy, but even there they are relied upon to consent to it. In fact, they are expected to consent and will be challenged if they fail to do so.

This situation is often referred to as the *futile care* problem.[18] Does a physician have to deliver an intervention that normally is used to save life but that in this case, because of the circumstances, he is convinced will fail? Sometimes physicians have reason to believe that the proposed intervention cannot work. This is often referred to as *physiological futility*. Generally we do not require a physician to deliver a treatment that cannot work, and we rely on the physician's professional medical judgment about whether it will work or not.

Often, however, physiological futility is confused with what can be called *normative futility*—the view that even though an intervention might produce an effect, it is an effect that is of no value. Increasingly, we are agreeing that health professionals should not be assumed to be experts on the value of the effects treatments produce. Suppose, for example, that the exploratory surgery had a chance of working but would leave Mr. Rushton in pain, bed-ridden, aphasic, and uncomfortable? Many of us would conclude that, on balance, the intervention is not worth it, i.e., that it leaves the patient so compromised that it does him no good.

That seems to be part of the basis for Dr. Lufty's opinion. However, if Mr. Rushton understands that that is the expected outcome but considers it a valuable enough life to pursue, then who is Dr. Lufty to override the patient's evaluation?

But Dr. Lufty is likely to go beyond this to say that the treatment does not even have this value because it cannot succeed. If it were 100% certain that it could not succeed, then he would have a point. But can Dr. Lufty or Dr. Stading determine with that level of certainty that the treatment will fail? It may turn out that the health care professionals cannot establish that the treatment is normatively futile but cannot establish with certainty that it is physiologically futile either.

Some commentators have claimed that there is a probability of success below which it is morally wrong for a physician to attempt treatment. Lawrence Schneiderman and Nancy Jecker, for example, have proposed that if a treatment has not succeeded in the last 100 similar cases that it should be labeled futile.[19] But surely that rule cannot work for all treatments regardless of the potential risks and benefits and regardless of the costs. Some treatments strive for such trivial benefits that we would exclude them from the standard of care even if they were successful somewhat more frequently. Others might offer so much potential benefit and be so inexpensive and easy to perform that they would be part of a standard of care if they succeeded even less often. Realizing that assessing benefits and harms is an inherently subjective judgment makes it impossible to establish some decision rule, that is, *a single, agreed-upon rule to be followed in a given circumstance,* such as the proposed 100 consecutive failures rule.

But does it follow that if the patient (or his valid surrogate) believes the effort is worth it that the health care team must then proceed? It might under the old ethic in which the welfare of the patient was the only morally relevant consideration. But we are moving in the direction of a more social ethic. As evidenced by the cases of Chapters 4 and 5, benefits and harms to other parties may be relevant. Moreover, justice in the distribution of health care resources may come into play.

A straight utilitarian would ask whether the same resources (time, energy, equipment, etc.) used somewhere else could do more good. If they would, then the conclusion would be that morally Mr. Rushton is not entitled to the service, even if he believes it would be for his benefit. An ethic that stressed the principle of justice in distributing resources would ask whether someone else had a stronger claim of justice to the resources than Mr. Rushton and would allocate the resources accordingly. Figuring out what a stronger claim of justice is will depend on which interpretation is given to the principle of justice. For example, if one believed that justice required that resources be allocated to the worst off persons first, then the key question would be who is the worst off among those who could get these resources? Since Mr. Rushton suffers from many chronic and acute problems it might seem that he is about as bad off as one could be from a medical point of view. If that were so, then he would have first claim, according to one who believes that resources should be allocated based on the principle of justice.

It is conceivable, however, that some other people might actually be considered worse off than Mr. Rushton. For one thing, he probably will die soon if he is not treated and probably can be kept reasonably comfortable during that process. If someone else were dying a slow, agonizing death, we might hold that that person could actually be worse off than Mr. Rushton and, according to the principle of justice, have a stronger claim on the resources. Some people believe that well-being needs to be assessed over a lifetime. Since Mr. Rushton has led a relatively full life, some might argue that youngsters with chronic or life-threatening problems might be worse off than Mr. Rushton from an over-a-lifetime point of view. Even if we must concede that we cannot prove that the surgery will fail or that the harms will exceed the benefits, there may still be moral reasons why a social ethic of health care might place limits on the use of resources in this way.

The lingering question, however, is whether these social ethical decisions should be made by Dr. Lufty or Dr. Stading (or by Mr. Rushton and his sister). It could be that in the future some limits will have to be placed on access to certain interventions that seem to have very low chances of success and very little possibility of producing what most of us would call benefits. But a case can be made that, if we do place such limits, they should be placed as a matter of social policy after long and careful public debate rather than by individual clinicians at the bedside who would have to make extremely difficult judgments without the benefit of careful public deliberation.

A case such as this one forces us to integrate the more traditional ethic of patient benefit with the newer ethic of patients' rights as well as the even newer ethic of social benefit and justice. Only by having some understanding of the full range of ethical principles and ethical theories will the pharmacist be prepared to deal with decisions like those confronting the pharmacist in this case.

Notes

1. Ramsey, Paul. *The Patient as Person*. New Haven, CT: Yale University Press, 1970.

2. Ramsey, Paul. *Ethics at the Edges of Life*. New Haven, CT: Yale University Press, 1978; Cohen, Cynthia, Editor. *Casebook on the Termination of Life-Sustaining Treatment and the Care of the Dying*. Bloomington: Indiana University Press, 1988; Veatch, Robert M. *Death, Dying, and the Biological Revolution*. Revised Edition. New Haven, CT: Yale University Press, 1989.

3. Bleich, J. David. "The Obligation to Heal in the Judaic Tradition: A Comparative Analysis." *Jewish Bioethics*. Fred Rosner and J. David Bleich, Editors. New York: Sanhedrin Press, 1979, pp. 1–44.

4. American Medical Association. Council on Ethical and Judicial Affairs. *Code of Medical Ethics: Current Opinions with Annotations, 2004–2005*. Chicago: American Medical Association, 2004.

5. President's Commission for the Study of Ethical Problems in Medicine and Biomedical and Behavioral Research. *Deciding to Forego Life-Sustaining Treatment: Ethical, Medical, and Legal Issues in Treatment Decisions*. Washington, DC: U.S. Government Printing Office, 1983.

6. Gervais, Karen G. "Death, Definition and Determination Of: III. Philosophical and Theological Perspectives." In *Encyclopedia of Bioethics*. Third Edition. Stephen G. Post, ed. New York: Macmillan, 2004, pp. 615–626; Youngner, Stuart J., Robert M. Arnold, and Renie Schapiro, Editors. *The Definition of Death: Contemporary Controversies*. Baltimore, MD: Johns Hopkins University Press, 1999; Wijdicks, Eelco F. M., Editor. *Brain Death*. Baltimore, MD: Lippincott Williams & Wilkins, 2001; Potts, Michael, Paul A. Byrne, and Richard G. Nilges. *Beyond Brain Death: The Case against Brain-based Criteria for Human Death*. Dordrecht/Boston: Kluwer, 2000.

7. President's Commission for the Study of Ethical Problems in Medicine and Biomedical and Behavioral Research. *Defining Death: Medical, Legal, and Ethical Issues in the Definition of Death*. Washington, DC: U.S. Government Printing Office, 1981, p. 2.

8. "The Law Concerning Human Organ Transplants" (Law No. 104 in 1997); Akabayashi, Akira. "Japan's Parliament Passes Brain-death Law." *The Lancet* 249 (June 28, 1997): 1895.

9. New Jersey Declaration of Death Act (1991). *New Jersey Statutes Annotated*. Title 26, 6A-1–6A-8.

10. For a sample of an advance directive see the following Websites: www.aging withdignity.org; www.gundluth.org; www.midbio.org; www.critical-conditions.org; www. hardchoices.com; http://fidelitywisdomandlove.org; also see Cantor, Norman L. "My Annotated Living Will." *Law, Medicine, & Health Care* 18 (Spring-Summer 1990): 114–122; Bok, Sissela. "Personal Directions for Care at the End of Life." *New England Journal of Medicine* 295 (1976): 367–369; Catholic Hospital Association. "Christian Affirmation of Life." St. Louis, MO: Catholic Hospital Association, 1982; Concern for Dying. "A Living Will." n.d.; and Veatch, Robert M. *Death, Dying, and the Biological Revolution*. Revised Edition. New Haven, CT: Yale University Press, 1989, pp. 154–155. For discussions of the ethics of advanced directives see Dyck, Arthur J. "Living Wills and Mercy Killing: An Ethical Assessment." *Bioethics and Human Rights: A Reader for Health Professionals*. Bertram Bandman and Elsie Bandman, Editors. Boston: Little, Brown, 1978, pp. 132–138; Buchanan, Allen. "Advance Directives and the Personal Identity Problem." *Philosophy and Public Affairs* 17, no. 4 (1988): 277–302; and Buchanan, Allen E., and Dan W. Brock. *Deciding for Others: The Ethics of Surrogate Decision Making*. Cambridge: Cambridge University Press, 1989.

11. McCloskey, Elizabeth Leibold. "The Patient Self-Determination Act." *Kennedy Institute of Ethics Journal* 1 (June 1991): 163–169.

12. Uhlmann, Richard F., Robert A. Pearlman, and Kevin C. Cain. "Physicians' and Spouses' Predictions of Elderly Patients' Resuscitation Preferences." *Journal of Gerontology: Medical Sciences* 43, no. 8 (1988): M1115–M1121; Hare, Jan, Clara Pratt, and Carrie Nelson. "Agreement between Patients and Their Self-selected Surrogates on Difficult Medical Decisions." *Archives of Internal Medicine* 12 (May 1992): 1049–1054; SUPPORT Principal Investigators. "A Controlled Trail to Improve Care for Seriously Ill Hospitalized Patients." *Journal of the American Medical Association* 274 (November 22/29, 1995): 1591–1598.

13. Dresser, Rebecca S., and John A. Robertson. "Quality of Life and Non-Treatment Decisions for Incompetent Patients: A Critique of the Orthodox Approach." *Law, Medicine, & Health Care* 17 (1989): 234–244; Buchanan and Brock, *Deciding for Others.*

14. Areen, Judith. "The Legal Status of Consent Obtained from Families of Adult Patients to Withhold or Withdraw Treatment." *Journal of the American Medical Association* 258 (July 10, 1987): 229–235; Veatch, Robert M. "Limits of Guardian Treatment Refusal: A Reasonableness Standard." *American Journal of Law and Medicine* 9, no. 4 (1984): 427–468.

15. Vorys, Yolanda V. "The Outer Limits of Parental Autonomy: Withholding Medical Treatment from Children." *Ohio State Law Journal* 43, no. 3 (1981): 813–829; President's Commission for the Study of Ethical Problems in Medicine and Biomedical and Behavioral Research, *Deciding to Forego Life-Sustaining Treatment.*

16. Moore, Maureen L. "Their Life Is in the Blood: Jehovah's Witnesses, Blood Transfusions, and the Courts." *Northern Kentucky Law Review* 10, no. 2 (1983): 281–304.

17. U.S. Department of Health and Human Services. "Child Abuse and Neglect Prevention and Treatment Program: Final Rule: 45 CFR 1340." *Federal Register: Rules and Regulations* 50, no. 72 (April 15, 1985): 14878–14892.

18. Miles, Steven H. "Informed Demand for 'Non-Beneficial' Medical Treatment." *New England Journal of Medicine* 325 (1991): 512–515; Veatch, Robert M., and Carol Mason Spicer. "Medically Futile Care: The Role of the Physician in Setting Limits." *American Journal of Law & Medicine* 18, nos. 1 and 2 (1992): 15–36.

19. Jecker, Nancy S., and Lawrence J. Schneiderman. "Medical Futility: The Duty Not to Treat." *Cambridge Quarterly of Healthcare Ethics* 2 (1993): 151–159.

Appendix

The Hippocratic Oath

I swear by Apollo Physician and Asclepius and Hygieia and Panaceia and all the gods and goddesses, making them my witnesses, that I fulfill according to my ability and judgment this oath and this covenant:

To hold him who has taught me this art as equal to my parents and to live my life in partnership with him, and if he is in need of money to give him a share of mine, and to regard his offspring as equal to my brothers in male lineage and to teach them this art if they desire to learn it without fee and covenant; to give a share of precepts and oral instruction and all the other learning to my sons and to the sons of him who has instructed me and to pupils who have signed the covenant and have taken an oath according to the medical law, but to no one else.

I will apply dietetic measures for the benefit of the sick according to my ability and judgment; I will keep them from harm and injustice.

I will never give a deadly drug to anybody if asked for it, nor will I make a suggestion to this effect. Similarly I will not give to a woman an abortive remedy. In purity and holiness I will guard my life and my art.

I will not use the knife, not even on sufferers from stone, but will withdraw in favor of such men as are engaged in work.

Whatever houses I may visit, I will come for the benefit of the sick, remaining free of all intentional injustice, of all mischief, and in particular, of sexual relations with both female and male persons, be they free or slaves.

What I may see or hear in the course of the treatment or even outside of the treatment in regard to the life of men, which on no account one must spread abroad, I shall keep to myself holding such things shameful to be spoken about.

If I fulfill this oath and do not violate it, may it be granted to me to enjoy life and art, being honored with fame among all men for all time to come; if I transgress it and swear falsely, may the opposite of all this be my lot.

Taken from Edelstein, Ludwig. "The Hippocratic Oath: Text, Translation, and Interpretation." *Supplements to the Bulletin of the History of Medicine* No. 1 (1943): 3. © 1943. Johns Hopkins Press. Used by permission.

Code of Ethics for Pharmacists: Preamble

Pharmacists are health professionals who assist individuals in making the best use of medications. This Code, prepared and supported by pharmacists, is intended to state publicly the principles that form the fundamental basis of the roles and responsibilities of pharmacists. These principles, based on moral obligations and virtues, are established to guide pharmacists in relationships with patients, health professionals, and society.

I. A pharmacist respects the covenantal relationship between the patient and pharmacist.

Considering the patient-pharmacist relationship as a covenant means that a pharmacist has moral obligations in response to the gift of trust received from society. In return for this gift, a pharmacist promises to help individuals achieve optimum benefit from their medications, to be committed to their welfare, and to maintain their trust.

II. A pharmacist promotes the good of every patient in a caring, compassionate, and confidential manner.

A pharmacist places concern for the well-being of the patient at the center of professional practice. In doing so, a pharmacist considers needs stated by the patient as well as those defined by health science. A pharmacist is dedicated to protecting the dignity of the patient. With a caring attitude and a compassionate spirit, a pharmacist focuses on serving the patient in a private and confidential manner.

III. A pharmacist respects the autonomy and dignity of each patient.

A pharmacist promotes the right of self-determination and recognizes individual self-worth by encouraging patients to participate in decisions about their health. A pharmacist communicates with patients in terms that are understandable. In all cases, a pharmacist respects personal and cultural differences among patients.

IV. A pharmacist acts with honesty and integrity in professional relationships.

A pharmacist has a duty to tell the truth and to act with conviction of conscience. A pharmacist avoids discriminatory practices, behavior or work conditions that impair professional judgment, and actions that compromise dedication to the best interests of patients.

V. A pharmacist maintains professional competence.

A pharmacist has a duty to maintain knowledge and abilities as new medications, devices, and technologies become available and as health information advances.

VI. A pharmacist respects the values and abilities of colleagues and other health professionals.

When appropriate, a pharmacist asks for the consultation of colleagues or other health professionals or refers the patient. A pharmacist acknowledges that colleagues and other health professionals may differ in the beliefs and values they apply to the care of the patient.

VII. A pharmacist serves individual, community, and societal needs.

The primary obligation of a pharmacist is to individual patients. However, the obligations of a pharmacist may at times extend beyond the individual to the community and society. In these situations, the pharmacist recognizes the responsibilities that accompany these obligations and acts accordingly.

VIII. A pharmacist seeks justice in the distribution of health resources.

When health resources are allocated, a pharmacist is fair and equitable, balancing the needs of patients and society.

Index